THE OMNIVORE'S DECEPTION

THE OMNIVORE'S DECEPTION

WHAT WE GET WRONG ABOUT MEAT, ANIMALS, AND OURSELVES

JOHN SANBONMATSU

NEW YORK UNIVERSITY PRESS

New York

NEW YORK UNIVERSITY PRESS
New York
www.nyupress.org

Library of Congress Cataloging-in-Publication Data
Names: Sanbonmatsu, John, author.
Title: The omnivore's deception : what we get wrong about
meat, animals, and the nature of moral life / John Sanbonmatsu.
Description: New York : New York University Press, [2025] |
Includes bibliographical references and index. | Summary:
"Shattering the conventional wisdom around animals, food, and
the environmental crisis, The Omnivore's Deception: What We
Get Wrong about Meat, Animals, and the Nature of Moral Life
offers the most powerful case yet for ending our exploitation of
animals for food, showing why "humane and sustainable
meat" is a contradiction in terms"-- Provided by publisher.
Identifiers: LCCN 2024039855 (print) | LCCN 2024039856
(ebook) | ISBN 9781479825967 (hardback) | ISBN 9781479833450
(paperback) | ISBN 9781479826001 (ebook other) | ISBN
9781479826018 (ebook)
Subjects: LCSH: Food of animal origin--Moral and ethical
aspects. | Animal welfare.
Classification: LCC GT2868.55 .S26 2025 (print) | LCC
GT2868.55 (ebook) | DDC 179/.3--dc23/eng/20250213
LC record available at https://lccn.loc.gov/2024039855
LC ebook record available at https://lccn.loc.gov/2024039856

The manufacturer's authorized representative in the EU for
product safety is Mare Nostrum Group B.V., Mauritskade
21D, 1091 GC Amsterdam, The Netherlands.
Email: gpsr@mare-nostrum.co.uk.

Manufactured in the United States of America

10 9 8 7 6 5 4 3 2 1

Also available as an ebook

For my son Emmanuel—always.

"When a man suspects any wrong, it sometimes happens that if he be already involved in the matter, he insensibly strives to cover up his suspicions even from himself. And much this way it was with me. I said nothing, and tried to think of nothing."

—Herman Melville, *Moby-Dick*

CONTENTS

Introduction 1

PART I: MEAT IN CRISIS

1. Apocalypse Now 19

2. Defending Your Dinner 39

3. The Omnivore's Deception 60

PART II: LIES OF DOMINION

4. Romancing the Farm 85

5. Freedom Is Slavery 109

6. Love Me, Beat Me, Kill Me, Eat Me 119

PART III: LIES OF KILLING

7. Murder, She Wrote 139

8. Harry Lime Disease 170

9. Blood and Soil 189

PART IV: BEYOND MEAT

10. Animal, Not Vegetable 221

11. Persons, Not Things 244

12. Two Ways of Looking at a Blackbird 262

Conclusion: After Dominion 277

Acknowledgments 289

Notes 293

Index 333

About the Author 347

INTRODUCTION

"I tried vegetarianism, once—not for the animals, for the environment."

I've lost count of the number of times I've heard someone say this over the years. The speaker is always anxious not to be misunderstood. While reducing or eliminating meat from one's diet to save the planet is seen as admirable, to do so to keep animals from being killed is to mark oneself out as an eccentric or moral scold. Society views as a fool or a sentimentalist anyone who would care so much about animals, particularly those we raise for food, as to wish to spare them the inconvenience of a violent death. Indeed, to exhibit exaggerated concern for mere animals when there are more important problems facing us, from global warming and war to racism and economic inequality, strikes many people not only as irrational but offensive, even an insult to our dignity as human beings. Nothing, surely, could be *less* important than the question of animals and meat.

But what if we were wrong? Wrong not only about animals and meat, but wrong too about the meaning and purposes of a human life? What if the question of our treatment of animals was not only *not* trivial, but the most important issue of our time?

I argue in this work that exploiting and killing other beings for human purposes is morally indefensible, and that we should abolish the meat, egg, dairy, and fishing industries. However, this book is no more about veganism, per se, than *Rosemary's Baby* is a movie about becoming a first-time mom. Rather, it is about civilizational error— about what happens when we organize our society, economy, and daily lives around a radical evil, then engage in self-deception to keep the truth of that evil from ourselves. The Omnivore's Deception, as

I call it in this book, is the idea that we can go on raising and killing other animals for food without harming animals, wrecking the planet's ecology, or ruining our souls. But, I argue, we can't.

Like everyone else around me, I grew up eating meat. Meat was not just another commodity, it was part of my identity. The roast turkey my mother spent hours basting in the oven seemed to anchor the Thanksgiving holiday, and the smell of steaks and burgers cooking on my father's backyard grill was no more incidental to my boyhood experience of summer than the smell of chlorinated swimming pools or the sound of crickets at night. Meat was in the air we breathed, and it was everywhere else too—in the movies and on TV, in restaurants and at school. In home room, we pledged our allegiance to the American flag and to the colorful wall poster from the Department of Agriculture depicting the Basic Four food groups. Milk, Meat, Vegetables/Fruits, and Cereals/Breads were categories seemingly provided by Nature herself, as eternal and immutable as the four seasons. In theory, every food group was important. But we all knew better. Though a close reading of the poster revealed beans and other legumes in the "meat" column, no meal was to be considered complete without the flesh of some animal. Eating our vegetables was the price of admission to the main attraction—some part of a once-living animal's body. For a long time, just where the meat on my plate came from remained a mystery to me. At four or five, when I asked my grandmother where hamburgers came from, she said they "grew on trees" and then hurriedly changed the subject. Even after I'd learned where meat "came from," it no more occurred to me to question our eating of animals than to question the rising or setting of the sun each day. Eating meat was no more a choice than putting on clothes in the morning. It was just something we did.

And, seemingly, always have done. Our species has been eating other animals since we diverged from our fellow hominins three hundred thousand years ago—first as scavengers, then as hunter-gatherers. Since then, we have been nothing if not ecumenical in our omnicidal appetites, killing and eating every creature within our reach, from woolly mammoths and wild pigs to pigeons, turtles, and swans. Humans eat iguanas and rabbits, octopuses and ostriches, horses and kangaroos, chimpanzees and monkeys, whales and sharks, grasshoppers and ants. (Eighty percent of humans today eat insects as part of their diet.) In Amazonia, we roast tarantulas alive in a fire. In North America, we eat mostly chickens, pigs, and cows, but also ducks, geese, turkeys, deer, bison, and dozens of species of fish, crustaceans, amphibians, and reptiles. In Korea and China, we eat millions of cats and dogs—the latter are beaten or strangled to death, or boiled alive.

The very longevity and ubiquity of our killing of other beings for food has long stood as the greatest proof of its moral rightness. Nothing, indeed, more quickly "settles" the dispute between the vegetarian and the meat-eater than the latter's assertion of self-evident fact and the supposed "naturalness" of our domination of other animals. The first zoological taxonomy we learn as infants is that of the farm. While still in our cribs, we learn that chickens *cluck* and cows *moo* and sheep *baaaa*. By four, we know that gorillas belong in the jungle and lions on the African savannah, while the natural habitat of pigs, horses, sheep, oxen, chickens, goats, and cows is the barnyard and pasture, behind fencing and barbed wire. Species that evolved over millions of years in different parts of the world—chickens in the jungles of Southeast Asia, cows in Africa and India, turkeys in Mexico—are depicted in children's books and nursery rhymes as belonging to the same natural order, as though Linnaeus had placed Farm Animals right alongside Kingdom, Phylum, Class, Order, Family, Genus, and Species.

Thus do we come to accept the idea that exploiting other beings for their ova, milk, fur, skin, labor, and flesh is the proper order of things. In the tautology of the meat system, we eat animals because we're entitled to do so, and we're entitled to eat them because we *do* eat them. Many animals thrive without killing and eating other beings— herbivorous species like horses, elephants, kangaroos, rhinoceroses, llamas, gorillas, and tortoises. But other animals of course prey upon others, and it's those species we choose to identify with. In our minds, we're "just another predator" meant to exploit and eat other species. When we kill other animals, therefore, we're merely expressing our inner natures. It follows that to reject animal agriculture, hunting, and fishing is in a sense to reject one's own *humanness*. Hence the exasperation with which the meat-eater greets the complaints of vegans, that "Hezbollah-like splinter faction of vegetarians," as celebrity chef Anthony Bourdain once described them, latter-day Puritans who seek to impose their abstemious, joyless lifestyles on an innocent and unsuspecting (or, these days, suspecting) public. In calling for an end to animal agriculture, vegans are guilty of a kind of metaphysical "category mistake." In misconstruing the reality of nature, that is, they misconstrue the nature of reality too. As Michael Pollan, the nation's foremost apologist for animal agriculture, claims, animal advocates who describe "domestication as a form of slavery or even exploitation" are "betray[ing] a deep ignorance about the workings of nature" and are engaged in a "quarrel . . . with nature itself."[1]

If there's any case to be made for our vast cruelties to other animals, however, it won't be found in arguments from nature. Animal agriculture, hunting, and fishing are not enduring metaphysical truths, but cultural practices. Breeding animals in the billions, raising them in confinement, and slaughtering them is no more or less natural than paying taxes, streaming Netflix, or burning witches at the stake. If we but chose to, we could shut down the slaughterhouses and recall our fishing fleets tomorrow. And in doing so we would no more be acting "against nature" than if we decided to ban opioids or to raise the minimum wage.

Even if it could be shown that our exploitation and killing of other species *was* natural, furthermore, that fact would tell us nothing about whether we ought to continue the practice. To argue that something is good or right on grounds that it is natural is to engage in a specious form of reasoning that philosophers call the "naturalistic fallacy." Properties of good and bad, that is, are not to be found in nature—rather, they are ascriptions of value that we give to things. Tooth decay, cancer, and *Yersinia pestis* (the bacteria that causes bubonic plague) are certainly natural. But that does not make them good. Some psychologists believe that aggression is natural in our species. If so, shouldn't we encourage aggression in society? If aggression is a "natural" trait, after all, it must therefore be good—and can one ever have too much of a good thing?

A popular version of the naturalistic fallacy concerns our physiological status as omnivores. The fact that we *can* metabolize the flesh of animals is adduced as evidence that we (a) are "meant" to, and therefore (b) are morally permitted to. However, the fact that we *can* eat just about anything—including beverages made with high-fructose corn syrup—tells us nothing about whether we *ought* to do so. Cannibalism too has been practiced by any number of cultures for thousands of years, but I cannot use that fact as an excuse for killing and eating my neighbor. Unlike the lion who eats the gazelle, humans aren't obligate carnivores, which means that we have a latitude of moral action that lions do not. If lions had a choice of whether to kill, and if they furthermore engaged in moral debates over right and wrong, then we might have reasonable grounds to level moral judgments against lion communities for continuing to hunt their prey. As neither situation holds, however, the problem is moot for lions in a way that it is not moot for us. It is for us to determine what values to live by, and to provide better or worse reasons for our practices and beliefs. Omnivorism is not a license to kill; it's an invitation to improve our moral characters, to act in accordance with our better natures.

While it is true that humans have been killing and eating other animals for a very long time, humans have also been killing one another for a very long time, too, yet few would consider that adequate justification for homicide. Neither the mere longevity of a practice nor its widespread acceptance can be used as justification to recommend it to us morally. As the sociologist Max Weber observed of the endurance of patriarchal relations, male dominance has long rested on "the belief in the inviolability of that which has existed from time out of mind."[2]

However, just because men have been dominating women for the last ten thousand years does not mean that men are entitled to do so for the next ten thousand. Nor are women obliged to go on accepting their social subordination forever. The very longevity of male dominance only strengthens the urgent case for ending it.

Arguments that appeal to the way things are to justify the way things should be are guilty of what philosophers call the "is-ought" fallacy. Such arguments appeal to our existing prejudices and beliefs, making them the weapon of choice in argument for those wishing to defend an unjust status quo, but the enemy of those seeking to reform society. Nothing indeed stands more in the way of social or moral progress than the received wisdom or "common sense" of society and the banality of an existing order. What *is*, what exists, is always easier to see and thus to believe in than what merely *ought* to be—some hypothetical state of affairs we can "see" only with our moral imaginations. During the period of modern slavery, it was difficult for people to envision a world without enslaved people or owners of slaves in it, but easy to stroll down to the London dockyards, or along the harbors of Jamestown or Providence, to watch the hulking slave ships being rigged for their next expeditions to Africa. In part, it was the quotidian nature of slavery, its apparent self-evidence as a thing of nature, that enabled it to persist for as long as it did in the ancient Middle East, in Africa, in Europe, in Asia. In 1842, when the British government asked the Emperor of Morocco to identify the steps he had taken to abolish the slave trade in his territories, he replied curtly that, as slavery was something "on which all sects and nations have agreed from the time of Adam," the acceptability of slavery therefore needed "no more demonstration than the light of day."[3] As the Emperor's reply suggests, an entire mode of civilizational development may be erected on corrupt foundations, yet survive and flourish for millennia owing in part to its very ordinariness.

We often condescend to past peoples and civilizations, smiling at their naive embrace of institutions and beliefs that, to us enlightened moderns, seem self-evidently immoral or corrupt. In reality, however, we are no more immune to colossal moral error than the Emperor of Morocco. Vis-á-vis our relations with other animals today, the most irrational and archaic beliefs and practices continue to be embraced as natural and right by the majority of persons, and with as much thoughtless credulity as our ancestors once held the Earth to be flat, or believed that demons sometimes invaded the bodies of young New England girls.

* * *

In a version of a joke told by David Foster Wallace, one fish turns to another and asks, "How's the water?" The second fish asks, "What is water?" *Speciesism,* the controlling theme of this work, is analogous to the water in Wallace's joke. Each day, we go about our business without giving a moment's thought to the medium through which we swim. It's just there, like the air we breathe, and being everywhere, it's thought to be nowhere. The fact that you have likely never heard the term "speciesism" before is only evidence of its total nature as the defining feature of our existence. The philosopher Peter Singer has described speciesism as an irrational "prejudice or attitude of bias" against other animals.[4] However, speciesism isn't merely a prejudice; it's a way of organizing our identity as human beings. Human supremacism, as we might also call it, sets the boundaries of our cultural institutions, modes of economic development, and moral and spiritual beliefs.

Few people have any idea of the true scale of our systems for killing animals, but we have effectively transformed the entirety of the Earth into our gulag and killing floor. Humans kill over 80,000,000,000 land animals and nearly 3,000,000,000,000 marine animals every year.[5] To effect this slaughter, we have extended over the surface of the globe a vast network of controls for breeding, surveilling, and exterminating our fellow creatures. Half the Earth's land surface is now devoted to agriculture, and 80% of that is devoted either to rearing animals for slaughter or to growing monocrops to feed them.[6] That makes the animal agriculture system the most extensive artifact ever built by *Homo sapiens*, dwarfing even our roadways and cities. The majority of the Earth's vertebrates have meanwhile become our captives. Measured in biomass, only 4% of mammals, excluding humans, now live freely in nature, with the rest in confinement awaiting human slaughter. Seventy percent of all birds too are our prisoners, living out wretched, abbreviated lives in the poultry industry.[7] Nature as it existed for countless millions of years, as a boundless realm in which sensuous beings dwelled in mutual interdependence with one another—facing hardship and predation, yes, but also joy, connection, and pleasure, all within a realm of freedom—has ceased to exist.

Each day, millions of fishing vessels aided by sonar and satellite data set out on search and destroy missions, scouring the ocean of what little remains of its conscious life. Only 3% of marine animals are thought to be free from fishing pressures; nine out of ten commercially exploited fish have vanished in just the last few decades, in a slaughter so indiscriminate that researchers at the Fisheries Centre of the University of British Columbia have compared it to "wars of extermination."[8] The collateral damage from these wars is responsible for much of the morbidity: every pound of netted wild shrimp, for example, results in five to ten pounds or more of dead "bycatch"—sharks, mantas, crabs, seals, turtles, dolphins, and other species who happen to be in the way of the trawler.[9] Scientists estimate that humans are killing 100 million sharks per year, pushing many species to the brink of extinction. Since I was in middle school in the 1970s, more than two-thirds of all sharks and rays have been wiped out.

For the individual beings caught up within this juggernaut of destruction, on land and at sea, suffering and trauma are the norm. Fish hauled out of the oceanic depths suffer "the bends" just as divers do when they surface too quickly: rapid decompression causes their swim bladders to explode, their eyes to be pushed from their sockets, and their stomachs to come out of their mouths. Baby pigs who fail to grow fast enough for farmers, termed "fall behinds," are grabbed by their hind legs and repeatedly dashed against the concrete floor, to smash their heads in. To induce chickens to produce more eggs before slaughter, farmers "shock" the birds by depriving them of food, water, and light. Billions of unwanted male chicks are sorted by low-wage workers onto conveyor belts, to be ground up alive or thrown into dumpsters to suffocate or die from dehydration. Improperly stunned cows in the United States are often dismembered and skinned alive while fully conscious, etc. These, however, are but a few of the thousands of cruel practices that we inflict on other sensitive beings as a matter of routine—forms of violence so extreme that, were they enacted on humans, we would describe them as atrocities or crimes of war.

Perhaps the most remarkable thing about this mass violence is how unremarkable it is taken to be, its very banality serving to confirm its imagined lack of moral or existential significance. The belief that human life alone has inestimable value and that the lives of other beings have no value apart from their utility for us—a vestige of a time when humans bought and sold one another as slaves and believed in divination by dreams—remains among the most enduring and closely guarded of our collective intuitions, a view as likely to be shared by the atheist as the religious fundamentalist, the university scientist as the village shaman. Whether one animal dies at our hands or a hundred million is seen to make no difference—the lives of the other animals are as weightless and inconsequential as air. In 2020, when minks in Denmark's fur industry became infected with COVID-19, the government ordered the killing of 17 million of the animals. Though minks are as intelligent, sociable, and emotionally sensitive as our own cats and dogs, they were put into gas chambers. Minks are aquatic animals who can hold their breath for long periods of time; many of the animals therefore survived the first gassing, struggling and suffocating, only to be gassed a second time. Animal welfare organizations objected only to the "unnecessary suffering" of the animals, not to the fact that they were being killed in the millions.

The killing of animals for food and other commercial purposes is not merely tolerated by society, but held to be the best, most ethical way to live a human life. Farmers, fishers, and others who make a living by exploiting animals are celebrated in our culture. Those who, on the contrary, decry our cruelties towards animals, or who merely refrain from eating them, are meanwhile treated with the sort of contempt reserved for pacifists in times of war. Few groups in society are as universally disliked as ethical vegetarians, vegans, and advocates of animal rights. One study indeed found that of all reviled groups in society, "only drug addicts were evaluated more negatively than vegetarians."[10] Libertarians denounce animal rights as a threat to free enterprise and individual liberty; Marxists dismiss veganism as "bourgeois." To walk away from the animal system is even seen as a betrayal of the human race. As the narrator of Chuck Palahniuk's satirical novel, *Lullaby*, remarks of an unkempt, self-righteous vegan-environmentalist named Oyster, "I say, he's a traitor to the species."[11]

Even to hint that there might be a better way to live a human life than causing terror and death to billions of our fellow creatures is to reveal oneself to be a kind of idiot. In *The Vegetarian Myth*, author Lierre Keith depicts vegans as literally brain-damaged, unable to form complete sentences owing to the supposed protein deficit in their diets. (As I myself have been a vegan for thirty years, you may want to be on the lookout for signs of my cognitive impairment.) Paranoia that vegans might pose an apocalyptic threat to humanity is meanwhile a recurring theme in science fiction, with novels like Palahniuk's *Lullaby* and Margaret Atwood's Mad Adam trilogy depicting vegan madmen who conspire to end civilization. In her book, *Animal, Vegetable, Miracle*, acclaimed writer Barbara Kingsolver engages in speculative fiction to blame vegans even for the imagined *non-existence* of the human race. "To envision a vegan version of civilization," Kingsolver writes, "start by erasing from all time the *Three Little Pigs*, the boy who cried wolf, *Charlotte's Web*, the golden calf, *Tess of the d'Urbervilles*. Next, erase civilization, brought to you by the people who learned to domesticate animals. Finally, rewrite our evolutionary history, since *Homo sapiens* became the species we are by means of regular binges of carnivory."[12]

If the existence of *Tess of the d'Urbervilles* justifies the past torment and slaughter of billions of animals, however, then by the same logic *Huckleberry Finn* and the sublime architecture of Monticello must presumably justify the miseries of the Atlantic slave trade. But arguments of this kind, which seek to defend an unjust system or way of life on grounds that it nonetheless yielded "good results," are intellectually dishonest and morally abhorrent. Notably, apologists for the meat economy credit our killing and eating of animals only with the achievements of civilization, never with its failures. But our domination of other species has not been the unalloyed good that it is often made out to be. Pastoralism led to warfare in the Middle East and East Asia, while animal domestication is thought to have served as the inspiration and model for ancient slavery. Furthermore, most of the deadly diseases ever to have plagued our species, including smallpox, cholera, diphtheria, influenza, measles, tuberculosis, AIDS, and Ebola, arose from our exploitation of animals for food.

While most people feel strongly that hurting animals is wrong, most also feel just as strongly that killing and eating them isn't. This cognitive dissonance can make meat-eaters uncomfortable around vegans at dinner time—research suggests that meat-eaters see veganism as a threat to their moral self-image and sense of group identity.[13] However, fear of being judged isn't the whole story. Contempt for vegans and animal advocates stems chiefly from the contempt in which we hold other animals themselves. The figure of "the animal" is a universal symbol of debasement in human culture, an ecumenical term of abuse as likely to be hurled by the left as the right. "These aren't people, these are animals," President Trump declared of undocumented immigrants in 2018, even as his critics were parading a giant inflatable "Trump rat" through American cities. After the Bolivian government massacred anti-government protesters at a gas plant in 2019, activists accused the country's leader of "killing us like dogs"; the next year,

Black Lives Matter protesters accused the police of treating them "like animals," prompting the New York City police union to accuse BLM protesters in turn of treating the police "like animals," too. Misogynists have long insulted women by comparing them to cows, pigs, cats, and other species; feminists have meanwhile described sexual predators like Harvey Weinstein as "pigs" (hence the Gallic version of the #MeToo movement—*#BalanceTonPorc*, or #OutYourPig).

Such usages are so ubiquitous that it is hard to imagine how humans might continue to animate their extraordinary hatred of one another without the category of the "animal" to serve as a universal currency of denigration. To call someone an "animal" is to imply that they are unworthy of respect, even unworthy of life itself. Hence the enduring use of animal metaphors as expressions of racial animus, and even as cultural preparation for genocide.[14] As Syl Ko observes, the "human-animal divide is indeed the ideological bedrock underlying the framework" of racism, with the figure of "the animal" serving as "the anchor of this system."[15] Yet speciesism is foundational to our identity in ways that defy even the obstinate fixtures of race and gender. As Sigmund Freud observed a century ago:

> In the course of his development towards culture man acquired a dominating position over his fellow-creatures in the animal kingdom. Not content with this supremacy, however, he began to place a gulf between his nature and theirs. He denied the possession of reason to them, and to himself he attributed an immortal soul, and made claims to a divine descent which permitted him to annihilate the bond of community between him and the animal kingdom.

Freud penned these words at a time when humans were busy slaughtering one another in the millions on the killing fields of Europe. Initially, Freud had greeted the outbreak of the First World War with patriotic fervor. But by 1915 he had become disillusioned by the war and was struggling to make sense of the instinctual needs and societal dispositions that had given rise to it. In "A Difficulty in the Path of Psycho-Analysis," Freud now sees our discomfort with other animals as rooted in our discomfort with our own animality. This "human narcissism," as he terms it, which leads us to view other sensitive beings as worthless biological inferiors, is a source of our aggression towards one another. As children, we see "no difference" between our own natures and those of animals. But by the time we have been socialized into adults, we have "become so far estranged from animals as to use their names in vilification of human beings."[16]

Whether we are entitled to this contempt, however, is another question. In *The Descent of Man* (1871), Charles Darwin denied that *Homo sapiens* was qualitatively superior to other species: the difference between our minds and theirs, he held, is "one of degree and not of kind," with many other species, too, exhibiting "high mental powers, such as the formation of general concepts, self-consciousness, etc." Even "senses and intuitions, the various emotions and faculties, such as love, memory, attention, curiosity, imitation, reason, etc., of which Man boasts," are also "found in an incipient, or even sometimes in a well-developed condition" in other animals.[17] More than a century of scientific research has since overwhelmingly confirmed Darwin's view. Complex consciousness, far from being an unusual or isolated phenomenon, turns out to be common across the animal kingdom, found not just in apes or mammals, but in avians, fish, reptiles, and invertebrates. Other animals exhibit psychologies and emotions similar to our own, and they are as vulnerable to trauma as we are. Virtually every significant cognitive capacity once thought to be unique to our own species has also been found in others. Tool use has been observed in New Caledonian crows, octopuses, and even insects. Chimpanzees outperform college professors on short-term memory tests. Elephants and ravens conduct funerary rites for fallen comrades. Cetaceans share traditions from generation to generation (the hallmark of culture). Pigeons are superior to humans in some measures of spatial reasoning, and can be taught to distinguish between the Impressionist styles of

Monet and Manet. Fish have feelings and learn from one another. Bees understand the concept of zero, and dream at night.

Every species has its own excellence, and ours is the ability to abstract from immediate context using language, a skill that enables us to build technologies and forms of life that other species cannot. Only humans, thus, have *Anna Karenina* and astrophysics. However, we possess no neurological or morphological structure that would separate us clearly from other animals. Furthermore, we have more in common with other animals than we believe, or choose to admit. Despite our many proven commonalities with other animals, however, we still behave as though we were living in a pre-Darwinian epoch, seeing ourselves as closer to the divine, or to some idealized conception of ourselves (the "thinking machine" is but the latest iteration), than to the merely "bestial." As a consequence, what few laws that exist to protect animals are meaningless. Animals are everywhere defined legally as property, rather than as autonomous beings with a right to their own lives or bodily integrity. Under our laws, to enter the world as a nonhuman is to be born *unworthy of life*.

Many people profess to love animals, and many genuinely do. An estimated two-thirds of American households keep at least one nonhuman companion, a fact that speaks to our desire to feel emotionally connected to other beings. However, our love for animals is partial. Americans keep about 150 million cats, dogs, birds, and horses as companions, yet each year kill and consume hundreds of times as many chickens, pigs, goats, cows, sheep, turkeys, fishes, and others. While we spend nearly $75 billion each year feeding, entertaining, and providing medical care for our companions, we spend at least twice as much to inflict violent trauma on billions of other animals. We thus love animals one moment, slaughter them the next, and fail to notice any discrepancy between the two modes of address. The same newspaper prints a heartwarming story about an animal rescuer or vegan chef one day, then about a cattle rancher or celebrity butcher the next. At the local hardware store, the bird feeders and birdseed can be found in the same aisle as the mousetraps and rat poison—just down from the cat toys and dog chews. Roberto is a meat-eater; his wife Michelle is a vegan. Paula likes volunteering at her local animal shelter; her husband likes shooting deer, then cutting off their heads and mounting them in his den. Often, the same person will exhibit opposite attitudes towards animals at once—like the hunter who grieves the loss of his dog from cancer, or the "bird lover" who donates to the Audubon Society, yet who dines on the bodies of chickens, turkeys, and ducks.

The contradiction between these two ways of living a human life—one lived in communion and love with animals, the other in violent contempt of their very lives—runs like an unmapped seismic fault beneath society, tracing the boundary of two irreconcilable value structures and modes of life. One might think that such blatantly contradictory attitudes and behaviors would provoke public debate or personal soul-searching. But the opposite is true. Since everything is permitted in our treatment of other beings—every kindness and every barbaric horror—our behavior towards animals is seen to be a matter of aesthetics or personal taste, not ethics. The case for respecting animals' lives and caring for animals is held to be no stronger than the case for subjecting them to trauma and death, and society makes no attempt to reconcile the two. Like waves of equal amplitude traveling in opposite phases, our contradictory attitudes and behaviors towards animals are thought to cancel each other out.

What is peculiar about this way of thinking about animals is that in no other domain of moral life would we accept such obvious contradictions in our values and behavior. No one would say that child abuse is "the same thing" as good parenting, or that throwing an elderly person down a flight of stairs is "neither better nor worse" than helping them across the street. Yet vis-à-vis other animals, one set of practices is held to be as good as another. To render these contradictory behaviors opaque to itself, society then resorts to Orwellian language, equating the enslaving of animals with freeing them, killing them with caring for them. Only in challenging these conceptual soporifics, I argue, can we hope to awaken from our deep moral slumber.

While I say a great deal about ethics in this work, however, I have not sought to provide a comprehensive account of the many moral theories that bear on the question of animal rights. By way of explanation, I would offer an analogy to climate change. The reason global warming gets worse and worse each year is not because we lack excellent scientific models or theories about the impact of carbon gasses on the atmosphere, but because powerful economic interests and entrenched cultural behaviors thwart meaningful change. By the same token, robust, principled arguments against our killing of other animals for food have existed for nearly 3,000 years, yet our treatment of animals today is worse than ever. Evidently, then, whatever else might be at the root of our systemic cruelties against other beings, it's unlikely to be a dearth of sound moral theories. For this reason I have chosen to focus less on philosophical theory than on the myths and forms of self-deceit that maintain us in our violent dominion—particularly the myth of the "enlightened" omnivore popularized by Michael Pollan and others.

A warning in advance: I have dispensed in this work with the euphemism and obliquity that other writers often use in addressing the violent nature of our relations with our fellow beings. This is not a book meant to console. Much of what I have to say will make you uncomfortable, and some of my claims will seem extreme. But difficult truths can make us uncomfortable, and the system I describe is itself extreme. That said, this is not a book without hope. As the ecology of our planet collapses—chiefly as a consequence of the animal economy—we face a choice between two different ways of relating to our fellow beings. The first, the one we know already, is based in ancient patterns of domination and violence. The second, as yet untried, would seek a deeper communion with animals through relations of compassion, respect, and love.[18] These two paths represent incompatible modes of life, even two different ways of being human, and we must choose between them.

PART I

MEAT IN CRISIS

1

APOCALYPSE NOW

When I was a boy growing up on the south shore of Massachusetts, my parents would drive my sisters and me out to the Point at Plymouth Beach, the terminus of a three-mile spit of coast jutting out along the edge of Cape Cod Bay. Once ensconced, we would spend the whole day, arriving in the morning and leaving at dusk. And wherever we went, the animal world, with all its mysteries of other-than-human sentience, rose up thrillingly to meet us.

Tiny quahogs squirted up from the mucky flats, burrowing at our approach, while piping plovers fretted the surf. Periwinkles left tiny contrails in the warm mud and clung like pebbles to slick ribbons of kelp. Wading into the water, we stepped gingerly lest we disturb the rare spiny skate concealed in the sand. Gobies and salt-water minnows darted beside us as we swam, while horseshoe crabs scavenged beneath us. At high tide, we explored the bone-white sand dunes or scrabbled across the barnacled rocks of the breakwater. We collected shells of mussels, razors, and whelks, or counted mermaid purses, the empty egg casings of skates that we found entangled in strands of drying seaweed. At low tide, starfish of brilliant hues would lie scattered along the shoreline. Living sand dollars, tawny and moist, quivered imperceptibly in our salty palms.

But that was then. Today when I visit the beaches of my native state, I find an intertidal world almost devoid of animal life. Hermit crabs and periwinkles can still be found in some abundance. But horseshoe crabs are rare, and it has been many years since I came across a living starfish. A pall, too, has settled over the forests and wetlands surrounding my childhood home. The painted turtles that once crossed the road in summer have vanished. So too have most of the snapping turtles, toads, garden spiders, salamanders, paper wasps, garter snakes, snails, and mantises common in my youth. Even the dead animals strewn on our roadways, casualties of automobile culture and its structural violence, have mostly disappeared.

But it isn't just my hometown—the same desolation is to be found everywhere. The animals of the Earth are dying. They are dying in the waters of the Antarctic and in the Himalayas, on the African savannas and in the fjords of Scandinavia, in the deserts of the Kalahari and under the canopies of the Costa Rican rainforest. The devastation is hitting with equal apocalyptic force across the phylogenetic spectrum. Species at risk of extinction include familiar ones like rhinoceroses, hammerheads, giraffes, tunas, orcas, polar bears, and elephants, and less familiar ones like the Arabian Oryx and the Desperate Leaf Chameleon. Two-thirds of all wild animals have perished since I was born. The Leatherback, a pelagic turtle the size of a small car, has seen its numbers plummet by more than 90% in recent decades. Population crashes of similar magnitudes have been observed in Pacific monarch butterflies, in brown bats, in King penguins. Even horseshoe crabs, denizens whose ancient forebearers populated the seas many millions of years before the dinosaurs, are suddenly approaching the brink of oblivion. Insects and other arthropods—an estimated 5 million species, constituting 97% of all animal life—are vanishing, destabilizing the whole terrestrial food web. Not since an asteroid slammed into the Yucatán sixty-six million years ago, bringing a sudden, violent end to the Cretaceous period, has animal life suffered a cataclysm of remotely similar proportions. There have been five mass extinctions over the previous half billion years—ours is the first to be caused by a conscious life form, our own.

That we are nearing a total collapse of the ecosystem is suggested by the growing scale and frequency of what scientists term mass mortality events, in which scores of animals die all at once, often without any clear etiology. In 2013–14, hundreds of millions of starfish in the Pacific

Ocean died from a mysterious wasting disease that caused their arms to shrivel and fall off and their bodies to dissolve into a sticky white fluid. Scientists had never seen anything like it—it was the first observed case of a "continental-scale collapse of a pivotal predator."[1] Many other mass die-offs have occurred since. Starlings in Rome, famous for their murmurations, collided in mid-air and plummeted to the ground, littering the streets of the Porta Pia with thousands of their tiny dead bodies. Two hundred thousand saiga antelopes in Kazakhstan, more than half the species, died in weeks. Mass strandings and deaths of dolphins and whales occurred in the Azov Sea, in Baja, off the coasts of Bangladesh, the Philippines, Tasmania, and San Francisco. Millions of kangaroos on Australia's western plains perished in agony from a mysterious hemorrhaging disease. In 2020, the *Moscow Times* reported that "an unexplained phenomenon" off the coast of Kamchatka had "wiped out 95% of marine life, including octopuses, seals, sea urchins and crabs."[2] Two months later, hundreds of thousands of migratory song birds suddenly dropped dead across the American Southwest; necropsies revealed muscle atrophy and kidney failure, suggesting that they had died of starvation. The worst recorded mass die-off occurred between 2018 and 2022, when a staggering 10 billion snow crabs perished in the Bering Sea, most likely due to warming of the ocean from climate change. As I write this, a global panzootic outbreak caused by avian flu—with origins twenty years earlier in the Asian poultry industry—is sweeping across the Earth, decimating hundreds of species from the Caribbean to Antarctica. "The scale of the mortalities is . . . something we've never seen before and there's no evidence that it's stopping any time soon," one virus ecologist warned.[3]

Frightened by what they see happening, scientists have taken to using terms like "biological annihilation" and "genocide" to describe our destruction of our fellow beings. What we euphemistically call the "extinction crisis" is indeed better described as *exterminationism*—a systemic, violent assault by our species on the identity and biology of all sentient life. The word "genocide" was coined by the Polish-Jewish jurist Raphael Lemkin in 1944 to name the policies of the Axis powers in occupied Europe. Lemkin described genocide as a form of war, but waged against defenseless populations rather than states or their armies. The perpetrator's goal in genocide isn't necessarily to kill every single member of the victimized group, but to obliterate its cultural and physical identity. Using tactics from legal disenfranchisement and theft of homes to ghettoization, starvation, and mass murder, the perpetrator of genocide sets out to destroy the targeted group's very "biological structure," its "elemental means of existence," Lemkin wrote. In like fashion, our species is waging a total war against the defenseless animal populations of the Earth.[4] It is war without end and without temporal or spatial limits, waged along innumerable fronts, from the fishing trawler and cattle feedlot to the luxury condo development and scientist's lab bench.

That it is also a war that we cannot hope to win—not without undermining our own conditions of existence—has been slow to dawn on us. Researchers at the Universidad Nacional Autónoma de México, Stanford's Center for Conservation Biology, and the Plant Science Department of the Missouri Botanical Garden, warn that our wholesale destruction of vertebrate species represents an "existential threat to civilization." In killing off other life forms, we are dismantling "humanity's [own] crucial life-support systems."[5] Despite similar urgent warnings from other leading scientific bodies, however, our destruction of animal life has provoked little public outcry or concerted government action. "Extinction" appears nowhere on the list of Americans' top polled concerns; few people seem aware of the extinction emergency, and even fewer could say with any confidence what is causing it. Our indifference to the fate of our fellow sentient beings is symptomatic of the underlying problem. For thousands of years, we have seen ourselves as the one indispensable species, the only being whose existence has meaning, value, or purpose. Now, having long behaved as if we were alone on the Earth, our solipsistic fantasies have run up against the objective ecology of our planet.

AUGURIES OF APOCALYPSE

Climate change is in part to blame for the widening catastrophe. While some animal species have shown resilience in the face of a warming planet, and some have even benefited from it, the overwhelming majority have not. Climate change means too much rainfall or not enough, too much heat or too little cold. Lakes and rivers are turning into dust beds, while record-shattering storms, floods, wildfires, and heat waves are destroying habitat and displacing or killing countless beings. A billion animals may have died in the 2019 Australian wildfires; since then, massive wildfires have ravaged millions of acres of forested habitat in Canada, California, Maui, Greece, Algeria, and Spain, killing untold billions more. In 2021, a heat dome over the Pacific Northwest killed an estimated billion marine animals; ocean temperatures of over one hundred degrees were recorded two years later off the Florida coast, wiping out coral ecosystems. Every climate disruption meanwhile ripples out across the food web, playing havoc with animals' metabolisms, nurseries, and food sources. Warmer and drier winters are causing bears to stop hibernating in the Pyrenees and Nevada. Penguins have turned up starving on the beaches of Ipanema. Elephants, who depend on their knowledge of rainfall and drought patterns to survive, no longer know when to set out for distant watering holes. Vanishing sea ice is forcing walruses and sea lions to huddle for safety along the Alaskan shore, leading to panicked stampedes that trample the young. Growing acidity of the ocean is thinning the shells of bivalves, which in turn is causing malnutrition in seabirds. Migrating songbirds, returning to Britain at their usual times, find that the insect larvae they depend on to feed their young have come and gone, because spring is arriving weeks earlier than normal—so their babies starve in their nests. Butterflies, moths, and birds are migrating to northern latitudes in search of food. But soon they will run out of "north."

But climate change is itself merely a symptom of a wider ecological calamity, the *coup de grace* to animal populations already reeling from centuries of violent depredation by humans. "As man proceeds toward his announced goal of the conquest of nature, he has written a depressing record of destruction directed not only against the Earth he inhabits but against the life that shares it with him." So wrote Rachel Carson in *Silent Spring* in 1962, long before most scientists had heard of global warming. Carson recounted the history of Euro-American violence towards animals—"the slaughter of the buffalo on the western plains, the massacre of the shorebirds by the market gunners, the near-extermination of the egrets." Now, animals were facing an even more far-reaching threat: indiscriminate spraying of DDT and other insecticides and pesticides was killing "practically every form of wildlife." And unless something was done to prevent it, soon a spring would arrive in which no birds sang.

Few books of the twentieth century proved as consequential as *Silent Spring*. The first popular scientific work to raise the specter of systemic ecological collapse, Carson's book helped spur the federal government to pass a series of landmark laws in environmental regulation. In 1970, President Nixon created the Environmental Protection Agency; two years later, the EPA banned the use of DDT in the US. In the same remarkable period, Congress passed the Clean Air Act, the Clean Water Act, the Federal Insecticide, Fungicide, and Rodenticide Act, and the Endangered Species Act.

But if Carson won the battle, she lost the war. *Silent Spring* was the first of two auguries of apocalypse that autumn; the second, arriving just weeks after Carson's book appeared at booksellers, was the Cuban Missile Crisis. Two generations later, nuclear war remains a terrifying but still only hypothetical threat, while the end times prophesied in Carson's book are already at hand. "Candidates for the 'DDT' of today" might be said to be neonicotinoids, a class of pesticides believed responsible for the deaths of billions of honeybees, or perhaps the chemicals in flame retardants, which scientists have now found "in everything from sea urchins to bobcats to Arctic foxes, and at alarming levels in endangered species such as red pandas, chimpanzees and killer whales."[6]

However, there are 70,000 other inorganic compounds produced by US chemical manufacturers each year: almost none are tested for safety and all wind up in the environment, causing genetic, metabolic, and neurological damage in countless species. Reptiles and amphibians, vanishing at a pace thousands of times greater than the background extinction rate, are particularly vulnerable to such chemicals. Scientists now routinely find them with multiple heads or with legs sprouting from their backs, like tormented figures out of Hieronymus Bosch.[7]

However, the problem isn't limited to toxic chemicals. Industrial civilization as such revolts against animal life. Light pollution is disrupting the courtship rituals of fireflies and the metabolism of many other species. Coyotes, tigers, elephants, and others who have lived diurnally for hundreds of thousands of years are suddenly turning nocturnal, sleeping during the day to avoid contact with humans. Even the din of civilization, the roar of air compressors, planes, pile-drivers, and highways, is lethal. Bluebirds, straining to listen out for predators above the nightly din, are exhibiting signs of PTSD—their chicks are emerging underweight and sparsely feathered. At sea, meanwhile, the ambient noise level has been compared by scientists to that of an airport runway. In addition to unceasing noise from millions of ship engines, petroleum companies charting oil and gas deposits fire seismic air guns for weeks at a time, sending deafening waves of sound crashing across the seascape, while powerful sonar blasts by Navy ships cause hearing loss and bleeding in the brains of cetaceans, leading to mass strandings.

There is simply no place of safety or refuge, however remote, where animals can escape the combined effects of industrialized development and human activity. Even the conservationist's patchwork quilt of protected wilderness areas, sanctuaries, and no-kill fishing zones— havens of last resort—offers protections more apparent than real. Wilderness zones cannot shield animals from a warming planet, acidification of the oceans, retinal damage from a thinning ozone layer, or long-term genetic damage caused by the millions of pounds of toxic waste, radiological agents, pharmaceuticals, and plastics dumped into the environment each year. (Up to 70% of the plastic debris polluting the ocean, causing the deaths of countless marine animals, is from the more than 600,000 tons of lines, nets, traps, and pots abandoned each year by the fishing industry.[8]) As the assault is systemic and global, piecemeal reforms amount to putting band-aids over failing organs.

Millions of people donate to environmental organizations each year in the expectation that their money will somehow right these wrongs. If nothing else, however, the extinction crisis has revealed the cruelly illusory nature of such efforts.[9] A half-century of environmental lobbying and government regulation have done nothing to interrupt an overall trajectory that can only be described as apocalyptic. Between 1980 and 2020, environmentalist behemoths like the Sierra Club, the National Wildlife Federation, the World Wildlife Fund, Greenpeace, and the Natural Resources Defense Council added millions of members, expanded their lobbying efforts, and raised record amounts of money. Meanwhile, during the same period, the planet's ecology was shutting down and its conscious life was being wiped out.

A DOUBLE HELIX OF DESTRUCTION: SPECIESISM AND CAPITALISM

The key to this paradox is to be found in the environmental movement's failure to name either of the two systems that lie at the heart of the crisis. The first is human supremacy, or speciesism; the second is capitalism.

Our species appears to have first begun exterminating others—including, most likely, the Neanderthals and other hominids—about 125,000 years ago: on every continent where early humans later settled, the extinction of large mammals soon followed.[10] "Size-selective extinction is a hallmark of human activity," observes biologist Felisa Smith. "In other words, when we're around, big animals die."[11] Were it not for our human predecessors, we would still be surrounded by woolly mammoths, giant sloths as large as elephants, and saber-toothed tigers.[12] Exactly what caused the early megafauna extinctions remains unclear, and some researchers suspect that climate fluctuations, rather than human hunting, were the primary cause.[13] Nonetheless, there has long been a pattern of human settlement followed by nonhuman population crashes. And by about 60,000 years ago, archaeologist Jon Erlandson suggests, widespread hunting, deforestation, and burning of vegetation had transformed the continents and "set the stage for human domination of the earth."[14]

With the shift from hunter-gatherer forms of human life to animal agriculture, a new orientation towards animals emerged. For the first time, humans began to exert direct control over the biology and reproduction of other beings. Though today we romanticize our pre-industrial relations with other species, imagining an idyllic era in which we practiced kinder or gentler forms of animal agriculture, such depictions are founded in myth. Confining and breeding animals entailed great violence, as oxen, goats, dromedaries, sheep, and other animals were castrated and hobbled, deprived of their liberty and their young, beaten or whipped to pull loads, and brutally killed. The process was also ecologically destructive. By the Bronze Age, intensive pastoral farming had led to widespread deforestation and interruption of the nitrogen cycle in parts of Europe.[15] Domestication had the further significance of diminishing the status of animals in our eyes, depriving them of their natural liberty and reducing them to the status of property and tools.

Animal husbandry, and with it, the idea of *dominion*, the foundational belief that other animals were put on the Earth for our exploitation and use, later set the stage for the second key inflection point in our relations with other beings—capitalism. While science journalists have vaguely blamed "industrialization" for the modern wave of extinctions, industrialization was itself an artifact of capitalism, accelerating ecocidal processes already unleashed by the new system of commodity production in early modern Europe.[16] The extinction crisis begins not with the steam engine or the cotton gin in the nineteenth century, but with mercantile capitalism, colonial expansion, and the Atlantic slave trade, in the sixteenth.

As feudalism gave way to capitalist relations in Europe, communal forms of peasant life that had persisted for countless generations were swept away. Nature, long viewed as a nurturing maternal figure imbued with mystery and the imprint of a divine Creator, was now reconceived as a lifeless machine obeying physical laws. A new model of "rational" control of nature—a masculinist conception closely tied to domination of women by men in early modern Europe—fit the needs of capitalist development, which required standardization of labor and materials.[17] Time itself was remade in the image of capital, as the need for accurate clocks for ship navigation—and, soon, to coordinate and police the work of wage laborers—segmented time into homogeneous fragments, without regard to the cycles of the natural world. In his utopian novel *New Atlantis* (1626), Francis Bacon depicted a futuristic society run by scientists whose total control over animals and nature would be used for "enlarging of the bounds of human empire" and "the effecting of all things possible." Together, Baconian science and capitalism were to turn this fantasy into reality, amplifying by orders of magnitude the ability of humans, or, more precisely, a small clique of them, to control and kill other sentient beings in service to a rapacious system of profit.

To survive in the marketplace, capitalists must produce goods as cheaply as possible, which in turn leads them to exploit human labor, animals, and natural resources as efficiently as possible. Nature is consequently devalued all the way down the line, as rivers, forests, and animals alike are treated as mere vehicles for the accumulation of private, short-term gain. Wetlands are filled in to build luxury condos, malls, and airports; rainforests are burned to graze cattle; mountains are dismantled, the toxic tailings from mines dumped downstream; rivers are diverted or dammed; corals are dynamited; forests are cleared for palm fruit plantations, etc. Because capitalism exists not to meet human needs but to generate profit, corporations meanwhile implant new consumptive desires in the populace. On a finite planet, however, capitalism's limitless proliferation of desires must inevitably outstrip what the Earth's ecology can sustain. It has been estimated that providing all humans with the same levels of consumption now enjoyed by middle-class Americans would require several additional Earths.[18] Authoritative reports on biodiversity losses concur that present levels of capitalist consumption are simply unsustainable.[19]

Together with unchecked human population growth, class inequalities under capitalism also exacerbate ecological pressures on animals.[20] The rural poor in Africa and Asia poach endangered animals to feed their families, or abduct them for export to scientific laboratories or the exotic animal market (for sale as pets or for use in traditional Chinese medicine); consumers in the wealthier global North meanwhile splurge on unnecessary goods, dine on the flesh of cows grazed on land carved out of the Amazon, and board planes for preferred vacation destinations. Carbon emissions from international tourism, already at record levels, are expected to grow by 40% in the coming years, as the world's air fleet doubles. Half of the world's plane emissions, though, are generated by the wealthiest 1% of travelers: the very rich consume hundreds of times more energy and goods than the poor, and their pollution is staggering.[21]

Concentration of wealth in the hands of the few also subverts democratic institutions, making it difficult for citizens to exert a restraining influence over the destruction of nature. Because politicians are beholden to the corporate interests that help get them elected, environmental regulations often die on the legislative vine, or don't get proposed at all. Even when environmental agreements do get signed, they often lack robust enforcement mechanisms—or any at all. In 2021, a group of nations met in Paris for the One Planet Summit to address the biodiversity crisis, agreeing to protect 30% of the Earth's animal habitats. However, the agreement had no enforcement mechanisms, and neither China nor the United States signed on.

In a sense, the ecological crisis can be seen as a conflict between the temporality of capital, whose time horizons extend only as far as the next quarter's profit-and-loss statement, and the time of nature, whose rhythms are timeless, and whose organisms, having evolved over the course of millions of years of exquisite adaptation and interdependence, are helpless before the ceaseless blows dealt them by the commodity system. Earlier extinctions of animal species at human hands probably resulted from a complex process of attrition. "Humans didn't need to go out and kill every last individual," explains Advait Jukar, a researcher with the Smithsonian National Museum of Natural History. "[A]ll you need is a stressed population and just enough hunting pressure to keep the fertility rate [below replacement levels]. Eventually, the population will collapse."[22] Much the same thing is happening now, except that it's happening everywhere at once and in a compressed period. The fact that two-thirds of all wild animals have died in the interval of less than a single human lifetime—a nanosecond in geologic time—suggests that capitalism is not merely "bad for the environment" but incompatible with the fundamental ecology of our planet.

Some scientists believe that the Earth has entered a new geological era, the Anthropocene, in which the planet's biophysical processes are being shaped primarily by *Homo sapiens*. Ecological Marxists have instead argued that it is capitalism, rather than "humanity" in the abstract, that is to blame for the widening rift between humans and the natural world.[23] However, *Homo sapiens* posed a lethal threat to its nonhuman neighbors long before capitalism arrived on the scene; furthermore, nature can only be reckoned cheap by capital if the lives of the other beings who dwell within it are first held to be without inherent value. Human dominion over animals must therefore be taken into account as a pattern of force in its own right. To ask whether capitalism or human supremacy is to blame for our predicament is thus to miss the point, which is that it's both.[24] Like entwined strands of DNA, the two systems form not so much distinct processes as elements of the same total structure of biological annihilation, a double helix encoding the end of terrestrial life.

THE ANIMAL ECONOMY AND THE RUIN
OF THE EARTH

These two entwined patterns of life have now reached their most lethal confluence in the meat and fisheries industries. Though it would occur to few of us to link the food on our plates to the collapse of terrestrial life, raising and killing animals for food is today the single most ecologically destructive force on our planet.

In 2009, officials at Nestlé, the largest food and beverage company in the world, met privately with US Embassy officials at the company's headquarters in Bern, Switzerland, to warn them that the Earth was "on a 'potentially catastrophic' course as billions of people in countries such as India and China begin eating more beef, chicken and pork like their counterparts in Western countries," leading to severe water shortages. By 2025, the world could "face a cereals shortfall of as much as 30 percent," leading to a humanitarian catastrophe. Nestlé warned: "It is clear that current developed country meat-based diets and patterns of water usage do not provide a blueprint for the planet's future."[25] Nestlé's view broadly echoed the conclusions of *Livestock's Long Shadow*, an influential study released two years earlier by the UN's Food and Agriculture Organization (FAO). Co-sponsored by the World Bank and the European Union, the report warned that animal agriculture was likely "the leading player in the reduction of biodiversity," "the major driver of deforestation," and "one of the leading drivers of land degradation, pollution, climate change, overfishing, sedimentation of coastal areas and facilitation of invasions by alien species." Numerous reports by other agencies have since confirmed the FAO report's findings. According to the World Wildlife Fund and London Zoological Society, half of the major drivers of biodiversity loss involve human exploitation of animals, including use of land "to raise livestock for meat, dairy, leather and wool products" and the killing of animals in the fisheries and aquaculture ("factory farming" of fish).[26]

The scientific evidence is clear: we cannot go on extinguishing the lives of billions of our fellow beings for food without tearing apart the very fabric of life itself. Compared to growing crops directly for human consumption, raising animals for food is grossly inefficient and ecologically destructive. Animal-based foods account for 90% of agricultural land use in the US, and almost 85% of greenhouse gas emissions in agriculture.[27] Animal foods also entail an enormous waste of water: it takes 1,800 gallons to produce a pound of beef, compared to 220 gallons to grow a pound of wheat; it takes 670 gallons of water to yield 3.5 oz of protein from dairy cheese, versus 91 gallons for potatoes and 24 for tofu.[28] (The insatiable water demands of the US meat, dairy, and egg industries are chiefly to blame for the dangerously depleted levels of our nation's aquifers, which supply Americans with 90% of their water.[29]) By contrast, a vegan diet requires less than half as much water, produces three-quarters fewer carbon emissions, cuts land use and water pollution by 75%, and reduces the loss of wildlife by two-thirds.[30] A global shift to a vegan diet would also free up 75% of the land now being taken up by agriculture: once reforested, that land could sequester up to 215 gigatons of carbon (GtC) over the next century, cooling the planet. Universal veganism would therefore be the safest way to geoengineer our way naturally out of the climate emergency.[31]

Despite these findings, proponents of organic regenerative agriculture still defend the meat economy, arguing that animal agriculture can be rendered "sustainable" through smaller, more biodiverse farms and more careful husbandry techniques. However, they have yet to provide any plausible scenario in which nearly 10 billion human beings (the projected population by 2060) are to be provided with flesh, ova, and milk from trillions of animals without shredding what remains of the web of life, let alone without subjecting animals to horrific cruelties. Pasture-raised ruminants produce even more greenhouse emissions, and require far more land, than animals raised in intensive confinement.[32] Not even under the rosiest scenarios offered by its proponents, in fact, would a reformed animal-based agriculture system approach the ecological savings of a plant-based one.[33] (The lowest-impact beef produces "six times more greenhouse gases" and requires "36 times more land" than plant protein, while the lowest-impact organic pork produces eight times more greenhouse gases "than the highest-impact plant."[34]) Veganic farmers have meanwhile shown that it is possible to produce high yields without synthetic fertilizer, pesticides, or animal inputs like manure, by employing nitrogen-fixing cover crops and organic compost from plant sources to maintain soil fertility.[35]

In light of such facts, a growing number of scientists have urged a shift toward a vegan diet. As omnivores rather than obligate carnivores, we can live and thrive without the flesh of other beings. Plant-based diets yield better outcomes for human health than animal-based ones: compared to meat-eaters, vegans suffer less from cancer, heart disease, hypertension, type 2 diabetes, obesity, and other ailments. (They may even live longer. One study in *JAMA* found that vegans have a 12% "lower risk of death from all causes compared with omnivores."[36]) Alex Honneld, the free-solo climber, Venus Williams, the former women's tennis number one, and Novak Djokovic, the best men's tennis player in history, are among dozens of high-performance athletes who have thrived on a vegan diet.[37]

Despite the ecological and health advantages of an animal-free diet, however, the animal economy remains the third rail of environmental politics. Even though animal agriculture is the second leading source of greenhouse gas emissions, surpassing cars, trucks, and planes combined, many climate activists have avoided the issue, out of fear of alienating potential supporters and inviting the wrath of the animal industry.[38] After the UN Food and Agriculture Organization published its *Livestock's Long Shadow* report in 2006, scientists who had worked on the original report "were censored, sabotaged, undermined and victimised for more than a decade," as punishment for writing "about the hugely damaging contribution of methane emissions from livestock to global heating."[39] Thanks to the power of the animal lobby, the most certain route to stabilizing our planet's ecology—ending our dependency on animals for food—thus remains the most taboo.

If we needed a further prudential reason to end our exploitation of animals, growing pandemic risk offers another. Animals raised in crowded conditions are so wretched and traumatized that farmers have to keep them plied with antibiotics just to keep them alive long enough to be slaughtered. Eighty percent of all antibiotics manufactured in the US today are fed to farmed animals; antibiotic-resistant strains of bacteria, called "superbugs," have proliferated as a result.[40] Three-quarters of all emerging diseases, meanwhile, are zoonotic in origin: scientists warn that habitat destruction, poaching, and animal agriculture are exposing us to millions of potentially lethal viruses carried by other species.[41] In 2024, avian flu infected millions of chickens and cows across the US, sickening dozens of farmworkers and creating the potential for a deadly global pandemic.

The prudent thing, then, would be to stop exploiting other animals for food. Instead, we are doing the opposite. Per capita meat consumption is rising, and more animals are being raised and killed for food than ever before, putting the meat industry on a collision course with the Earth's ecology. To ensure its continued dominance, the industry has now created the myth of a looming "protein" and "meat" crisis—despite the fact that we can easily satisfy our protein and other nutritional needs using plant sources alone. Venture capitalists have seized on the opportunity by investing in cellular meat products—animal flesh synthesized in vats—to meet projected meat demand. However, the technical hurdles to producing cellular meat at scale appear to be insurmountable.[42] Furthermore, agribusiness has no plans to scale back meat produced through conventional slaughter. When Cargill, the largest private company in the US, announced in 2017 that it was investing in "alternative" proteins like cellular meat, it also reaffirmed its "overarching commitment to animal protein" by announcing a new $600 million investment in factory farming.[43] Even as the market in vegan foods and "alternative protein" expands, therefore, the total number of animals killed for food isn't expected to decline.[44] A trillion more birds and mammals, and up to sixty times that many marine animals, will die at human hands in the next twenty years, unless we put a stop to it. The trouble is, we don't want to stop it. We cling to a sinking ship, rather than risk swimming to a distant but visible shore.

VICTIMS OF HUMAN EMPIRE

For the dying beings of the Earth, it is cultural as well as biological survival that is at stake, the extermination of unique ways of life and structures of experience that have survived for millions of years. The disoriented bears wandering our city streets, the foxes and skunks sheltering under our porches, are the equivalent of displaced persons and stateless citizens, refugees of our war. Torn from the once-predictable rhythms of nature, and driven across a perilous landscape fragmented by highways, feedlots, shopping malls, airports, and sprawling development, or confined in airless agony inside fetid warehouses awaiting slaughter, the animals have become strangers in their own land. The Earth is no longer their home—we have taken it from them. If asked, we would disavow any intention to exterminate other species outright. But we must ask ourselves what we do intend, then, when we appropriate their lands by clearing forests and damming rivers, or slay their young, or burn them alive in their dens and warrens, or haul them out of the ocean depths to be suffocated on our ships—in short, when we treat them "like animals."

Not far from where I live west of Boston lies a kettle pond formed 10,000 years ago by the Laurentide ice sheet as it withdrew across the eastern portion of North America. It was here, at Walden Pond, that Henry David Thoreau built and lived in a small cabin in 1845, that he might "front only the essential facts of life." Reading Thoreau's account in *Walden* of his encounters with owls, squirrels, groundhogs, chickadees, and other denizens of the Concord woods—many of whom, like the sparrow who alights on his shoulder to regard him as he labors in his garden, seem as curious about him as he is about them—one gets the impression of a biotic community in fullest flower. Yet by the time Thoreau settled into his cabin to begin his sojourn, New England had already been depopulated of most of its animal life, through deforestation, the killing of millions of animals for the fur trade, and exterminationist campaigns by local authorities to eliminate reviled species like wolves. *Walden* was therefore as much a requiem for nature as a celebration of it. In a journal entry in March 1856, Thoreau laments that he finds the book of nature "mutilated," its pages "torn out":

> I spend a considerable portion of my time observing the habits of the wild animals, my brute neighbors. . . . But when I consider that the nobler animals have been exterminated here—the cougar, panther, lynx, wolverine, wolf, bear, moose, deer, the beaver, the turkey, etc. . . . Is it not a maimed and imperfect nature that I am conversant with? Do not the forest and the meadow now lack expression . . . ? When I think what were the various sounds and notes—the migrations and works and changes of fur and plumage which ushered in the spring and marked the other seasons of the year—I am reminded that this life in Nature . . . is lamentably incomplete. I listen to a concert in which so many parts are wanting.[45]

Though not a vegetarian, Thoreau was a deeply conflicted omnivore who ate little meat, was skeptical of the need for animal agriculture, and did not like hunting. In *A Week on the Concord and Merrimack Rivers*, Thoreau describes feeling ashamed after he and his brother kill a pair of squirrels during their journey. "Who could commit so great a crime against a poor animal, who is fed only by the herbs which grow wild in the woods, and whose belly is burnt up with hunger?" Filled with remorse, the men discard the squirrels' tiny bodies, uneaten, having lost their appetites. Elsewhere, Thoreau asks: "Who hears the fishes when they cry?"[46]

Today, Walden is a popular tourist destination, with a large parking lot and air-conditioned visitor's center. A recent highway expansion and housing development destroyed thousands of trees outside the

Walden reservation, dealing a further blow to the few wild animals left in Concord. Meanwhile, the voices that Thoreau strained to hear have grown even fainter, and fewer people are straining to hear them—or noticing when they fall silent. On Cape Cod, I find beachgoers bowed over their phones as if in prayer, while children stroll along the water's edge checking Instagram accounts, oblivious to the sound of the waves and the cry of the gulls. In *Walden,* Thoreau warned us against becoming "tools of our tools." But even he could not have envisioned a state of technological alienation as complete as the one that afflicts us today.

It is no accident that animal life should be disappearing at the very moment that technology has overrun our culture, imposing its machinic structure over all waking life. Capitalism has constructed a second, artifactual nature around us, a virtual world pitted against the primary, indispensable one. With each passing day, we are losing contact with the texture of the living world, and failing to register the loss. Some years ago, I sat in a darkened theater watching *Interstellar,* director Christopher Nolan's sci-fi film about a space mission to colonize planets in a distant galaxy after an ecological apocalypse renders Earth uninhabitable. What struck me most was the behavior of the film's characters. Though all the other animals had disappeared, no one mentioned their absence: it was as if they'd never existed at all. As if to console themselves for a loss they never knew, a connection to the animals they never had, the characters in the film instead formed relationships with their machines—robots that spoke flawless English and wisecracked easily with their human overseers.

It has become disconcertingly easy for us to imagine such futures, "ethnically cleansed" of animal life, yet crowded with companionate machines that supposedly behave and think "like us." Like our fascination with UFOs and rumors of alien visitations, our obsession with robots and artificial intelligence suggests nothing so much as malignant self-love, the narcissist's fascination with his own reflection. Love of the machine is but the flipside of our indifference to the flesh and blood beings who live alongside us—the extraordinary beings we slaughter in mountainous heaps and discard as so much trash. In *Interstellar*, there is a telling scene of self-apotheosis in which humans traveling back in time rescue *Homo sapiens* from a wrecked Earth through advanced technology. In the film's re-imagining of Michelangelo's painting of Adam reaching out to touch the hand of God, an astronaut slips through a hole in space-time to touch a spectral human hand from the future. The message is, we have met the divine and it is us. God is dead; but our machines shall render us unto gods.

As beings who dwell in language, we have long found it easier to believe in the superfluidity of our own imaginations than in the fixity and necessity of the natural order we evolved from, and without which we cannot live. Now, our technological dreams have outrun our moral imaginations. Shortly before his death, the physicist Stephen Hawking added his voice to the chorus of futurists calling for our species to begin looking around for another planet to colonize, now that we have ruined this one. "We are running out of space," Hawking warned, "and the only places to go to are other worlds." But such calls for colonizing other planets, beyond their sheer implausibility, have about them the odor of moral and spiritual obscenity. If we cannot learn to live harmoniously with other conscious life forms, let alone with ourselves, then surely we have no business setting up shop somewhere else.

To hope that there is another planet waiting in the wings for us is anyway to misconstrue what ails us. It is not outer space but the inner reaches of conscience that we need to explore; not other star systems, but new ways of living a human life. We are animals, not gods, and what we do to the other beings we therefore do to ourselves, too. In his memoir, Raphael Lemkin noted the destructive effect of genocide not only on its victims, but also on those who perpetrate it. "I realized that such persecution cannot go on endlessly," he wrote. "Those who destroy others also destroy themselves—if not bodily, then in their souls."[47] There is no spacecraft, even in our imaginations, fleet enough to carry us beyond the certain knowledge that we have turned a once-thriving world into ash and bone. And all in defense of meat.

2

DEFENDING YOUR DINNER

On a Sunday morning in March 2012, home subscribers to the *New York Times* awoke to find an unusual invitation on their doorsteps. In the paper's magazine was an announcement for a contest entitled, "Defending Your Dinner: An Open Contest for Hungry Ethicists." Readers were urged to send in essays explaining why we are justified to eat animals, with the winning essay to be published in a later issue of the magazine.[1] First, though, the winner would have to run a gauntlet of "some of the most influential thinkers to question or condemn the eating of meat."

There were to be five judges. Philosopher Peter Singer was famous for his book *Animal Liberation*. Novelist Jonathan Safran Foer had written a book against meat, entitled *Eating Animals*. Both Mark Bittman, the leading food columnist at the *Times*, and Andrew Light, a policy analyst, had published works highlighting the role of animal agriculture in climate change. Finally, there was journalist Michael Pollan, a vocal critic of industrialized animal agriculture. It was this "veritable murderer's row of judges" that would choose the winning essay.

The contest could not have been more timely. Scientists had warned for years that raising billions of animals for slaughter had become a significant driver of the methane and CO_2 emissions responsible for global warming. Now, as freak storms, historic floods, wildfires, and droughts began to command headlines, the link between animal agriculture and the climate was becoming harder to ignore. Only the week before, the nation had suffered a record-shattering heat wave that had pushed temperatures in New England, the Midwest, and the

Great Lakes region up to forty degrees higher than normal. Nature itself seemed to be urging Americans to reflect on their dietary habits.

As news of the *Times* contest spread, however, conservative pundits denounced it. "The premise is that eating meat is bad," fulminated Rush Limbaugh, the far-right broadcaster. "It destroys the planet, causes climate change, kills you. So what they want is somebody to write in and tell 'em why that's wrong. Can you believe we've come to that, that there's a contest for the best entry on why to eat meat? . . . *The New York Times* intends to put people who eat meat on trial. *The New York Times* intends to stigmatize people who eat meat."[2] In reality, rather than challenge its readers to question their views about meat or our relations with animals, the *Times* had instead invited them to rally around their existing habits and beliefs. The editors hadn't asked readers *whether* it was ethical to eat meat, but *why it was*. Far from seeking to "stigmatize" meat-eaters, then, the paper had set out to reassure them.

Still, Limbaugh had a point. Merely by holding the contest, the *Times* had implicitly conceded an argument that ethical vegetarians had been making since the time of Pythagoras: that our killing and eating of animals was neither an immutable fact of nature nor necessary for our survival, but a choice fraught with moral and even existential significance. Now the public was being asked to justify that choice. For the first time, meat had come into doubt.

HOW MEAT BECAME "MEAT"

While it is tempting to think of meat as just another commodity, its cultural significance goes far deeper than that. In *Meat: A Natural Symbol*, Nick Fiddes notes that killing and eating animals "provides perhaps the ultimate authentication of human superiority over the rest of nature."[3] To consume other conscious beings after violently ending their lives is to exert power over life itself. Because of its potent cultural mystique, *flesh* has long assumed an outsized role in the human imaginary, out of proportion to its actual role in our nutrition. Though we think of our ancestors as chiefly eating meat, the evidence suggests that vegetables, legumes, nuts, fruits, grains, and rice have made up the bulk of human calories for millennia. There's a reason the Bible calls bread, rather than beef or mutton, the "staff of life," a staple to lean on for survival in hard times. "Hominins were probably predominantly vegetarian," concludes Amanda Henry, an expert on the dietary ecology of Pleistocene hominins at the Max Planck Institute for Evolutionary Anthropology.[4] Only about 3% of chimpanzee diets consists of the flesh of other animals, a fact that may be indicative of our own ancestral past.[5] Even in the US today, with unprecedented rates of per capita meat consumption, 70% or more of Americans' daily food calories come from plant sources.[6]

Our ancient dependence on a wide variety of foodstuffs to satisfy the bulk of our nutritional needs explains why the word "meat" itself—from the Old English *mete*, for "food"—for nearly a thousand years of common usage denoted any substantial foodstuff, not just the flesh of animals. As late as 1971, the *Oxford English Dictionary* still defined the word "meat" as, "Food in general: anything used as nourishment for man or animals; usually solid food, in contradistinction to drink," hence a synonym for "meal, repast, or feast." While the OED also defines meat as the flesh of animals, the term's primary definition refers to "the edible parts of fruit, nuts, eggs, etc.; the pulp, kernel, yoke, and white, etc., in contradistinction to the rind, peel, or shell"—hence the expression, "getting to the meat of the matter." Once-common usages of the word "meat" cited by the OED include a dish of "crumbled bread and oatmeal," "meat-giver" (one who provides food), "meat-while" ("the time of taking food, meal-time") and even "meat-lust" (signifying not an erotic attachment to bacon, but merely "an appetite for food"). A child sent by her parents to "collect meat for the cattle" would have been asked to gather provender, not carcasses. Such "green-meat," as it was termed, referred to any "grass or green vegetables used for food or fodder"—whether eaten by domesticated animals or by humans. Similar usages of plant meat survived into the early twentieth century, as in a recipe for "nut meats" that appeared in the *Boston Evening Transcript* in 1900. Even "meatless," a term we now associate with vegetarianism, for centuries meant simply to be "without food."[7]

If today we've forgotten these once-common usages of "meat," it's because powerful industries have spent a century convincing us that only foods derived from animals are properly nourishing ones. Amid declining sales of dairy and beef, and growing interest in veganism, the meat, dairy, and egg industries are now pushing state and federal legislation to prohibit the use of "meaty" words in the marketing of plant-based foods. Missouri enacted the nation's first "real meat" law in 2018, making it illegal to sell plant-based products using meat-like words; Louisiana and Mississippi passed virtually identical bills the following summer. Similar legislation is now pending in more than half the nation's states. In an Orwellian reversal, backers of the new bills claim that the marketing of tofu burgers and vegan sausages amounts to deceptive advertising, since "everyone" knows that "meat" refers exclusively to products made from the bodies of animals. A similar falsification of the history of English usage is occurring too with "fake milk" bills targeting non-dairy beverages made from soy, almond, and oat. Urged by the Louisiana Cattlemen's Association, the Louisiana legislature passed a bill making it illegal to sell as "milk" anything that doesn't come from a "hooved mammal." The Food and Drug Association meanwhile proposed that milk be defined as the "lacteal secretion . . . obtained by the complete milking of one or more healthy cows." As Chris Galen, vice president of the National Milk Producers Federation, declared: "You don't got milk if it comes from a nut or a seed or a grain or a weed." But referring to the secretions of nuts, seeds, and grains as "milk" has in fact been common since at least the fifteenth century. The OED thus cites "the milk of cocoa nuts," the milk of figs, and the "milks of wild-poppies, garden-poppies, dandelions, hawk-weed, and sow-thistle."

The irony is that the animal industry wouldn't now be having to police the English language, or to outlaw tofu hot dogs, if it hadn't itself unleashed such catastrophic environmental, health, and ethical problems that it has become necessary to stabilize meat and dairy as cultural objects. The problems embedded in the structure of the animal economy have become so dire that the very idea of meat must everywhere be defended—from federal district court to the pages of the *New York Times*.[8]

ANIMALS AND EMPIRE IN THE NEW WORLD

The crises of the animal economy begin not with the factory farm, but with the economic compulsions of a rising capitalist class in early modern Europe, whose interests were bound up with the enclosure of peasant lands, financial speculation, and foreign trade and plunder. The need for land and resources to fund imperial commercial expansion led European powers to establish footholds on every inhabited continent. The resulting racial polity placed economically advantaged whites of the North on top, and the peoples of the global South, depicted as "subhuman," on the bottom.[9] Millions of people in Africa were ripped from their cultures by Europeans and transported across the ocean for use as slave labor in the New World; Native peoples in the Americas were meanwhile subjected to zoonotic disease, warfare, and forced labor. Crucially, European expansion depended too on the ruthless exploitation of nonhuman animals, in a frontier ethos that pitted "civilized" white culture against "wild" animals and "savage" Indigenous human communities alike. Political authorities subjected bears and wolves to extermination drives—their cubs and pups were bludgeoned to death, shot, or burned alive in their dens. Meanwhile, hundreds of millions of other animals were killed for profit.

For centuries, the exploitation of animals for food, whale oil, fur, and other purposes constituted the main economic output and export economy of the American colonies. As environmental historian Troy

Vettese observes, "demand from European milliners for furs spurred early corporations like the Hudson's Bay Company" to explore and subdue North America. "Corporations and merchants contracted out hunting to Indigenous peoples, transforming beaver fur into a commodity that could be exchanged for kettles, beads, guns, horses, and knives."[10] The colonists also exported thousands of tons of cod and salmon, and by the late seventeenth century had established a permanent whaling settlement on Nantucket. Between 1835 and 1872 alone, the whaling industry slaughtered 300,000 cetaceans, driving humpbacks, blue whales, and North Atlantic right whales to the brink of extinction.[11] Stroll the streets of Nantucket, Salem, or New Bedford today, and you will see stately mansions built with the blood of whales butchered for oil and spermaceti.

It was the introduction of cattle to the Americas, however, that would one day end up destabilizing the Earth's ecological order. Colonization of the Americas probably could not have taken place at all, or occurred as rapidly as it did, had the Europeans not brought horses and cattle with them across the Atlantic.[12] Both species provided the conquerors with significant advantages in mobility and force projection, serving not only as a means of transportation but as a mobile food supply. Horses had the further advantage of terrorizing local inhabitants who had never imagined the existence of animals capable of being ridden into war.[13] Cattle ranching later made it possible for white settlers to establish footholds in Indigenous territories. By the nineteenth century, the wide-open spaces of the American West and Southwest had attracted capitalist interest in large-scale animal husbandry. If Cotton was King in the American South in the 1830s and 1840s, the Cattle Baron had emerged as the new economic aristocracy of the West and Southwest by the 1870s. Control over vast herds of cattle, sheep, and horses came to symbolize the greatness of the United States, bound up with civic ideals of liberty and imperial national myths of the open frontier. The roundup, rodeo, and cattle drive became romantic emblems of the restless, surging power of the American nation. White rural masculinity meanwhile became bound up with America's spiritual identity as the land of the free—an ethos later exploited by the Leo Burnett advertising agency in its Marlboro Man advertising campaign, which associated cigarettes with cowboys lassoing calves and driving horses and cattle.[14] These mythologies of the rural West were to become enmeshed with automation and the ruthless mechanization of animal agriculture. Today's high-tech meat industry, with its genetically engineered chickens and sheep implanted with computer chips, ironically has its origins in cowboy culture.

THE BUTCHER TO THE WORLD

As capitalism concentrates wealth, it also concentrates the mind. And by the late-nineteenth century, some of the best minds were put to work to render animal production more efficient and profitable. In 1862, Congress created the US Department of Agriculture—a first step towards concentrating agricultural knowledge at the federal level. Two months later, President Abraham Lincoln signed the Morrill Land Grant Act into law, giving states authority and land to create new institutions of higher learning focused on military science and agricultural knowledge. The scientific management of animals begins here, in the formation of the land grant colleges. Henceforth, the capitalist state would work hand in hand with industry and academia to streamline the industrial-scale production of animals for commercial purposes. Improvements in transportation meanwhile created new spatial scales of animal exploitation. In 1845, Asa Whitney presented his plan for a continental railway to Congress; twenty-five years later, thousands of miles of track had been laid across the country. Rail technology revolutionized modern warfare, making it possible for both sides of the Civil War to ship thousands of troops to remote battle sites across the South. It also revolutionized ranching, making it possible to transport cows, sheep, horses, and pigs for slaughter across great expanses of the continent.

Chicago became the hub of this new animal economy. By the 1860s, the city had become a national transportation hub and thriving commercial center, its outskirts used as a staging ground for the mass killing of animals brought by several rail lines. With the incorporation of the Union Stock Yard & Transit Company, or "the Yards," in 1865, Chicago became the fulcrum of a national and international meat economy, "The Butcher to the World." Over the next several decades, 400 million more animals were stabbed, bled to death, and dismembered in Packingtown. Conditions at the Yards were chaotic and filthy, as tens of thousands of exhausted, sick, and frightened sheep, cows, pigs, and goats were crowded together within a few hundred acres of pens and feedlots.[15] The appalling labor conditions of meatpacking workers, most of them East European immigrants and some of them children, soon became a major concern of the American labor movement.

In 1904, the Amalgamated Meat Cutters Union in Chicago held a strike for better pay and safer working conditions, leading to strike-breaking efforts by the four meat companies with a monopoly over the Yards. After four thousand workers rioted, the editor of the Kansas-based socialist magazine *Appeal to Reason* asked a young journalist in New York named Upton Sinclair to travel to Chicago to write an account of the meat workers' struggle. Sinclair spent the next six months living in Packingtown, bearing witness to its abominable conditions. Workers labored in filthy, dark, dangerous conditions ten hours a day, six days a week. To relieve themselves, workers either urinated in the corner or defecated in buckets right alongside the carcasses of slaughtered animals. (There was no soap or water.) To extract more value from the workers' labor, the Big Four meatpacking companies sped up the pace of the killing and cutting lines, leading workers to lose fingers or hands. Workers fell screaming into boiling lard vats, to be maimed for life or killed outright. To thwart union organizing efforts, meanwhile, companies employed replacement workers and resorted to violence and intimidation.

A fictionalized account of Sinclair's experiences was serialized in *Appeal to Reason* in 1905. The protagonist of Sinclair's story was

Jurgis Rudkus, a young immigrant from Lithuania who becomes injured at the Yards and loses his job, home, and family (a frequent enough occurrence on the lines). Later, Jurgis attends a socialist rally where he listens raptly to a stirring speech by a leftist politician modeled on Eugene Debs; Sinclair would himself later go on to run twice for Congress on the Socialist Party ticket (both times without success). Published the following year as *The Jungle*, Sinclair's book became a national sensation. It was the first time many Americans had been exposed to the killing of animals on an industrialized scale. Henry Ford is usually credited for the first assembly line; but semi-automated production was first employed in the "disassembly lines" of the Chicago slaughterhouses. Sinclair's account of terrified pigs being shackled to a giant vertical wheel to be "processed" is worth quoting at length:

> They had chains which they fastened about the leg of nearest hog, and the other end of the chain they hooked into one of the rings upon the wheel. So, as the wheel turned, a hog was suddenly jerked off his feet and borne aloft. . . . At the same instant, the ear was assailed by a most terrifying shriek. . . . The shriek was followed by another, louder and yet more agonizing. . . . Meantime, heedless of these things, the men upon the floor were going about their work. Neither squeals of hogs nor tears of visitors made any difference to them; one by one with a swift stroke they slit their throats. There was a long line of hogs, with squeals and life-blood ebbing away together; until at last each started again, and vanished with a splash into a huge vat of boiling water.
>
> It was all so very businesslike that one watched it fascinated. It was porkmaking by machinery, porkmaking by applied mathematics. And yet somehow the most matter-of-fact person could not help thinking of the hogs; they were so innocent, they came so very trustingly; and they were so very human in their protests. . . . Each one of these hogs was a separate creature. Some were white hogs, some were black; some were brown, some were spotted; some were old, some were young. . . . And

each of them had an individuality of his own, a will of his own, a hope and a heart's desire; each was full of self-confidence, of self-importance, and a sense of dignity. . . . Now suddenly [Fate] had swooped upon him, and seized him by the leg. Relentless, remorseless, it was; all his protests, his screams, were nothing to it—it did its cruel will with him, as if his wishes, his feelings, had simply no existence at all; it cut his throat and watched him gasp out his life. . . . The carcass hog was scooped out of the vat. . . . It was then again strung up by machinery, and sent upon another trolley ride; this time passing between two lines of men. . . . One with a swift stroke cut the throat; another with two swift strokes severed the head, which fell to the floor and vanished through a hole.[16]

Sinclair doubtless intended this passage as an allegory for the exploitation of the men of different races and nationalities who had come to America—each too with "a will of his own, a hope and a heart's desire"—only to be chewed up and discarded by the system. But passages like this also invited sympathy for the pigs. Cows "processed" at the Yards fared no better. One government inspector at the time, Adolphe Smith, writing for *The Lancet*, described cows being struck in the head with a mallet, then tumbled into the basement of the building, where workers then hoisted them by their hind legs with ropes. Some animals jumped up and broke away, leading the men to chase after them and try to shoot them with a pistol. When Smith asked why the animals couldn't be fitted with a leather head piece with a nail, so that the latter could be driven into their skulls, killing them instantly, he was told that there wasn't time. "Indeed," he wrote, "so great is the hurry that the unfortunate animals are frequently not given time to die." While dangling in the air, fully conscious, the cows were stabbed in the throat, as men chased after them to catch their hot blood in giant buckets as it gushed out. "The machinery carries forward the animals that are hooked on it regardless of their agony."[17]

The Jungle became the most talked-about novel of the young century, with critics comparing its impact to that of Harriet Beecher Stowe's

Uncle Tom's Cabin. Sinclair himself was disappointed at the book's reception, however, fearing that its anti-capitalist themes had been overlooked. As he famously complained, he had "aimed at the public's heart" but "by accident" had "hit it in the stomach."[18] What had indeed most scandalized the public weren't the degraded conditions of the laborers, nor the corruption exhibited by the meat company (a lightly fictionalized portrait of Armour & Co.), but the disgusting, unhygienic conditions in which the nation's meat was produced. People had known for centuries that diseases originated in farmed animals; by the late nineteenth century, Louis Pasteur and other scientists in the new field of bacteriology had meanwhile formed a clearer picture of the role germs played in spreading illness. Public health officials were therefore alarmed by conditions at the Yards. Animals arrived at slaughter diseased and covered in maggots; their dismembered bodies were then bathed in a pathogenic environment of sawdust, spit, blood, and fecal matter. Workers with tuberculosis coughed on themselves and on the bodies of the animals they had just slaughtered; many workers became infected with skin diseases. It was enough to turn anyone's stomach.

After meeting personally with Sinclair, President Teddy Roosevelt appointed a commission to investigate monopolization of the meat-packing industry and its consequences for food safety. Within months, Congress had passed the Pure Food and Drug Act and the Meat Inspection Act, providing the first federal guarantee of the "cleanliness and wholesomeness of animal products."[19] Despite government reforms, however, the new federal meat inspection system left many of the pathologies of the industrialized meat system intact. To this day, many of the animals caught up within its apparatus of destruction are stabbed, skinned, and dismembered while still conscious; meanwhile, workers in the slaughterhouse industry, many of them immigrants and some of them children as young as thirteen, continue to labor in dangerous conditions.[20] In 2023, the *New York Times* profiled a young immigrant from Guatemala named Marcos Cux, an eighth grader who had just turned fourteen when his lower arm was ripped to shreds while he was working a deboning machine at a Perdue plant.[21] The paper found that hundreds of other migrant children were being exploited by Perdue, Tyson Foods, and other leading meat companies. Children and adults alike suffer repetitive stress injuries, cuts, bacterial infections, and workplace abuse in slaughterhouses. Many also suffer psychological trauma from killing animals—a form of PTSD known as "moral injury," unique to perpetrators of violent harm to others.[22]

In the decades following publication of *The Jungle*, however, government assurances of food safety calmed the public, and the system of industrialized animal agriculture continued to expand. The Second World War proved a turning point. The distribution of meat to American soldiers around the world effectively established a new global meat economy, as cheap animal commodities circulated widely throughout Europe and the Pacific theater, anticipating the trade routes that were soon to become central to America's booming postwar economy. After Japan's surrender in 1945, factories that had churned out millions of pounds of ammonium nitrate for bombs and explosive shells now began churning out the same nitrogen-rich compound for use as fertilizer by US agribusiness, mostly to grow crops to feed animals.

In the 1950s, American consumption of animals increased dramatically, as expanding markets abroad and record wage growth at home enabled millions of Americans to afford mass-produced commodities like appliances, cars, homes—and meat. The agricultural colleges created a century earlier by President Lincoln now bore commercial fruit in newly sophisticated sciences of crop agriculture and animal husbandry. The Green Revolution of the 1950s-60s led to a doubling and even trebling of agricultural production, thanks to synthetic fertilizers, new high-yield cereals, and selective breeding of animals.[23] For centuries, animals bred for food had had relatively little "meat on their bones," owing to poor nutrition, disease, and imperfect breeding. Now, animals' biological processes were made to conform to the principles of scientific management. Scientists increased meat yields by exerting minute control over every aspect of animals' lives in captivity, from insemination and pregnancy to diet, medical care, and metabolism. So-called "factory farming"—the rearing of animals in intensive confinement—made possible new scales of animal production. Chickens were treated as throw-away objects, described in the technical literature as "egg-laying machines," while cows were corralled into giant feedlots and raised on corn and soy. Billions of animals could now be "processed" at great speed by low-paid, low-skilled workers.

By mid-century, animal meat had become associated with prosperity and consumer choice. In 1954, a salesman named Ray Kroc was so impressed by the efficiency of a small restaurant chain run by the McDonald brothers in San Bernadino, California, that he took over the franchise and made it into a national chain. By 1958, McDonald's had sold one hundred million hamburgers.[24] Three years later, the Chicago Mercantile Exchange added pork bellies to its futures market, underscoring the enormous new power of the meat industry. By the early 1960s, Americans were consuming nearly twice as much meat per capita as Europe and the rest of the developed world.

Meanwhile, the problems identified by Upton Sinclair in *The Jungle*—worker exploitation, monopolization, and brutality towards animals—had receded into the background. It was easy to forget "how the sausage is made" amid robust economic growth and a dangerous Cold War. From the perspective of agribusiness and its powerful animal industry lobbies, it was boom times. Fast food culture, new supermarket chains, sophisticated advertising techniques, and government subsidies, price supports, and tax breaks for industry, together produced explosive demand for meat, eggs, and dairy. As children hummed McDonald's jingles, the rich got richer and animals died in ever greater numbers, their cries and screams muffled behind slaughterhouse walls. The dynamics unleashed by capitalism centuries earlier had culminated in a malignant homeostasis, with increases in the production of animals matched by ever-growing rates of consumption.

Everything was going like clockwork.

THINGS FALL APART

In 1963, Universal Pictures released Alfred Hitchcock's science fiction horror film *The Birds*. Based on a story by the English writer Daphne Du Maurier, the film depicted a series of escalating attacks by birds against the people of Bodega Bay, a small coastal town in northern California. The attacks in the movie are set in motion with the arrival in town of Melanie Daniels, a wealthy socialite who has driven up from San Francisco to play a prank on Mitch Brenner, a man she'd met earlier in a pet store while buying love birds. By the end of the film, the attacks have left scores of people dead, Melanie is in a catatonic state, and a bird apocalypse looms on the horizon.

Since every villain needs a motive, Hitchcock provided the birds with one. Though few moviegoers noticed, Hitchcock and his screenwriter Evan Hunter had sprinkled ironic references to the poultry and pet industries throughout the script, satirizing our unexamined dominion over animals. (The besieged characters in the film wonder aloud "why" the birds would ever *want* to harm them.) In a remarkable five-minute monologue for the movie's trailer, Hitchcock described the film as a "lecture" on "our good friends" the birds, and on their "age-old relationship with man." With mock seriousness, Hitchcock described the many ways that humans have honored the "noble history" of the birds—like killing them with shotguns, slaughtering them for women's hats, and raising them in confinement for food. Displaying an egg, Hitchcock praised the innovations of the factory farm. "Thousands of years ago," he said, "Man was satisfied merely to steal an egg from a nest and use it for food. Now he has perfected this process by imprisoning each hen in a separate cage, and by scientifically manipulating the lights so that she doesn't fall into the rut of the old 24-hour day. Thus he can induce the bird to reach fantastic heights of egg production." Hitchcock later said that *The Birds* was intended "as a reversal of the age-old conflict between men and birds. Here the human beings are in cages and the birds are on the outside," with the birds assuming the ironic role of the aggressor.[25]

By coincidence, six months before Universal Studios released *The Birds* in theaters, Rachel Carson had published her own "lecture" on birds in *Silent Spring*, warning however of a very different sort of bird apocalypse. That Carson's book and *The Birds* were released within mere months of one another shows the degree to which, by the early 1960s, the public was already becoming dimly aware of the impacts of industrialized society on animals and nature. From this period on, scientists, conservationists, and animal advocates would push for reforms in a variety of ecologically damaging industries—including animal agriculture.

The following decade was a period of enormous social and cultural change. The Civil Rights, antiwar, and women's movements upended existing political and social conventions, drawing attention to pervasive inequalities in society; the counterculture, meanwhile, loosened attitudes towards recreational drug use and created an opening for franker attitudes towards sex. (Alex Comfort's bestselling *The Joy of Sex* appeared in 1972; *Rubyfruit Jungle*, Rita Mae Brown's novel celebrating lesbianism, appeared the following year.) Growing public awareness of the environmental crisis now also awakened interest in the cognition and experiences of other animals. Hollywood films like *Born Free* (1966)—the story of Elsa, a lioness befriended by Joy and George Adamson in Kenya—and *Dr. Doolittle* (1967) highlighted complex emotions and intelligence in other species; films like *Planet of the Apes* (1968) and *Day of the Dolphin* (1973) meanwhile deflated human pretensions to being the only "intelligent" animal on Earth. Such films mirrored emerging scientific research challenging the dominant view of animals as behavioral machines. In 1969, the same year Jane Goodall published her account of living among chimpanzees, psychologist Louis Herman founded the Kewalo Basin Marine Mammal Laboratory in Honolulu to study dolphin intelligence and communication.

It was amid this cultural upheaval that food policy expert Frances Moore Lappé in 1971 published *Diet for a Small Planet*, advocating global vegetarianism as a solution to world hunger, food insecurity, and the unsustainable nature of industrialized animal agriculture. Lappé documented in detail how a "grain-fed-meat-centered diet" wasted land and fresh water resources, ruined the soil, and polluted the environment with pesticides and nitrogen run-off from animal waste. Monopolization in the meat industry had meanwhile led to enormous concentrations of economic power and to the loss of millions of small American farms. International grain traders like Cargill profited the most, while the global poor suffered from food insecurity. Lappé included a guide to vegetarianism and a set of recipes for cooking "meatless meals." Over the next decade, *Diet for a Small Planet* sold more than two million copies.[26]

Two years after Lappé's book hit the bestseller lists, the philosopher Peter Singer published an essay in the *New York Review of Books* in which he made the ethical case for universal veganism. Singer, a utilitarian, later expanded his essay and published it in book form as *Animal Liberation* (1975). Traditional utilitarianism held that we should act in such a way as to maximize the pleasure or happiness of the greatest number of people, while minimizing their suffering; Singer now extended this principle to include all sentient beings. Not to give equal consideration to the suffering of other animals, he argued, amounted to moral hypocrisy and even "speciesism" on our part—a "prejudice" in favor of our own species. Since practically all forms of human exploitation of animals cause them terrible suffering, we are morally obligated to end virtually all of our uses of animals, including in agriculture and scientific research. To bolster his case, Singer provided numerous examples of animals suffering horrifically at human hands. To keep dairy cows lactating to produce milk for the dairy industry, cows were impregnated again and again, then their calves were torn from their mothers' sides and thrown into the veal industry, where they were chained in total darkness and made to lie in their own filth in stalls too small to turn around in. Tens of millions of hens were crowded into tiny battery cages, periodically starved to shock their systems into producing eggs. Pigs, as intelligent and emotionally sensitive as dogs, were scalded to death inside hair-removal tanks.

The examples Singer gave of animal torture inside the nation's labs were equally horrific. Singer described the maternal deprivation experiments of primatologist Harry Harlow, who had raised baby monkeys alone inside a stainless steel chamber, then introduced a mechanical "monster" mother to assault them with cold air and steel spikes whenever the baby would try to cling to her. Other infants were thrown into a "well of despair" without even a surrogate mother for company—to induce "helplessness and hopelessness." Singer described dogs burned with blowtorches to study burn trauma, rabbits blinded to test cosmetics, goats and sheep shot with assault weapons by the military, kittens and dogs placed in heat chambers and cooked alive. Scientists joked openly about the helplessness of their victims; one restraint device used to impregnate female animals was called a "rape rack" in the scientific literature.[27] Singer showed that most animal experiments were in fact useless, failing to provide any clear benefit to humans.

One of the readers impressed with Singer's book was a young woman named Ingrid Newkirk, who convinced her boyfriend, Alex Pacheco, to start a new animal advocacy organization. People for the Ethical Treatment of Animals, or PETA as they called it, became the first organization to oppose all forms of animal exploitation, from zoos and circuses to factory farms, puppy mills, and vivisection. Over the next decade, PETA would become the largest animal advocacy organization in the world, using lobbying, grassroots activism, public education, sensationalism, and undercover video exposés of shocking cruelties in laboratories, factory farms, and the fur industry to challenge the system of human supremacism.

Ironically, however, one consequence of PETA's growing notoriety and success was to eclipse the long history of ethical vegetarian thought and animal advocacy that had preceded it. Though many people have come to see veganism and animal rights as the recent, faddish conceit of middle-class Americans and white hippies, principled objection to our exploitation and killing of other species in fact first arose thousands of years ago in Asia. Adherents to Jainism in India have practiced vegetarianism since at least the sixth century BCE, and some Buddhists sects have abstained from eating flesh for at least 1500 years. (The Buddhist Laṅkāvatāra Sūtra, written in about the fifth century, denounces meat-eating as a form of "terror" against animals, maintaining that if "meat is not eaten by anybody for any reason, there will be no destroyer of life."[28]) The first vegetarian restaurants thus appeared not in Haight-Ashbury in the 1960s, but in China in the thirteenth century, following the spread of the Mahayana Buddhist principle of *ahimsa*, or universal compassion for all suffering beings.[29]

In the Western tradition, the earliest dissent to the human killing of other beings for food dates back to Pythagoras, the mathematician whose theorem we learn in grade school, and the first person to call himself a philosopher, or "lover of wisdom." Pythagoras appears to have objected to the eating of other animals chiefly out of a belief in the transmigration of souls—the idea that our souls get "recycled" into other bodies, including those of other animals, after we die. However, the vegetarian sects that sprang up after his death depicted the slaughtering of animals as a moral evil, as well—as suggested in Ovid's depiction of Pythagorism in *Metamorphoses*:

> Wicked as human bloodshed, to draw the knife
> Across the throat of the calf, and hear its anguish
> Cry to deaf ears! And who could slay
> The little goat whose cry is like a baby's,
> Or eat a bird he has himself just fed?
> One might as well do murder; he is only
> The shortest step away.[30]

Later philosophers of antiquity, notably Plutarch and Porphyry, denounced human violence against animals in similar terms. Many centuries later, Leonardo DaVinci, an ethical vegetarian, would write with feeling of the "[e]ndless multitudes of these [animals who] will have their little children taken from them ripped open and flayed and most barbarously quartered."[31]

Two thousand years after his death, Pythagoras's name was still synonymous with refraining from flesh, with "Pythagorism" even showing up as the butt of anti-vegetarian jokes in Shakespeare's plays—as in *Twelfth Night*, when Feste tells the unfortunate Malvolio (a pompous servant shut up in a cellar under false pretenses): "Remain thou still in darkness: thou shalt hold the opinion of Pythagoras ere I will allow of thy wits, and fear to kill a woodcock, lest thou dispossess the soul of thy grandam." Not until 1847 did British social reformers in fact first begin calling themselves "vegetarians." Famous ethical vegetarians since have included George Bernard Shaw, Frantz Kafka, Mary Shelley, Mohandas Gandhi, Leo Tolstoy, Rosa Parks, and Jane Goodall.

By the 1970s, then, when Peter Singer's *Animal Liberation* appeared on the scene, the ethics of eating animals had already been a matter of recurring philosophical debate for many centuries (Singer himself had in fact borrowed some of his arguments from the English social reformer Henry Salt, whose book *Animals' Rights* was published in 1892). Nonetheless, Singer's book, along with Lappé's *Diet for a Small Planet*, introduced many Americans to vegetarianism and animal rights for the first time.

Over the next twenty years, a raft of scientific studies established that vegan and vegetarian diets conferred significant health benefits, while consumption of meat, eggs, and dairy led to higher rates of cardiovascular disease, stroke, cancer, and other ailments. During the same period, thousands of people became ill from eating contaminated animal foods. In 1985, nearly 200,000 people in northern Illinois were sickened by milk contaminated with salmonella.[32] In early 1993, 600 people fell gravely ill after eating burgers at Jack in the Box restaurants in Washington, Idaho, and California; four of them, including three children, died.[33] Five years later, hot dogs and packaged meats sold by the Sara Lee Corporation became contaminated with *Listeria monocytogenes,* resulting in eight deaths and several miscarriages.[34] There were dozens of such incidents.

At the turn of the new century, attorney Roger Roots observed that it was "questionable" whether any of the federal regulations to ensure the safety of the nation's animal food supply were working. "Indeed," Root wrote, "the stated goals of meat-packing regulation may be impossible to achieve. The microscopic world of bacterial pathogens most responsible for meat-borne illness are beyond the feasible reach of government inspectors on a general scale."[35] As if to underscore Roots's point, an outbreak of *E. Coli* poisoning the next year caused the ConAgra Beef Co. to recall 19 million pounds of contaminated meat—a record. At about this time, Americans meanwhile began hearing about two public health threats from meat that sounded like storylines out of a sci-fi horror film. One was a brain-eating disease called bovine spongiform encephalopathy (BSE), or mad cow disease. Caused by a folded protein called a prion, BSE caused cows infected with the disease to become insane, lose control over their bodily functions, and then die, as their brains disintegrated. The same thing happened to humans unfortunate enough to eat cows infected with the disease. In 2002, BSE was discovered in a twenty-two-year old woman in Florida who had contracted the disease after eating beef in Britain. The next year, a cow slaughtered in Washington State tested positive for BSE, causing Japan to impose a ban on US beef products. Overnight, Japanese imports of American beef plummeted from more than $1 billion per year to zero.

Even as the beef industry scrambled to allay public concerns over mad cow disease, reports began circulating about a second ominous disease, this one tied to the poultry industry. In 1878, an Italian scientist named Edoardo Perroncito isolated a lethal strain of influenza then killing domesticated fowl outside Turin. In the 1990s, the disease, avian influenza, began infecting chickens and humans in China following explosive growth of the Asian poultry industry. Unlike the prions of mad cow disease, which can only be contracted by consuming the flesh of an infected animal, the H5N1 virus that causes avian flu can be transmitted through the air and through contact with the blood or other bodily fluids or flesh of infected animals. Public health experts warned that the proximity of humans to stressed and sickened birds crowded together in cages had created the possibility of a global pandemic. David Nabarro, an epidemiologist at the World Health Organization, warned that if the H5N1 virus mutated into a form transmissible between humans, the resulting global pandemic could kill up to 150 million people.

On the centennial anniversary of *The Jungle*, critics rued how little had changed in the meat industry since first publication of Sinclair's book in 1906. From the standpoint of industry, the animal economy was a smashing success. During the postwar period, per capita global meat consumption had doubled, and the market was still rapidly growing in China and other emerging economies.[36] But storm clouds had gathered on the horizon, and the industry could no longer ignore them.[37] Raising and eating animals had conclusively been shown to be devastating for the environment, dangerous to human health, an inferior source of nutrition, a leading cause of food insecurity, a waste of natural resources, and cruel to the sensitive beings trapped inside its apparatus.[38] Some scientists began calling for the reduction, or even elimination, of animal foods to save the planet. Between 1998 and 2003, sales of vegetarian products in the US doubled, and Zagat-rated vegan restaurants began appearing across the country, not just in bohemian enclaves like Berkeley or Austin, but in places like Columbus and southside Chicago.[39] It seemed as though Americans might at last be willing to rethink their troubled love affair with meat.

Then along came Michael Pollan and his bestselling book, *The Omnivore's Dilemma*. And meat suddenly got its game back.

3

THE OMNIVORE'S DECEPTION

The September 11, 2001, terrorist attacks on the Twin Towers in New York and other targets across the eastern US led America to a very dark place. The attacks shocked a nation that had come to think of itself as invulnerable, putting it on an urgent war footing. President George W. Bush announced a "War on Terror" without temporal or spatial limits. In the coming years, the US would deploy nearly two million soldiers to the Middle East. Hundreds of thousands of Iraqi and Afghan civilians, and thousands of US soldiers, would wind up dead, and torture would become a widely used instrument of US foreign policy. At home, meanwhile, mental health experts noted a jump in rates of depression, anxiety, and post-traumatic stress. More than a million Americans who had quit smoking started up again. Hate crimes against Arabs, Muslims, and Sikhs skyrocketed. The Patriot Act eroded civil liberties, granting the National Security Agency and other intelligence agencies extraordinary powers to monitor the private communications of American citizens. As the country lurched further to the right, Fox News, riding high after the 2000 election, extended its audience of conservative viewers. Millions of people became interested in survivalism and paramilitarism for the first time. "When the asteroid hits and civilization crumbles, you'll be ready," went the ad copy for the new Hummer H2, a hulking 6,500-pound behemoth modeled closely after the US Army's Humvee. "You give us the money, you get the truck, and nobody gets hurt."[1] Hummer sales soared, as did sales of cigars, violent porn, and guns.

It was in this oppressive atmosphere, in the early years of America's War on Terror, when life became overshadowed by national trauma, paranoia, and a violent bunker mentality, that author Michael Pollan sat down to write a book meant to restore the nation's waning faith in meat. A journalism professor at Berkeley, Pollan had been the author already of several bestsellers, including *The Botany of Desire* (2001), a lyrical account of how plants had cultivated humans through horticulture as much as we had cultivated them. An elegant prose stylist whose nonfiction ranged widely and with erudition over natural history and culture, Pollan now turned his attention to the nation's broken food system. Pollan had ended *Botany of Desire* with a paean to animal agriculture; just months after the September 11 attacks, he had published an influential article in the *New York Times Magazine*, "Power Steer," about the ecological impacts of industrialized animal agriculture. Now, in 2006, on the centennial anniversary of *The Jungle*, Penguin Press issued Pollan's *The Omnivore's Dilemma: A Natural History of Four Foods*. Like Upton Sinclair, Pollan had set out to document the problems of industrialized animal agriculture. Unlike Sinclair, though, Pollan had set out to redeem the idea of meat.

After the Second World War, Pollan showed, corporate control of agribusiness and a rising standard of living had enabled a vast expansion of the animal agriculture system. To provide Americans with cheap meat, a handful of corporate behemoths were now raising billions of animals in crowded conditions that were dangerous to public health, inhumane to the animals, and unsustainable. Decades of government subsidies to agribusiness were partly to blame, having fostered a destructive monoculture system, mostly based on corn, that was dependent on petroleum-based fertilizers. Where millions of small family farms had once dotted the American landscape, a handful of giant corporate conglomerates now dominated. Monopolization of food production had damaged rural ways of life, depleted the soil, and estranged us from the land. Distortions in agricultural production had also led to pathologies in our consumption habits, inuring us to cheap but tasteless processed foods. Fast food culture had replaced the home-cooked meal and the pleasures of leisurely communion with others over a well-laid table.

Pollan's goal was to help Americans overcome their "national eating disorder," as he termed it. For too long, we had allowed nutritionists and animal rights zealots to make us suspicious of our food. As biological omnivores, we were capable of eating a wide range of foodstuffs. Why then not celebrate that diversity, and resist the homogenization of food imposed on us by agribusiness? It was time to stop hanging on the words of the moralists and fear-mongers—vegans and fussy nutritionists—and return to the "pleasure and tradition" of eating. Hence the "dilemma" of Pollan's title, which focused chiefly on the question of eating animals. We could continue eating meat, eggs, and dairy from animals raised on factory farms, contributing to environmental degradation, animal abuses, and further communal losses. Or we could give up animal products and join the cult of vegetarians. But both choices were repugnant. What, then, was a conscientious meat-eater to do?

Pollan claimed to have found a narrow passage between the rock of the factory farm and the hard place of vegetarianism. The solution to our broken industrialized food system was to be sought in smaller-scale animal farming. By employing traditional as well innovative farming techniques, small independent producers were already showing a way to minimize the ecological harms of agriculture while providing consumers with delicious, locally grown produce and meat, eggs, and dairy. Meanwhile, the animals benefited from more humane living conditions, grazing outdoors rather than in feedlots or battery cages. The new agriculture was a "win-win" for everyone—for farmers, consumers, animals, and the Earth.

With this reassuring message, Pollan stepped nimbly into the growing breach between Americans' heads, hearts, and stomachs. While earlier critics, too, had warned the public about the dire impacts of industrialized agriculture, they had advocated vegetarianism and veganism as the solution to the crisis.[2] And that wasn't a message most Americans wanted to hear. Decades of advocacy by animal rights groups, and urgent warnings by environmentalists about the ecological impacts of the animal industry, had barely dented Americans' eating habits. In 2006, only 1–2% of the American public identified as vegetarian or vegan, and Pollan was uninterested in moving the needle on that score. Instead, he positioned himself as the bearer of glad tidings for the millions of meat-loving consumers who, though concerned about the environment and vaguely uneasy over reports of animal cruelty, had no wish to overturn their dietary habits. By buying products from smaller farms, Pollan said, we could reclaim our connection to the land, while savoring delicious food again. Meat-eaters could feast on steaks made from "grass-fed" cows and pork from "humanely" slaughtered pigs, while facing down the hard stares of vegans. We could have our meat and our consciences, too.

The Omnivore's Dilemma vaulted onto the New York Times Bestseller List. Acclaim for Pollan's book was universal. Critics hailed it as "brilliant," "revolutionary," and a "passionate journey of the heart." Pollan suddenly became the nation's most sought-after speaker on food issues, interviewed on TV and radio and in documentaries like *Food, Inc.*, where he was treated as a national sage. Universities and colleges assigned *Omnivore's Dilemma* as required reading for incoming students. When Pollan expanded on his arguments in another bestseller, *In Defense of Food*, the Humanities Center at the University of Wisconsin made his new book the center of a university-wide reading curriculum. The university's Chancellor personally invited UW's forty thousand students, faculty, and alumni to participate. The capstone of the program was a campus visit and lecture by Pollan himself. Seven thousand people flocked to hear Pollan and his "defense" of food. Improbably, the mild and faintly patrician Pollan had become a rock star.

But timing is everything. By the early 2000s, an informal alliance had already developed between urban food activists, environmentalists, small-scale animal farmers, and the billion-dollar organic foods industry to sell the public on a "new" animal agriculture, one ostensibly more sustainable and humane than the old. *The Omnivore's Dilemma*, itself a product of these forces, was to provide this emergent coalition with the rhetorical and intellectual scaffolding it needed to consolidate a new common sense around food—the myth of the Enlightened Omnivore.

LOCAVORES AND OMNIVORES ASCENDANT

In 2005, the year before *Omnivore's Dilemma* appeared in bookstores, three young women in San Francisco—Jessica Prentice, Dede Sampson, and Sage Van Wing—circulated a manifesto promoting locally grown, organic foods by small-scale producers. The idea was that buying locally grown produce and products from locally raised animals would reduce "food miles," or the distance it took for food to travel from farm to table, thus reducing carbon emissions and keeping resources within the community. By buying locally, consumers would also be in closer contact with producers, supporting local farmers. And food grown organically and locally was fresher and more nutritious.

In fact, the ideals of the locavores were not entirely new. Public interest in "whole" and healthy foods can be traced back at least to the early nineteenth century; with industrialization of the nation's food supply, concerns about food safety became even more acute. In the 1930s, historian and philosopher Lewis Mumford warned against the fallacy of equating mechanization of agriculture and commodification of food with social progress, observing that while canning and refrigeration made sense "as a means of distributing a limited food supply over the year, or of making it available in areas distant from the place originally grown," using "canned goods . . . in country districts when fresh fruit and vegetables are available comes to a vital and social loss." Anticipating later locavore objections to excessive "food miles," Mumford observed that there was "no virtue whatever in eating foods that are years old or that have been transported thousands of miles, when equally good foods are available without going out of the locality."[3] At the time of these observations, socialists, labor activists, and community organizers were meanwhile developing cooperative businesses, including food co-ops, as a way to meet social need.

Later, in the 1960s and 1970s, with the rise of the counterculture and environmental movements, food activists set up thousands of food cooperatives across the nation, built around principles of decentralized authority, agroecology, organic foods, and progressive politics. With the more difficult operating environment facing small businesses in the 1980s, however, co-ops eventually lost their former left-leaning and activist sensibility.[4] Many were to be taken over or forced out of business by the Whole Foods Corporation. By century's end, half of the organic food industry's $7.8 billion in sales were taking place not in community-run food enterprises but in conventional supermarkets (a trend Pollan criticized in *Omnivore* as "Supermarket Pastoral" and "industrial organic").[5] The economic policies of the Reagan Administration had meanwhile displaced thousands of smaller-scale farmers and strengthened the hand of corporate agribusiness. In response to these developments, farmer-poet Wendell Berry and other proponents of a new "rural renaissance" developed a populist agrarianism that romanticized small-scale animal farming.

Emerging in parallel with this new agrarianism, locavorism was intended as a way to push back against the corporate stranglehold on the nation's food system. However, the locavore position was contradictory. Buying locally may not always make sense from a social justice perspective—it might be better to purchase goods from a struggling workers cooperative in another country, say, than from a local company engaged in exploitative labor practices. Also, reducing "food miles" only makes ecological sense when all else is equal, which is seldom the case. Transportation, even across long distances, represents only a sliver of resource use in food production—what matters more are the resources expended in growing the food.[6] It might thus be more resource-intensive to produce a tomato locally than to have one shipped from another state where the climate and resources are more conducive to efficient production. Furthermore, if producing and buying locally is so important, shouldn't our other commodities be produced locally, too? Yet locavores continued buying computers, appliances, books, and cars manufactured on the other side of the globe—without calling for producing such goods locally. The Maine deer hunter who claimed to be "shopping locally" and "organically" by killing deer might thus do so with a Mauser rifle imported from Germany, firing cartridges manufactured in South Dakota, after travelling hundreds of miles to kill his preferred "game." Locavores also made convenient exceptions to their rules. In *Omnivore's Dilemma*, when Pollan prepares a "locally-sourced" meal after paying a visit to Polyface Farm in Virginia, he permits himself to purchase Belgian chocolate for the meal, on grounds that Virgina doesn't produce its own.[7] (Pollan writes: "I also needed some chocolate for the dessert I had in mind. Fortunately the state of Virginia produces no chocolate to speak of, so I was free to go for the good Belgian stuff, panglessly.") Celebrity chef Jim Weaver, midway through his book extolling the virtues of locavorism, similarly admitted that he buys organic meat shipped to his neighborhood in Brooklyn aboard a refrigerated truck from the Midwest—a distance of over 1,000 miles.[8]

Despite these contradictions, locavorism appealed to food activists and consumers wanting to push back against corporate domination of the food system. Springing up as it did in the troubled period following the September 11 attacks, the movement offered the balm of community and connection for a nation still divided by war, promising a "return" to a simpler mode of life. In 2007, the Oxford American Dictionary named "locavore" its Word of the Year. Though the word had not appeared once in *Omnivore's Dilemma*, Pollan's book became a rallying point for locavores and other cultural and commercial forces, galvanizing a sensibility decades in the making. Like Carson's *Silent Spring* (1962), Jonathan Schell's *The Fate of the Earth* (1982), about nuclear war, and Bill McKibben's *The End of Nature* (1989), about global warming, *Omnivore's Dilemma* marked a cultural watershed, changing the way many Americans saw the world. In contrast to these other works, however, Pollan asked little of his readers beyond a change in their personal eating and buying habits. Dovetailing with a broader neoliberal shift in politics and society, *The Omnivore's Dilemma* spoke more to Americans' pastoral dreams and consumer desires than to a need for legislative remedies or sweeping new policies. The crisis of agriculture could be overcome without disturbing society, the economy, or our existing beliefs. Simply by supporting local farmers, seeking out fresh foods, and sitting at table with family and friends for luxurious meals, we could all be food revolutionaries.

That Pollan's book in fact had a libertarian cast was signaled in the titles of his book's three sections, *Industrial, Pastoral, Personal*, a narrative structure that briskly conveyed the reader from the realm of economic and government policy to the reader's private shopping cart and local farmer's market. Decades earlier, at a very different inflection point in the nation's cultural politics—at the apogee of the New Left and the counterculture—Lappé's *Diet for a Small Planet* had by contrast attempted to move food policy debates "out of the realm of individual ethics" and into "the international political economy of agriculture," as researcher Julie Guthman puts it.[9] Pollan had now done the opposite—taking global political economy and reducing it to "consumer choice." Coming as it did, however, during a period marked by national trauma and by broad neoliberal retreat from the public sphere, *Omnivore's Dilemma* was the book that many people needed at the time, a gripping summer beach read that both terrified and consoled. Like Immanuel Kant's aesthetics of the sublime—the experience we get observing some powerful natural phenomenon, like a great storm, but from a safe distance—*Omnivore's Dilemma* allowed readers to peer into the abyss, without however the abyss peering back into them. Reading about the horrors of the factory farm system was bearable, so long as one could also read about the "good" meat system that would soon replace it.

THE PLEASING STORY OF "GOOD" MEAT

A year after *Omnivore's Dilemma* appeared, another book about animal agriculture hit national bestseller lists. *Animal, Vegetable, Miracle,* by writer Barbara Kingsolver, offered a nonfiction chronicle of a year in the life of the Kingsolver family as they grew crops and raised animals for slaughter on a small organic farm in Appalachia. Like Pollan, Kingsolver lamented the damage inflicted by corporate agribusiness on rural communal life, and she too advocated smaller-scale, family-run farms. Like Pollan, too, Kingsolver sought to defend animal agriculture against the moral claims of vegetarians and animal advocates. To underscore their belief that animals have no value in themselves, apart from the uses we make of them, both authors had personally killed dozens of birds and mammals in the course of researching their books. Pollan described cutting the throats of thrashing chickens and shooting a pig with a rifle; Kingsolver described killing turkeys and other animals on her farm. Kingsolver, however, said she preferred the word "harvest" to "killing," on grounds that while the latter was "a culturally loaded term," *harvesting* instead "implies planning, respect, and effort." Cutting animals' throats or decapitating them with a hatchet was "a lot less fun than spending an autumn day picking apples off trees," she admitted. But it was "a similar operation on principle and the same word." Animal advocates were, therefore, hypocrites to object when farmers "cut off the heads of lettuces," but not when they chopped the heads off "crops that blink their beady eyes."[10]

The two books proved enormously influential, helping to solidify an emergent public consensus around the role of animals in a sustainable food system. (To this day, *The Omnivore's Dilemma* is widely taught in colleges and universities and is part of the required core curriculum for middle schools and high schools in states across the nation.) For decades, the public had been told that animal products were contraindicated with public health, ecological sustainability, and animal welfare. Now they were told that there were *two* animal economies, one bad (industrial "factory farming") and the other good (small-scale animal farming). A "new meat" renaissance now spread like wildfire, as millions of consumers began buying beef from "grass-fed" cows and building backyard chicken coops. Journalists and media executives enthusiastically promoted the myth of "humane" and "sustainable" animal production; sympathetic profiles of cattle ranchers, hunters, farmers, aquaculture entrepreneurs, and butchers appeared in thousands of articles, films, blogs, and news stories. In 2007, celebrity chef Wolfgang Puck announced "that he would use eggs and meat only from animals raised under strict humane standards."[11] Articles like, "Veal to Love, without the Guilt," about chefs "serving veal once more, finding the grain-fed meat more flavorful," appeared in the *New York Times*. Magazines like *Modern Farmer* made animal husbandry appear chic to young urban professionals. Documentary films romanticizing animal agriculture, like *Sweetgrass*, *The Greenhorns*, and *Kale vs. Cow*, found eager audiences in theaters and on Netflix. In 2009, the video game *Farmville*, enabling players to raise and sell virtual farmed animals on their cell phones, became the #1 best-selling game in the world.

The science of animal husbandry, formerly satirized in novels like Jane Smiley's *Moo*, suddenly became hip. At my alma mater in Western Massachusetts, Hampshire College, students were invited to participate in a multidisciplinary laboratory at the college's Farm Center, learning how to exploit sheep "sustainably." Though long a fixture on the campus, the Center in past years had played only a modest role in the life of the college. Now, though, as the mania for animal husbandry swept the country, faculty from different disciplines began to partner with the Center. A cognitive science professor trained students in "observing, coding, and analyzing animal behavior," while a film professor showed them how to unite "artistic and agricultural development" by videotaping sheep. From a psychologist, students learned to apply Jacques Lacan's psychoanalytic "concept of desire and the Other of language" in studying the birth of baby lambs during Lamb Week.[12]

There would be no talk of Lacan weeks later, however, when the lambs were taken from their mothers and sent to the slaughterhouse.

Thousands of Americans who had been seeking a more "authentic" relation to nature meanwhile began to seek out opportunities to kill animals with their own hands—raising and slaughtering chickens in their backyards, hunting deer, or enrolling in DIY workshops and classes on killing and dismembering pigs and sheep. Publishers began churning out hundreds of books with titles like *Meat Eater: Adventures from the Life of an American Hunter* and *Raising Steaks: The Life and Times of American Beef*. A new genre of women's nonfiction sprang up, featuring memoirs by professional women who had walked away from well-paying jobs to herd cattle, castrate sheep, and slaughter pigs as a form of empowerment (the topic of a later chapter).

This same cultural tidal wave overwhelmed the animal advocacy movement itself. For years, a struggle had raged between "welfarists" in the movement, who sought to improve the conditions in which animals were exploited, and "abolitionists," who opposed the exploitation and killing of animals as such. The new meat culture now turned the tide toward the welfarists. Months after *Omnivore's Dilemma* appeared in print, animal advocate and filmmaker James LaVeck warned that the animal industry had begun to co-opt the movement. In 1991, the American Cattlemen's Association (ACA) had hired the corporate PR firm Mongoven, Biscoe & Duchin (MBD) to formulate a strategy to defuse the animal rights and vegan movements. MBD partner Ronald Duchin laid out a three-pronged approach for the cattle industry: (1) to isolate the moral idealists in the movement; (2) to "educate" idealists to become "realists," so that they would soften their approach to industry; and (3) to convince "opportunists" in animal advocacy to work directly with industry. By "opportunists," MBD meant activists who had attached themselves to the animal movement for "visibility, power, followers, and perhaps, employment." The best way to control such opportunists, Duchin explained, was "to provide them with at least the perception of a partial victory."[13]

By the early-2000s, LaVeck now showed, an alliance had formed between powerful interests in animal agribusiness, on the one hand, and mainstream animal welfare groups like the Humane Society of the United States (HSUS), on the other. Some "idealists" had changed their former views, "adopting a more 'realistic' position," in "a textbook application of Duchin's turn-idealists-into-realists formula." These new converts to the industry's position now advocated the "humane" or "compassionate" killing of billions of animals for commercial purposes. "Eerily," LaVeck observed, "these newly transformed idealists even begin to refer to themselves as 'realists,' and to those who hold on to their own former values for non-participation as 'purists' and 'absolutists,' [or as] 'selfish' or 'self-righteous' in their 'moral rigidity.'"[14]

In 2006, in a story entitled, "Meat Labels Hope to Lure the Sensitive Carnivore," the *New York Times* reported that Whole Foods Market was "preparing to roll out a line of meat that will carry labels saying 'animal compassionate,' indicating the animals were raised in a humane manner until they were slaughtered."[15] The following year, the big animal welfare organizations began inviting organic animal farmers to their conventions, promoting "humane" meat. Wayne Pacelle, then-president of the HSUS, now joined forces with John Mackey, the libertarian, union-busting owner of Whole Foods, to create the Global Animal Partnership program (GAP)—an Orwellian effort that brought together the world's largest retailer of organic meat and the world's largest animal welfare organization under the same roof. Pacelle, a free market apostle, invited Mackey and the Missouri hog producer Joe Maxwell—a killer of some 50,000 pigs a year who believed that God had given other animals to humans to dominate—to sit on the Humane Society's executive board.[16] In 2016, Pacelle published *The Humane Economy*, arguing that capitalism was making things better for animals every day. Two years later, Pacelle was forced to resign from the HSUS under a cloud of sexual abuse allegations—one of several opportunists in the corporate-welfarist wing of the movement, including Nick

Cooney of Mercy for Animals and Paul Shapiro, a former vice president of HSUS, forced out of the movement over allegations of sexual misconduct. Most subsequently found work doing lucrative business with industry.[17]

Marketed under store banners promising "A Hearty Helping of Animal Compassion with Every Order," meat, eggs, and dairy products at Whole Foods achieved explosive sales growth. Consumers who had previously reduced their meat and dairy consumption out of environmental concerns now felt comfortable buying "grass-fed" beef and "cage free eggs." The press gleefully reported that some vegetarians were becoming meat-eaters again, now that they could eat animals without compromising their moral principles or environmental concerns. In Cambridge, Massachusetts, the Clear Conscience Cafe promised diners an opportunity to experience the pleasures of meat, but without the bitter moral aftertaste.

THE "DEFENDING YOUR DINNER" CONTEST WINNER

It was in this altered cultural landscape that the *New York Times* ran its "Defending Your Dinner" contest in 2012. Six years had gone by since Pollan had published *The Omnivore's Dilemma*, five since Kingsolver had published *Animal, Vegetable, Miracle*. From the start, the *Times* contest had been conceived not as an opportunity for moral reflection on our violent exploitation of animals, but as a victory lap for enlightened omnivorism, a movement that the *Times* had itself been promoting for over a decade.

To readers unfamiliar with debates in animal ethics, the five experts assembled by the *Times* seemed to form just the imposing "gauntlet" the paper had promised. But the opposite was true. Though all of the judges had previously criticized factory farms, not one was opposed to the killing of animals for food—so long as it was done "humanely" and "sustainably." Jonathan Safran Foer had concluded his book *Eating Animals* with cautious support for small-scale animal agriculture, and had gone on to promote "humane" meat through a nonprofit called Farm Forward. *Times* food critic Mark Bittman supported a "flexitarian" diet that included meat and fish. Policy expert Andrew Light wanted to reform animal agriculture, not do away with it. Even philosopher Peter Singer was open to "painless" exploitation and killing of farmed animals. Finally, there was Michael Pollan: no one had done more than he to promote the myth of "sustainable and humane" animal agriculture. The *Times* had assembled a "murderer's row" of heavy hitters, all right. But they were batting for the home team. Running this line-up, meanwhile, was *Times* journalist Ariel Kaminer, the contest's organizer, who just the year before had written a breezy account for the *Times* about her experience selecting a turkey for slaughter. In an article entitled, "The Main Course Had an Unhappy Face," Kaminer had mocked the bird's fear and vulnerability:

> She was a beautiful bird, a Bourbon Red turkey whose rich brown feathers were flecked with white, and she had spent her days roaming free around an organic farm that overlooked the Hudson River. But as I stood watching her, she did not seem happy. Instead, with her almond eyes downcast, her subdued manner suggested a kind of forbearance.
>
> Perhaps she sensed I was not there to make friends. In truth, I was there to kill her.[18]

There were other informed critics who the *Times* might have invited as judges instead, ones however who believed "ethical meat" to be a contradiction in terms. Philosopher Tom Regan had long called for abolishing animal agriculture. Breeze Harper had recently published *Sistah Vegan*, a book linking the oppression of Black Americans with exploitation of nonhuman animals. Catharine MacKinnon, a leading feminist law scholar, had compared the domination of animals by humans to the domination of women by men. South African writer J. M. Coetzee, winner of the Nobel Prize for Literature, had compared our treatment of animals to genocide. There were many other such critics. But the newspaper had only wanted judges who could be counted on to return the "right" verdict, one that bestowed legitimacy on the meat economy.

The essay that ended up winning the contest, "Give Thanks for Meat," by Jay Bost, appeared in the *Times* magazine two months later. A writer and farmer, Bost argued that raising animals for slaughter was justified so long as it served the interests of the wider biotic order, what the naturalist and hunter Aldo Leopold had called "the land ethic." Bost defined "the ethical" as "living in the most ecologically benign way." And grazing cows and eating them, he argued, could be more ecologically beneficial than a plant-based diet. Bost gave the example of "living among dry, scrubby grasslands in Arizona," where "eating meat . . . [was] the most ethical thing you can do other than subsist on wild game, tepary beans and pinyon nuts." Nothing was otherwise better than a "well-managed, free-ranged cow . . . to turn the sunlight captured by plants into condensed calories and protein with the aid of the microorganisms in its gut." Bost represented the latter as a formula: "Sun → diverse plants → cow → human." That equation was preferable to "the fossil-fuel-soaked scheme of tractor-tilled field → irrigated soy monoculture → tractor harvest → processing → tofu → shipping → human."

Bost's essay summed up the fraudulent themes that proponents of enlightened omnivorism had promoted for years, such as the idea that raising animals for slaughter is a more "natural" way of producing food than growing crops, and that consumers had to choose between "oil-soaked processed foods" like tofu, on the one hand, and sustainable animal agriculture, on the other. For meat to be ethical, Bost maintained, it must be based on three principles. First, it was necessary to "accept the biological reality that death begets life on this planet and that all life (including us!) is really just solar energy temporarily stored in an impermanent form." Second, we must "combine this realization with that cherished human trait of compassion and choose ethically raised food, vegetable, grain and/or meat." Finally, we must "give thanks."

None of Bost's arguments held up under scrutiny, however. Bost had ignored the scientific consensus that transforming plant matter into animal protein is a grossly inefficient use of land, water, and energy. His metaphysical formula, "Sun → diverse plants → cow → human," had hence inserted a wholly unnecessary animal input—*cow*—where none was indicated or needed. Bost had also neglected to mention that cows grazed on pasture produce considerably *more* climate-altering methane than cows confined on feedlots.[19] Feeding billions of humans the flesh of cows raised on pasture is, moreover, impossible—there just isn't enough Earth to go around. In an op-ed published in the *Dallas News* just weeks before Bost's essay appeared in the *Times*, historian James McWilliams had dismissed the idea that "grass-fed, free-range" beef could replace beef from cows raised on feedlots. "A tract of land just larger than France has been carved out of the Brazilian rain forest and turned over to grazing cattle," he noted. "Nothing about this is sustainable." McWilliams went on to observe that if all the cows in the United States were to be raised on grass, they would take up "almost half the country's land," not including "space needed for pastured chickens and pigs."[20]

Bost had meanwhile built his case for ecologically sustainable meat around the grasslands of Arizona. Eating locally grazed cows, he claimed, was the "most ethical" way to eat in that context. Like other locavores, however, Bost had arbitrarily separated out food consumption from the wider system of commodity production of which our foods form only a part. If it was wrong, though, to buy a veggie burger made of millet grown in Iowa, then surely it was also wrong to buy a Toyota made in Japan, a fishing pole assembled in Vermont, or an orange grown in Florida. Shouldn't Arizonans make their clothing out of palm fronds and shoes out of cactus hides, smelt their own iron ore, and build their own semiconductor chips—perhaps out of pinyon nuts? And what about tomatoes, peanuts, chocolate, and other foodstuffs? None were native to Arizona, yet Bost planned to go on eating them.

Finally, Bost had dodged the problem his essay was supposed to address—the ethics of eating animals. Since we don't need to kill animals for food, what justifies our continuing the behavior? In place of an argument, Bost had instead posed a rhetorical question: "Am I willing to divide the world into that which I have deemed is worthy of being spared the inevitable and that which is not worthy?" For him, the answer was "yes": all human life fell into the category of "the worthy," while all other animals fell into the category of the *unworthy*. Bost had not bothered to justify this ugly sentiment; he had merely reduced the question of killing animals to a matter of personal preference. Ethics, however, requires more from us than this, insofar as it concerns the question of how *everyone* ought to conduct their lives, not just ourselves. If we are debating the ethics of elder abuse, say, and I tell you, "Well, it should be left up to each of us to decide," you would rightly accuse me of having fled the field of moral debate. This is effectively what Bost had done. He merely *liked meat*. As for Bost's gnomic assertion that "death begets life," that is only true in the banal sense that, if no one ever died, the Earth would soon run out of space and resources. But that was no argument in favor of reproducing and raising billions of animals in order to kill them.

The judges awarded Bost first place, anyway. Proponents of the new meat economy at the *Times* had wanted a rousing valedictory on behalf of enlightened omnivorism, and Bost had given it to them.

THE "HUMANE" MEAT MYTH

Nearly two decades after publication of *The Omnivore's Dilemma*, 99% of meat, eggs, and dairy today still comes from animals raised in intensive confinement. Investigations by animal rights groups have meanwhile shown that animals raised even in smaller-scale, so-called "humane" operations are often subjected to horrific cruelty. "Pasture-fed" cattle are branded with red-hot irons; "free-range" chickens are crowded in the thousands on the dirt floors of giant warehouses; chickens and pigs on organic farms are either put into gas chambers or shipped off to the same mechanized slaughterhouses as animals from industrialized facilities, to suffer the same degradation and extremity. At the Hudson Valley Foie Gras company in Ferndale, New York—"the humane choice for purchasing foie gras," the company claimed—an undercover video exposé revealed workers "violently grabbing ducks by their wings and necks and then shoving metal pipes down their throats," while birds with open, suppurating wounds suffered in small wire cages "without proper veterinary care." So swollen were the birds' livers from forced feeding that the organs had begun pushing up against the birds' lungs, making it difficult for the animals even to breathe, causing them to hyperventilate.[21]

Other "compassionate" companies have done no better. After the Chipotle Mexican Grill restaurant chain publicly committed itself to sourcing from "humane" animal suppliers, the company took out billboards boasting that it was "Pro-Chicken," even premiering a television show on Hulu about a fictional animal activist who seeks to improve conditions on factory farms—"Farmed and Dangerous."[22] Thanks to such efforts, the company's sales of conventional and "high welfare" meat more than tripled. Later investigations, however, revealed that Chipotle was secretly switching suppliers when it suited its purposes, sometimes sourcing animals from places like Harris Ranch—the largest cattle feedlot in California. In 2018, a former Chipotle manager turned whistle-blower told the press that chicken parts would sometimes arrive from "the big factory farms."[23] When other activists conducted an undercover investigation of another Chipotle supplier, a Whole Foods "Humane Certified" egg-laying facility, the activists found "birds starving, crowded, and collapsed on the floor of a filthy industrial shed."[24] Both the Humane Society and PETA nonetheless gave Chipotle awards for its "animal welfare" policies, and the animal welfarist group Compassion in World Farming honored Chipotle with a "Good Sow Commendation in Pig Welfare" award. Just as James LaVeck had warned, the "opportunists" within the animal advocacy movement had won.

Chipotle's customers were meanwhile learning the hard way that "high welfare" animal products had failed to mitigate the biohazards of the animal economy. In 2015, nearly 150 Chipotle customers in Boston became seriously ill from a norovirus, most likely caused by improper handling of uncooked flesh at the restaurant. Over the next three years, a thousand other Chipotle customers, in Virginia, California, and Ohio, also fell ill. In 2020, following a Justice Department investigation, the company agreed to pay $25 million in fines for violating federal laws protecting the public from adulterated foods—the largest settlement of its kind.

As documented in the film *Seaspiracy*, the fish industry has meanwhile perpetrated its own "humane" hoax on the public, with companies hiding their indiscriminate slaughter of marine life behind the euphemism of "sustainable" practices. Despite urgent warnings by scientists that the oceanic ecosystem is on the verge of collapse, however, per capita consumption of fish has continued to grow: in 2021, per capita fish consumption in the US reached its highest level ever.[25] Billions of tilapia, salmon, and other fish are meanwhile being raised in crowded, filthy tanks in the aquaculture industry—"factory farms" for fish—where they suffer so much stress and trauma that, like intensively farmed cows, pigs, and chickens, they must be fed antibiotics to survive the ordeal long enough to be killed, at a fraction of their natural lifespans.

In a 2006 article about Whole Foods' "animal compassion" campaign, *Times* reporter Andrew Martin noted that "[w]hile the animal-welfare labels are proliferating, it remains unclear whether they appeal to anyone other than a niche market of animal lovers, particularly since the meat and eggs are as much as twice as expensive as products that do not carry the labels."[26] Certified "high welfare" animal products today remain an expensive niche market, while doing little if anything to improve the living conditions of the animals or to reduce demand for meat from factory farms. Because "enlightened" omnivorism trivializes ethical objections to animal exploitation, the discourse seems only to have whetted the public's appetite for new animal products, whether from "humane" sources or otherwise. But just as one wouldn't expect to cure a nation of alcoholics by offering them organic bourbon or artisanal Scotch, it was folly to have believed, as proponents of the new omnivorism did, that offering consumers "grass-fed" bison and "artisanal" pork would somehow wean them off meat from animals raised in industrial conditions. In 2021, Americans ate more than 220 pounds of meat per person, an all-time record[27]; meanwhile, the US model of intensive animal confinement has been exported to developing economies of Eastern Europe, China, India, and elsewhere. As for the tens of billions of beings languishing today in the gulag archipelago of animal agriculture, their suffering has gone wholly unrelieved.

The federal government, far from seeking to ameliorate farmed animals' wretched conditions, itself remains a leading perpetrator of violence against them.[28] In 2015, the *New York Times* conducted an investigation of the US Meat Animal Research Center in Clay Center, Nebraska, a government facility whose purpose is to help "producers of beef, pork and lamb turn a higher profit," using "surgery and breeding techniques to re-engineer the farm animal to fit the needs of the 21st-century meat industry." The investigation revealed a decades-long pattern of "illness, pain, and death" at the facility, with ewes made to give birth "unaided, in open fields where newborns are killed by predators, harsh weather and starvation" and genetically engineered pigs made to produce litters so huge that the mothers inadvertently crush their piglets to death. Cows, who normally gestate a single calf, have been "redesigned" to produce twins and even triplets, birthing calves so "weakened or deformed" that many die outright, in numbers that "even meat producers have been repulsed" by. One veterinarian who worked at the Center recounted the case of a juvenile female cow forcibly immobilized so that a succession of six bulls could rape her, for a study measuring "sexual libido" of bulls. Normally, "a single bull [would be placed] in with a cow for 15 minutes. But these bulls had been in there for hours mounting her." Throughout the ordeal, the "cow's head was locked in a cage like device to keep her immobile." "Her back legs were broken," the veterinarian told a reporter. "Her body was just torn up." The veterinarian was so disturbed seeing the cow suffer that he sought permission to euthanize her. But because the scientist in charge couldn't be tracked down, the cow died in agony over the course of hours.[29]

Since the Center's founding in 1964, more than 500,000 animals have suffered and died in similar circumstances. Yet their suffering has been a drop in the boundless sea of the animal economy, which exterminated trillions of other animals in the same period. Meanwhile, the handful of state laws prohibiting battery cages for hens or the confinement of nursing pigs in farrowing crates (an estimated 10 million piglets are crushed to death each year in the US alone due to such crates) have made no meaningful difference in the lives or fates of the animals we raise for food.

If enlightened omnivorism has neither slowed the pace of killing nor mitigated the suffering of animals, however, it has nevertheless succeeded in providing new forms of legitimacy for the industry, reinforcing the public's view of animal agriculture as a benign institution. Every one of the biggest animal exploiters—Tyson Foods, JBS, Cargill, Hormel, Smithfield—now markets itself as committed to "animal welfare" and to "compassionate" and "sustainable" animal products, even while utilizing the same intensive confinement practices of old. For the consumer, meanwhile, there is no practical way to distinguish meat from animals raised in accordance with (largely meaningless) "high welfare" standards and meat raised in conventional ways but marketed as "humane."[30] Few Americans, anyway, care enough about animals to invest time investigating companies' claims of sustainability or "compassion" in depth.[31] A public told that animals shouldn't suffer "unnecessarily," but also that they can be killed in the billions without moral difficulty, cannot be expected to take animals' interests seriously. One study indeed found that consumers who "transition to eating welfare-labelled meat" may be *less* likely to eliminate meat from their diet."[32] Even consumers who make some effort to buy the "right" animal products—seeking out "local" chicken at the farmer's market, say—have no hesitation dining at a steakhouse with friends, or taking their children to McDonald's to eat animals raised on feedlots in North Dakota or Texas. "Flexitarianism" and "Meatless Mondays"—positions whose moral seriousness might be compared to pledging not to be racist on Tuesdays or to commit assault on Sundays—only reinforce the prevailing view that animals' lives and interests are so trivial as not to be worth bothering about.

In 2000, George W. Bush campaigned for the US presidency as a "compassionate conservative."[33] After the September 11 attacks, the same compassionate conservative invaded two countries and secretly set up CIA torture camps in Cuba, Poland, Romania, Afghanistan, and at the Abu Ghraib airbase in Iraq. The notion that "compassion" could be reconciled with Bush's vicious policies—like cutting the budget for poor children's school lunches or engaging in war crimes—was mirrored during the same period in the specter of the "compassionate" killer of animals. In the autumn of 2006, President Bush acknowledged the existence of the CIA's torture sites; months earlier, as *The Omnivore's Dilemma* was appearing on bookshelves, *Harper's* magazine published "A Carnivore's Credo" by Roger Scruton, in which the conservative British philosopher—an old-school misogynist who still referred to feminists as "harpies"—urged "conscientious carnivores" to rally around "compassionate farming," on grounds that God had put animals on the Earth to serve us and answer to our needs.[34] Two years later, Catherine Friend published *Compassionate Carnivore: Or, How to Keep Animals Happy, Save Old Macdonald's Farm, Reduce Your Hoofprint, and Still Eat Meat*, a bestseller arguing that animals could be killed with love.[35] "Compassionate" omnivorism, with its promise of a "kinder, gentler" animal husbandry, would now embrace the most conservative values of all—a return to ancient principles of natural hierarchy and violent dominion.

PART II

LIES OF DOMINION

4

ROMANCING THE FARM

Peering into the ethereal blue light of our laptop on a night flight, or sitting slumped over our desk waiting for the clock to strike five, who hasn't wondered if we wouldn't all be better off living a simple life in the country, off the grid? Freed of the soul-destroying demands of email and other encumbrances of technological life, we might lounge on verdant hillsides watching sheep placidly graze, like shepherds in a Maxfield Parrish painting. Under the warmth of a lazy sun, the pall of fragmented, hurried time would lift like a chilly morning fog. At last we could feel at home in the world, at one with nature and at peace with ourselves. . . .

Yearning for a return to pastoral simplicity, an escape from the stresses of society, is to be found in some of our oldest myths and stories, from the Garden of Eden to Virgil's Arcadia. With modernity, our longing for a more authentic form of life became more achingly acute, as science and the waning of religious belief led to the disenchantment of nature, a purging of its mystery and wonder. Today we feel estranged from the ebb and flow of the seasons, from the land and from the other animals. Few of us would wish to give up the conveniences of civilization, like penicillin, MRIs, or hot showers. But few of us, either, would miss traffic jams or the twenty-four-hour news cycle, to say nothing of polluted rivers, toxic waste, and global warming. We thus feel pulled between giving in and giving up—between buying a new flatscreen TV and home-schooling our kids in a yurt.

Millions of consumers have seized upon "enlightened" omnivorism as the middle ground between these extremes, a way to experience a more "authentic" relation to food and to nature, yet without having to surrender their iPhones or ribeye steaks. Call it the New American Pastoral. With its wistful longing for a bygone era when small-scale animal farms dotted the landscape, enlightened omnivorism is as much a spiritual *cri de coeur* of the middle classes as it is a quest for healthier foods, a supposed answer to "the sentiment of a heartless world, and the soul of soulless conditions."[1] From the start, however, locavorism and "ethical" omnivorism were creatures less of hardscrabble rural farmers than of relatively well-off urban professionals yearning for authenticity. As locavore Jenna Woginrich explains of her decision to abandon her office job in the city to buy an animal farm, in her memoir *Made from Scratch: Discovering the Pleasures of a Handmade Life*, "all I want in the future is to sit on a hill and look at sheep. I'll know I've made it in this world when I can perch on a grassy overlook, pull out my fiddle, and play a Scottish reel for the flock."[2]

Pastoralism, or the raising and keeping of goats, sheep, camels, cattle, llamas, etc., for human use, dates back to the Neolithic period about 12,000 years ago, when the first sedentary human communities organized themselves around agriculture and domestication. Though pastoralism is often idealized, herding cultures were patriarchal and rooted in cruelty, not only to nonhuman animals but to humans too. Even by modern standards, many nomadic pastoralists were remarkably violent: the highest per capita slaughter of human beings in warfare was effected by Mongolian pastoral marauders under the command of Genghis Khan, in the twelfth to thirteenth centuries.[3] It is no small irony, then, that while many of the most ardent advocates of the "new" pastoralism identify with liberal ideals, the pastoral and agrarian myths they evoke in the name of liberation are thousands of years old, harkening back to a time when human beings lived in tribal communities, believed in gods and spirits, and enslaved one another without compunction. Beneath the enlightened omnivore's patina of "progressivism" today in fact lurk deeply conservative themes, including nationalism, faith in an unfettered free market, and nostalgia for a past untroubled by claims of social justice.

GRASS *DHARMA*—OR WHY THERE WILL BE
NO FREE LUNCH

We return once more to the book that played a pivotal role in defining the new sensibility around farms and food, *The Omnivore's Dilemma*. If Michael Pollan's book obtained to a certain genius, it was in the way its author skillfully retooled ancient pastoral myths of animal husbandry for the needs of twenty-first century capital. Millions embraced Pollan's belief that the problems endemic to capitalism and corporate animal agriculture could be overcome through better free markets and smarter animal husbandry. In short, the crises of agriculture could be overcome without us really having to change anything at all.

Pollan's idea of a self-sustaining animal farm as the cure for a corrupt and corrupting food system was in fact not new. The notion that agrarian life is superior to other forms of life, and that moral virtue clings to the farmer's character as stubbornly as loam to his trousers, goes back to the founding of the American republic.[4] The author of the first survey of the state of American agriculture, published in 1775, though criticizing New England farmers for overplanting corn each year (without taking the time to alternate crops to allow the soil rest), nonetheless admitted that New Englanders were "a very happy people" who, though living mostly without "luxuries," had produced "men in a state of great ease and content, possessing all the necessities of life."[5] Later books, like *The Practical Farmer: Being a New and Compendious System of Husbandry* (1793) and *Nature and Reason Harmonized in the Practice of Husbandry* (1823), argued that farming should be conducted in scientifically informed ways to work with nature rather than against it. Similar themes carried well into the twentieth century. In 1940, E. B. White, the celebrated essayist (and, later, author of *Charlotte's Web* and other beloved children's books), reviewed a bestselling book called *Practical Farming for Beginners*. Written by a farmer named H. A. Highstone, the book purported to instruct readers on how to run a "self-sustaining farm" so that one might "produce *all* one's needs." White, a hobbyist farmer himself, gently poked fun at Highstone's "formula for subsistence farming," particularly his warning not to purchase any grains lest "your whole structure topple." According to the advertising blurb, White wryly noted, Highstone's book would "be welcomed by 'an increasing number of American people who, fed up with the pressure of city living, are going back to the land for their livelihood.'"[6]

It was this same hoary theme that Pollan brought to life again in *The Omnivore's Dilemma*. Rather than grains, however, *grass* was the motif of his pastoral hymnal. Pollan devoted a third of his book to the subject. In chapters entitled "All Flesh Is Grass" and "Grass: Thirteen Ways of Looking at a Pasture" (a nod to Wallace Stevens's famous poem, "Thirteen Ways of Looking at a Blackbird"), Pollan elevated grass to the status of a supreme metaphysical principle, invoking foxtail grass and prairie grass, switchgrass, needlegrass, tall-grass, timothy grass, little bluestem grass, and "nourishing grass," "precious little grass," and "miraculous" grass. Grass gives human life meaning, perhaps even its purpose, since it is through its medium that nature transmutes the blood of slaughtered animals into human life.[7] Because cows graze on grass, and we eat cows, in a sense we are made of grass too. Unlike corn and other monocrops, Pollan argued, grass stands outside the poisonous influence of the free market, because grass "is not a commodity" and "can't easily be accumulated, traded, transported, or stored, at least for very long."[8] Animal agriculture was therefore unique in offering "one long, beautiful, and utterly convincing proof that in a world where grass can eat sunlight and food animals can eat grass, there is indeed a free lunch."[9]

In its monomaniacal obsession with a single genus or species, Pollan's grass *dharma* has few rivals in modern arts and letters. "Grass" and its permutations ("grassy," "grassland," etc.) appear more than 300 times in *The Omnivore's Dilemma*, more frequently than "Moby-Dick" appears in Melville's story about a sea captain's obsession with a white whale—eighty-two. What makes this odd is that neither grass nor cows is necessary for successful agriculture, a healthy diet, a thriving ecosystem, a flourishing human life, or, really, anything else. Far from being a virtuous or self-sustaining cycle, the practice of grazing cows for consumption on pasture is in fact one of the least efficient and most ecologically damaging ways to satisfy our dietary needs, a wasteful practice requiring massive amounts of water and deforested land.[10] Nor does grass stand outside capitalist relations. Hay—grass sold as fodder for domesticated animals—is a nearly $20 billion annual market in the US alone, five times greater than the market in apples and oranges combined. More importantly, grass is grown not in outer space but here on Earth, which is to say, on land—one of the scarcest and most expensive commodities on the planet. So there is no free lunch, after all.

Pollan's talents as a prose stylist are considerable, however, and it was easy for his legions of readers, particularly those eager to keep meat on their plates, to be swept up in his ecstatic vision of grass, cows, and humans living in karmic harmony. As a rhetorical strategy, however, it could only have succeeded in the United States, where animal husbandry has long been intertwined with national myths of the West, the prairie, and the Open Road.

Since colonial times, the domination of animals has been central to our nation's identity. Settler culture was bound up with clearing wilderness and emptying the land of the Indigenous peoples who dwelled in North America prior to European colonization. With westward expansion, the frontier became defined less and less by dense forestland and more and more by the open spaces of prairie and cultivated pasture. The image of the farming homestead resting lightly on the Plains—the Little House on the Prairie—became a utopian emblem of white sovereignty and self-sufficiency. In the twentieth century, this vision of the boundless prairie merged with the myth of the Open Road, as motorists were invited by the automobile industry to view car travel as a way to escape the fetters of small-town life. Enshrined in Jack Kerouac's *On the Road* and in countless Hollywood films, the iconic "road trip" became associated with communion with the land

and nature, even as automobile culture fragmented habitats, polluted water, soil, and air, and killed and maimed wild animals in the billions. Both mythologies, of the Open Road and of the grassy plain peopled with cows and cowboys, spoke to the restlessness of capital, converging in an aesthetic that reflected the surging powers of an entrepreneurial nation. Under wide open skies, surrounded by prairie and fields of corn and wheat, a citizen might experience the harmony of two discordant ideas of the American nation—the ceaseless flow of capital, goods, animals, and people, on one side, and the infinite expanse of nature, on the other.[11] And mediating these vast forces of the national sublime was the lone figure of the white farmer, heroically tending his livestock.

THE MEAT GOSPEL OF JOEL SALATIN

Had *Omnivore's Dilemma* been a dry academic treatise on the problems of industrialized agriculture (and there had already been many), it is unlikely it would have achieved the extraordinary success that it did. But at the heart of Pollan's book lay a "relatable" story of two macho men heroically triumphing over a corrupt Babylon of commodified, processed, and (as it were) sissified food. One was Pollan himself, who interspersed criticisms of agricultural policy with lively descriptions of his personal experiences as a modern-day "hunter-forager" and gourmand; the other was Joel Salatin, a Christian entrepreneur *cum* farmer, whom Pollan elevated to near-mythical proportions.

Thanks to dozens of books and films, many people are familiar with Joel Salatin and Polyface, the farm Salatin runs in the unincorporated township of Swoope in Augusta County, Virginia. Salatin has taken inspiration in part from the writings of J. I. Rodale, the guru of organic agriculture who called for minimizing external inputs like synthetic fertilizer while maximizing "outputs" (profits). While Salatin and his wife grow fruits and vegetables, their core business revolves around raising sheep, rabbits, cows, chickens, turkeys, and pigs for meat, eggs, and milk. The idea animating Polyface, the "farm of many faces," is to raise diverse animals and plants in a "holistic" and "sustainable" way.

It is no exaggeration to say that if Joel Salatin hadn't existed, Pollan would have had to invent him; as Johnson had his Boswell, Salatin has his Pollan. Though Salatin had long been a hero among afficionados of small-scale animal farming, it took Pollan's devotional account of Salatin and his mythic farm to propel him to national fame as the icon of the "new" animal husbandry. Here was a man who not only walked the walk of sustainability, but who stood up against the unholy trinity of Big Ag, federal bureaucracy, and veganism. Without Salatin as the larger-than-life figure of home-grown rural virtue and American gumption, and without Polyface itself as the model of the nouveau pastoralism, Pollan's critique of the predations of corporate agriculture would have lacked both human scale and a workable note of religious awe. Tagging along behind Salatin on his sprawling farm, Pollan portrays the farmer as a latter-day pastoral saint, an embodiment of the enduring character of the American nation. Even Salatin's straw hat is pregnant with significance, for it "bespoke independence, sufficiency, even ease," signifying "a political and aesthetic stance, one descended from Virgil through Jefferson with a detour through the sixties counterculture."[12]

Pollan's reference to Thomas Jefferson was by no means incidental to his storytelling, for it is in Jefferson's writings that we find the most fully elaborated view of the American agrarian myth, including its familiar notion that democracy grows in the soil tilled by the hard-working farmer. The self-sustaining farm frees the farmer from dependency, and dependency, Jefferson reminds us in *Notes on the State of Virginia*, "begs subservience and venality, suffocates the germ of virtue, and prepares tools for the designs of ambition." Nowhere in history, by contrast, do we find a case in which "the mass of cultivators" had succumbed to "[c]orruption of morals." The virtues of the farmer are not merely ethical but spiritual. "Those who labour in the earth are the chosen people of God, if ever he had a chosen people,"

Jefferson wrote; they are those "whose breasts he has made his pe-culiar deposit for substantial and genuine virtue."[13] Today, Jefferson's religious conception of farmers as the "chosen people of God" is still wending its way in American culture, as proponents of animal agricul-ture invoke religious imagery and the "sacred" language of providence, epiphany, and "conversion" in their depictions of animal husbandry and slaughter.[14]

Jefferson's notion of farming as civic religion reaches its apogee in Pollan's hagiographic treatment of Salatin. For Salatin, running Poly-face is literally God's work. A dyed-in-the-wool evangelical Christian educated at Bob Jones University—the far-right Christian college that views homosexuality as an abomination, and that not long ago banned racial mixing at the school dance—Salatin justifies the killing of animals by citing passages from the Bible to portray his farm as "ex-actly the model God used in building nature."[15] The image of God the builder segues into the figure of Salatin as free market savior—God's earthly representative in spreading the Word of private animal enter-prise. Author of several entrepreneurial books with titles like *Pastured Poultry Profit$*, Salatin describes himself as "a Christian libertarian environmentalist capitalist lunatic," and the moniker sticks. Pollan, though, prefers to compare him not to Rockefeller or Carnegie, but more grandiosely to Martin Luther. While "it was the printing press that allowed the Protestants to break off and form their own commu-nities" during the Reformation, Salatin tells him, "now it's the Inter-net, splintering us into tribes that want to go their own way."[16] One day, the world will "wake up" and find that locavores have taken over. "It won't happen overnight, but it will happen, just as it did for those Catholic priests who came to church one morning only to find that, my goodness, there aren't as many people in the pews today."[17]

Pollan gamely plays up Salatin's sense of divine mission, describing the customers who line up to buy Salatin's fleshy goods as "Polyface's four hundred parishioners."[18] Even the dead piles rotting in the heat of Salatin's farm—the corpses and fragments of slaughtered animals—

exude quasi-religious significance, as a way to "transubstantiate" a "mass of blood and guts and feathers into a particularly rich, cakey black compost."[19] Promoting his carnivorous gospel, Salatin sounds at times like Reverend John Winthrop, the spiritual leader of the Puritans, who compared the Massachusetts colony to a City on a Hill, the righteous Christian community serving as exemplar to a corrupt world. Even Winthrop's declaration that "the eyes of all people are upon us" finds a distant echo in Salatin's farm, an island of grace in a sinful world, whose "many faces" are offered to the world as part of a mission to redeem animal husbandry from big government.

For the pastoral fable Pollan needed to tell, it was important that his protagonist's "deliberate and hard-won" independence be shown to have arisen organically in the rural soil of the United States, beyond the reach of corrupt foreign influences, like native wild rice flourishing beside a polluted riverway. In a letter in 1795, Jefferson confesses that he "never liked" public life, and reports that he has returned to his estate "with infinite appetite, to the enjoyment of my farm, my family and my books, and . . . determined to meddle in nothing beyond their limits." Notwithstanding his contributions to diplomacy, Jefferson favored an isolationist politics, confiding his private wish that the new states "practice neither commerce nor navigation, but . . . stand with respect to Europe precisely on the footing of China. We should thus avoid wars, and all our citizens would be husbandmen."[20] Salatin, likewise, is staunchly isolationist, disinterested in the world outside his electrified paddock. The Salatins live in a "remarkably self-contained world," Pollan notes approvingly, their outlook circumscribed by a small-town newspaper that "devoted more space to local car crashes than the war in Iraq."[21] Like Jefferson, who favored the free market but resisted foreign entanglements, the Salatins don't know what is going on in the rest of the nation and world, and they don't care. Jefferson described the metropolis as a source of "degeneracy" and as "a canker which soon eats to the heart" of the republic's "laws and constitution," warning that "the mobs of great cities add just so much to the support of pure government as sores do to the strength of the human body."[22] Two centuries later, Joel Salatin, anti-cosmopolitan to his core, pointedly asks Pollan, "Why do we have a New York City? What is it good for?"[23]

Pollan portrayed the Salatins as free not only of cosmopolitan influences, but of the taint of modernity too. The Salatins "had largely detached their household from industrial civilization"; Polyface was "as far from . . . industrialized agriculture as it is possible to get without leaving the planet."[24] In reality, far from cutting himself off from industrialization, Salatin has made canny use of high technology, finance capital, and mass media to leverage his island of grace into an enterprise bringing in $2 million in sales each year, while relying on the Internet, diesel-powered trucks, "space age, microchip, electric fencing," and a gas-powered scalding tank kept at precise temperatures for burning away the hair on dead pigs.[25] He also uses the most advanced high-tech batteries "to power the electrified paddock fence" on his farm.[26] The four thousand chickens Salatin keeps have no liberty, but are pulled around the property in portable electric fencing known as "net corrals." And they are the same genetically altered animals manufactured by corporate industry, bioengineered to grow quickly to such enormous sizes that their hearts, lungs, and legs would eventually give out from the weight of their monstrous breasts, if Salatin didn't kill them first.

FROM FARMS TO MILITIAS

In fine, Pollan's portrait of Salatin as a simple Christian shepherd tending his flock, unfettered by the *technics* of a decadent civilization, was merely part of Salatin's own self-mythologizing. As a literary conceit, though, it succeeded in lending a mystical aura to Polyface, serving to justify its main bit of business—the mass killing of animals. It also distracted readers from Salatin's conservative worldview, which was strikingly at odds with the liberal sensibilities of *Omnivore's* mostly urban, middle-class readers. Salatin and his family say grace at every meal, abstain from alcohol and caffeine, quote Scripture, and subscribe to traditional gender roles. As Pollan approvingly observed, "much about dining with the Salatins had . . . the flavor of a long ago time and faraway place in America." When the Salatins sit down to eat, they do so in "exactly the sort of farmhouse kitchen—wood-paneled and decorated with all things quaint and hearth-like, up to and including the neatly framed needlepoints—that countless kitchens in American suburbs and sitcoms have been striving to simulate." Pollan described Salatin's retreat from the world as "an achievement," saying his "independence" from the world constituted "a politics and economics and way of life both deliberate and hard-won."[27]

But a politics of disengagement from the world is arguably no politics at all. Or rather, it is an anti-politics, a retreat from what the philosopher Hannah Arendt called the "space of appearances" where citizens argue over the values that ought to define their common life together. In place of a meaningful conception of civic engagement and political life, Salatin has instead substituted the unregulated free market and a fetish of private consumption. "All we need to do," he told Pollan, "is empower individuals with the right philosophy and the right information to opt out en masse."[28] For the customers who drive hundreds of miles to buy Polyface's products, Pollan averred, "buying a chicken from a local farmer" is "a kind of civic act, even a form of protest."[29]

To the extent that Salatin has any politics at all, it is plainly libertarian.[30] "If I were President," Salatin has said, "there wouldn't be an Education Department."[31] Calling federal regulation the "single biggest impediment to building a viable local food chain,"[32] Salatin has also said that the government has no business regulating the production or sale of food products.[33] ("We do not allow the government to dictate what religion you can observe, so why should we allow them to dictate what kind of food you can buy?" Buying food from whomever one wishes, without government rules about safety or public health, ought to be a "constitutional right."[34]) Though worried that Big Ag is intent upon destroying the little guy in agriculture, Salatin, who served as an invited guest speaker at the 2020 Libertarian National Convention, opposes federal regulation even of corporate monopolies, resisting laws that could level the playing field for smaller-scale farmers, on grounds that "we ask for too much salvation by legislation." Salatin suggests that small-scale animal farmers instead model themselves on Native Americans. "They didn't care if there was a Washington, D.C., or a Custer or a USDA; just leave us alone . . . [Today we're] going to have to refight the Battle of the Little Big Horn to preserve the right to opt out. . . ." Today, "we're in a war with the bureaucrats."[35]

An author more alive than Pollan to the ways in which rural conservatism has fueled some of the most virulent authoritarian movements of the nineteenth, twentieth, and now twenty-first centuries, from the antisemitism of the agrarian Populists to Trumpism, might have found Salatin's right-wing outlook troubling.[36] But Pollan was careful not to press Salatin too far on his political views. While skepticism towards politicians or federal bureaucracy can be a healthy thing, Salatin's "paranoia," as Pollan himself termed it, suggests something more disturbing—a fundamental hostility toward the very notion of a shared democratic life, if not sympathy for authoritarianism.

In interviews, Salatin has attributed his aversion to political life to the personal circumstances of his family during his childhood. Salatin's father moved the family to Venezuela after the Second World War, where he worked as the accountant of a major oil company before buying a 1,000-acre chicken and dairy cow farm there. The elder Salatin carved grazing lands out of the rainforest and soon cornered the poultry market, thanks in part to what his son Joel later described as a pleasing environment of "totally free market . . . without government regulations."[37] All went well until 1958, when pro-democracy leftists overthrew the dictatorship of Gen. Pérez Jiménez—an anti-Communist oligarch who terrorized and murdered his opponents—and later confiscated the Salatin family business as part of their effort to redress inequalities in land ownership. The Salatins fled back to America—an early trauma that convinced Salatin of the twin evils of government and leftism.

Against this backdrop, Salatin's colorful language of being "at war" with federal authorities seems rather less innocent. The same language has been used for decades by the militia movement and other far-right groups in the South and Midwest to portray the US government as a threat to Americans' liberty. Rural right-wing networks, composed of aggrieved white men from rural communities who identify closely with ranching and hunting culture, are testing the limits of federal authority, sometimes by threat of arms. In 2014, Cliven Bundy, an anti-government cattle rancher associated with the sovereign citizen movement, engaged in an armed stand-off with federal authorities over longstanding unpaid grazing fees from his herd in Nevada. Two years later, Bundy's son Ammon occupied the Malheur National Wildlife Preserve in Oregon with other heavily armed protesters to promote the view that the federal government had no right to own or to manage public lands (a common lament of ranchers), which instead belong to the states. This same sensibility, with its view of the federal government as an illegitimate authority imposing its "globalist" agenda on farmers and ranchers, helped prepare the ground for the assault on the US Capitol by a pro-Trump mob on January 6, 2021.

More and more, we see links forming between animal farming and reactionary politics. In Europe, government attempts to scale back greenhouse gas emissions in animal agriculture have been met with anger and sometimes violence by farmers, a growing number of whom are gravitating toward nationalist parties of the far right.[38] (One local leader in the German neo-Nazi Heimat Party, speaking at a recent farmers' protest, decried "climate ideology" and "gender madness."[39]) Meat has also become a flashpoint in the US culture wars, with right-wing politicians defending meat-eating and ranching. Republicans are seeking to pass federal legislation to suppress animal welfare standards, while accusing vegans of anti-American conspiracies.[40] "Florida is fighting back against the global elite's plan to force the world to eat meat grown in a petri dish or bugs to achieve their authoritarian goals," Republican Governor Ron DeSantis warned in 2024, as he signed legislation banning sales of lab-grown meat in his state. "Our administration will continue to focus on investing in our local farmers and ranchers, and we will save our beef."[41] As Julie Guthman observes in *Agrarian Dreams*, the American populist agrarian ideal has long been "based on particular class, race, and gender privileges, as well as a deep-rooted cultural conservatism."[42]

Locavorism and its close European cousin, the Slow Food movement, have both held out the promise of a return to familial connection, community, and local place as antidotes to alienation. As Jim Weaver, the locavore chef and a Slow Food proponent, puts it, living the "good life" means living a life of "love . . . of oneself, of one's friends, of one's family, of one's food."[43] No one could argue with that. But when private interests get split off from public and political concerns, they can become reactionary. Sitting down at table with others to enjoy a savory meal may be one of life's pleasures, but it remains a luxury that many working class and poor families don't have. The locavore's disengagement from a broader politics, meanwhile, all but ensures that the fundamental structures that lead to inequality and ecocide go unchallenged. The locavore saves the world not by addressing imbalances in global trade, an unjust division of labor, the militarized national security state, or ownership of production by a wealthy elite, but by buying expensive "pasture-raised" flesh.

While there is nothing wrong with shopping at one's local farmer's market or wanting to join a CSA, the liberal principle of buying and producing locally can segue into the illiberal notion of taking care of "one's own" first, at the expense of others more distant but with more urgent needs. At times, the locavore's fetishization of native plants and animals can even shade into *nativism*, an animus towards those who "don't belong" to one's nation or community. Of Salatin's right-wing, anti-animal rights views, scholar Vasile Stănescu observes that sustainable animal agriculture discourse often flirts with "a deeply disturbing strain of conservatism, provincialism, xenophobia and anti-immigrant sentiment."[44]

After the American Revolution, Jefferson spoke approvingly of popular aversion to European "sophistication, aristocracy, luxury, elegant language, etc." (as historian Leo Marx summarizes American opinion at the time). It was during this period that the slogan "Buy American!" was first heard in the streets—the belief "that crude local products were preferable (on moral grounds, of course) to European finery."[45] Echoes of Jefferson's populist localism still show up in American agrarian politics, with boosters of locavorism tying animal agriculture to nationalism. Farmer Catherine Friend, for example, in a chapter entitled "The Fuzzy Patriots" in her book *Sheepish*, cites an article in *Marine Corps News* about the benefits of using wool to clothe US soldiers then fighting in Iraq and Afghanistan, boasting that "if you shear off that fleece, underneath you'll find centuries of red, white, and blue." "Everyone we talk to expresses strong desire to bring their products back to the United States," *Sheep Industry News* reported, "and promote the fact that they are all domestic."[46]

In 2020, the bloom finally came off the Salatin rose when journalist Tom Philpott published a searing article in *Mother Jones* that punctured the myths surrounding the born-again farmer. For years, Philpott admitted, he and "a host of white food politics writers" had "glorified" Salatin and ignored his right-wing views, "chalking up his occasional bursts of illiberalism to a sort of rough-hewn eccentricity." Salatin instead had proven "less a beacon to a sustainable future than an example of Black and Indigenous erasure and nostalgia for a mythologized agrarian past." Vegan critics had in fact tried to draw attention to Salatin's ugly views for years, without success. In 2019, however, there had been a public dust-up between Salatin and a Black farmer named Chris Newman. In the back and forth that ensued in the alternative farming press, Salatin denied that "America is systemically racist," insisting instead that "the failure in the Black community is dysfunctional collapse in the family." The problem isn't racism, he said, but "fundamental social breakdown," namely, the fact that "75 percent of Black boys grow up without a father in their lives." Salatin offered "that the BIPOC [Black, Indigenous, and people of color] folks who feel America offers them no opportunity should give up all modern conveniences and return to their tribal locations and domicile."[47]

Had Salatin been running a veganic farm rather than an animal enterprise, it is unlikely that the alternative press would ever have lionized him. Nor would Pollan's liberal readers have so easily turned a blind eye to Salatin's reactionary views. But left-leaning foodies were happy to bracket their politics in their eagerness to embrace the Salatin myth of "humane and sustainable" animal husbandry. Many, too, were sympathetic to Pollan's depiction of vegans and animal advocates as "animal rightists," as he termed them—a smear calculated to link animal advocacy in his mostly liberal readers' minds with conservatism.[48]

FROM LOCAVORISM TO DONALD TRUMP

In 2016, when Donald Trump ascended to the White House on a campaign to put America first, running on a nationalist and nativist program, he had the enthusiastic support of American farmers. Farmers overwhelmingly voted for a presidential candidate who openly called Third World countries "shitholes," boasted about grabbing women by their genitals, and allied himself with white supremacists. Farmers' support for Trump put paid to the notion that there was anything inherently progressive about agrarian culture. In its electoral postmortem, *Modern Farmer*, the flagship publication of boutique meat culture and DIY animal husbandry, identified the issues that had drawn farmers into Trump's camp. One was the Water Rule of the United States, a critical part of the Clean Water Act intended to mitigate pollution of waterways by animal agriculture. While environmentalists supported the bill, the Farm Bureau opposed it as "federal 'over-reach,'" warning that its "impact on farmers and ranchers will be enormous." Farmers also opposed Democratic presidential candidate Hillary Clinton's plan to raise the minimum wage and healthcare benefits, on grounds that it would have forced them to spend more to improve the lives of farmworkers, including undocumented workers. They also disliked Clinton for her support of Obamacare and for promising to raise the Estate Tax that President George W. Bush had killed during his administration. Farmers viewed Trump favorably, too, because of his promise to uphold the Biofuels Tax—an environmentally dodgy government subsidy to corn producers. "The common thread here," *Modern Farmer* observed, "is that all these issues can be portrayed as attempts by an intrusive government to regulate and ruin the lives of farmers."[49]

Anti-government sentiment among farmers has only grown in the years since, endangering human health and safety. In 2024, as the highly pathogenic H5N1 virus spread rapidly throughout the chicken, dairy, and beef industries, creating the potential for a global pandemic of avian flu, US farmers refused to cooperate with federal efforts to monitor spread of the disease. Farmers declined to let inspectors from the CDC or FDA onto their properties, and they ignored requests to use electronic IDs to monitor the health of cattle. "Don't let them fool you," one Twitter user wrote. "These E-ID tags have nothing to [do] with animal disease & everything to do with control."[50]

Jefferson's romantic image of the simple farmer undoubtedly had some truth to it at the time, since most small farmers then produced only what they needed to live, with little left over for luxury goods. Nor was Jefferson wrong to associate the small farmer with a certain independence of mind and spirit. Many of the New England militiamen who swarmed the British in the spring of 1775, bloodying them on their hasty retreat back to Boston from Lexington and Concord, were precisely the yeoman farmers Jefferson had in mind, and their militant embrace of liberty, personal and civic, became legendary. But that was nearly three centuries ago, and much has changed since. Today, farmers seem no different from other people I know, neither more nor less wise or virtuous than carpenters, construction workers, or professors. And though their political views run the gamut, from libertarians like Joel Salatin to the utopian anarchists at Acorn Community Farm in Virginia, on the whole they tilt more right than liberal or left. There is nothing revolutionary, or even democratic, about farming culture today.

Though Jefferson's conception of farmers as the bedrock of colonial-era democracy was not wrong, it ignored white colonial expansion, the extermination of Native peoples, and the enslavement of millions of people of African descent. (In praising the virtue of white farmers, Jefferson neglected to mention that most of the agricultural labor of the South was performed by enslaved Blacks, including on his own plantation at Monticello.) These earlier traumas continue to haunt the agrarian imaginary today. Locavorism remains an overwhelmingly white movement; and in its obsession with the breeding, keeping, and killing of other species, it is literally backward-looking, drawing on principles of "natural" domination that should have been abandoned centuries ago.

In 2008, Pollan approvingly cited an editorial in *The American Conservative* that praised locavorism as "a conservative cause if ever there was one."[51] A number of critics have in fact noted the conservative thrust of the "new" food politics. As *The New Yorker* journalist Dana Goodyear observed of the locavore fad for raw cow's milk: "The new wave of refined American cuisine has a regressive side, wrapped up in nostalgia for an imagined past."[52] Pollan's own attacks on veganism and animal advocacy have been of this flavor. The worst thing about those who eschew meat, he implied in *Omnivore*, was their refusal of *tradition*—"Thanksgiving turkey . . . franks at the ballpark, and family traditions like my mother's beef brisket at Passover."[53]

The association of meat with tradition has long been used by corporate agribusiness as a selling point for meat; more and more, the trope is interwoven with a libertarian rhetoric of consumer freedom. Judith Capper, a self-described "sustainability" consultant to the American Cattlemen's Association, has attacked the "Meatless Mondays" campaign of the Humane Society of the United States on grounds "that meat-eaters [should] be afforded the same courtesy as vegetarians or vegans—to choose foods according to their individual or religious beliefs." In a nod to the National Rifle Association, Capper asks: "Give up meat on Mondays? As Charlton Heston would say: only when you pry it from my cold dead hands."[54]

That a frankly reactionary politics lurks even in the thickets of the progressive sectors of the sustainable animal agriculture movement can be seen in the work of Lierre Keith, a back-to-the-land farmer who attacks animal rights. While cultural conservatives are often said to want to turn the clock back to the 1950s, that is nothing for Keith, who wants to turn the clock back to before the Neolithic period 12,000 years ago. Keith and her frequent collaborator, Derrick Jensen, argue that we should do away with agriculture and return *Homo sapiens* to its "original" hunter-gatherer state. Would Keith listen to the demands of insufferable vegans, or "would I learn the grammar of my great-grandparents, and feed the trees with the bones of animals that lived beside me?" Would she eat "the food of our ancestors," or would she eat tofu?[55]

THE MYTH OF A "RETURN" TO SMALL-SCALE ANIMAL FARMS

American readers of *The Omnivore's Dilemma* were told that, by buying local chicken and organic pork, they could triumph over twin threats to their liberty—on one side, agribusiness and its enablers in the federal bureaucracy, and on the other, militant vegans who sought to impose their emasculating cosmopolitanism on a helpless nation. But Pollan's proposal for an Animal Husbandry 2.0—replete with browse-and-click online markets and "pasture-grazed" sheep tagged with RFID bar codes—was never a workable, or just, solution to the crisis of the animal food economy. However laudable the goals of locavorism—decentralized markets, closer farmer-consumer bonds, communal meals—the movement from the start misapprehended the nature of animal exploitation within the capitalist system, particularly the symbiotic relation between small- and large-scale agriculture.

Consumers who seek out "sustainable" beef and "cage-free eggs" do so in the vague expectation that they are buying from the kind of small farm run by Dorothy's aunt and uncle in *The Wizard of Oz*. Yet ecological limits and the economics of the free market alike make widespread small-scale animal production impossible. Even Salatin's Polyface farm is a sizable operation. In a single season, Pollan notes, "Salatin's grasses will have been transformed by his animals into some 40,000 pounds of beef, 30,000 pounds of pork, 10,000 broilers, 1,200 turkeys, 1,000 rabbits, and 35,000 dozen eggs."[56] Given these numbers, typical of a small- to medium-sized farm, there is no chance that a farmer will "get to know" each of the animals on his or her farm, let alone treat them with compassion or respect. Meanwhile, it will always be cheaper and more efficient in a profit-based economy to take our pound of flesh from an animal raised on a factory farm than on a smaller, organic one.

As aesthetically pleasing as smaller farms may be, market forces are tugging in the opposite direction, putting irresistible pressure on small farmers to fold their enterprises into bigger entities. In 2016, struggling family farmers in North Dakota reluctantly formed an alliance with corporate agribusiness to overturn a 1932 law prohibiting all but resident families from owning farms in the state. Local proponents argued "that the farming and ranching business in North Dakota needs to evolve to stay competitive: Dairies and pig farms have declined in recent years, prompting many people to argue that the industries could use a boost." As local rancher Katie Heger explained: "We have this picture in our head of the Hollywood farm, with the dairy cows, a couple of pigs, a couple of chickens. . . . There are very few farms that are like that. Farming and ranching is a business. So if we're looking at sustaining agriculture in the state of North Dakota, we need to look at how we can build business."[57]

To picture the future of animal farming is indeed to picture small farms being absorbed into bigger ones, even conglomerates. OBE, the largest exporter of organic animal goods in Australia, is indicative. An industry coalition of forty organic beef producers, OBE herds 100,000 animals, using a computerized "electronic identification system" as part of the company's "quality traceability system." At the end of their short lives, all of these animals receive the same violent fate as that of animals on non-organic farms—a journey of up to a thousand miles, sometimes in harsh weather conditions, to a killing center.[58] In the US, Niman Ranch offers another cautionary tale. Founded by rancher Bill Niman with his wife and partner, Nicolette, Niman for years traded under the motto, "the best-tasting animals around." For years, the liberal press lionized Niman Ranch, holding it up as a supposed model of sustainability and "humane" animal agriculture. Then in 2006 the Nimans lined up "a parade of investors" to hire a "new management team . . . led by Jeff Swain, who had been at the company that produces Coleman Natural Beef."[59] By the following year, Niman's new owners reported that they were "processing" 3,200 pigs and 400 cattle every week—over 150,000 animals per year—and generating annual sales of $85 million.[60]

The marketing of "sustainable" animal products has proved a boon chiefly to multinational corporations, as the pastoral aesthetic drives First World consumers to buy meat from "grass-fed" cows in the Third World. The Brazilian company JBS, the largest beef producer in the world and the single largest driver of destruction of the Amazon— its suppliers are burning down the rainforest to graze cattle—found that shifting from soy and corn cattle feed to grass helped buffer the company from volatility in world commodity markets.[61] "Brazil is in a sweet spot for the next 18 months," raved an analyst at ING Groep NV, the Dutch multinational bank. "Brazilian cattle are grass-fed so you don't care about [the price of] corn."[62] Driven by First World demand, JBS SA announced a quarterly profit in 2012 of $160 million, its highest in five years. The fact that "grass-fed" cows produce *more* climate-changing methane than cattle fed soy or corn is hidden from American consumers, who believe they are "doing the right thing." Pollan's grass *dharma* has shaped world commodity markets, and not for the better.

In short, small-scale and large-scale production are merely differ-ent segments within the same global market. The capitalist economy is happy to accommodate smaller-scale farming, even as the agribusi-ness giants accumulate staggering new levels of wealth and influence. Talk of a "return" to the small farm therefore amounts to wishful thinking—nostalgia for a bygone mode of production.[63] We can no more go "back" to a simple agrarian existence than return to a time of kings and queens, when society was built with the skilled labor of bricklayers, seamstresses, and blacksmiths. Industrialization rendered artisanal labor and small-scale animal agriculture obsolete over a cen-tury ago, and expensive workshops in *charcuterie* won't alter that fact.

Meanwhile, the most "enlightened" omnivores and locavores re-main opportunistic in their eating habits—buying meat, cheese, or eggs from factory farms whenever it is more convenient to do so. After visiting a Concentrated Animal Feeding Operation (CAFO) and see-ing the animals crowded together there in misery, their hides caked with their own bacteria-laden feces, even Michael Pollan freely admits in *The Omnivore's Dilemma* that after "the stink of this place is gone from my nostrils, I will eat feedlot beef again."[64]

KILLING AS COMMUNION

Whenever we board an airplane or click "buy" on Amazon, we partici-pate in a lethal chain of cause and effect that undermines the ecology of our world. The clothes on our back, sewn by poor women labor-ing in sweatshops in Bangladesh and Pakistan, are made with fabrics derived from petroleum; our cars and computers are built with ele-ments plundered from several continents. Overcoming these and myriad other environmentally and socially destructive practices will require a radical transformation of states and economies, and funda-mental changes to our way of life. Only with such a transformation, to a post-capitalist economy, is there any hope of healing the rift between *Homo sapiens* and the rest of the natural world.[65] Proponents of the new omnivorism, however, take their stand against capitalist modernity not by organizing against the rich and powerful, but by enacting violence against animals, helping cows and sheep and chickens to die on boutique organic farms to atone for the sins of factory farming.

In recent years, neoliberal austerity policies have gutted labor unions, weakened state protections for the vulnerable, widened social inequalities, and destabilized the ecological order. With the waning power of the individual in society—an artifact of the widening gap between ordinary people and the super-rich, on the one hand, and of the imposition of social controls about which the ordinary person has only a faint inkling, on the other—capitalists have now taken advantage of our vulnerability to sell us *authenticity* as the antidote to the ills of society. Appeals to the "romance" of animal agriculture, in this context, amount to attempts to commodify our despair. The fragmentation and commodification of animals' bodies is presented to the public as a curative for the corrosive effects of the free market on community and daily life. *Dissociation* from animals and nature is marketed as *connection* and *relation*, while the *killing* of animals is depicted as *affirming life*.

Proponents of the "new" meat have in short embraced violence as a way to transcend the contradictory nature of modernity. In New York, a yeshiva student studying to be an Orthodox rabbi is learning to butcher live chickens, as a way of overcoming a "disconnection from our food sources," a disconnection that causes "numerous environmental and social ills."[66] At a "whole hog" butchering class in San Francisco, one participant explains that while he was initially disturbed by the smell of death, the experience "was the connection to my food I really wanted to capture." (Students are advised to show up to class with "rain gear and boots, because there's going to be blood."[67]) Killing animals, in short, is presented as a way to overcome the anonymity of our modern transactions with the natural world. When journalist Ariel Kaminer seeks out a halal butcher to kill a turkey before her eyes, she does so, she explains, in order to be "part of the broader cultural effort to escape the climate-controlled, linoleum-lined artificiality of supermarket shopping, in which meat magically appears all ready for your oven and animals are characters in children's story-books."[68]

But there are many other ways to experience a meaningful sense of connection with animals short of destroying them. Scientists like Jane Goodall have forged lifelong friendships with the beings they study, without harming them. Ordinary people, too, can feel a connection to animals by birding, hiking in a canyon, swimming in the sea, camping in the wilderness, or photographing local fauna. Even our close attachments to our cats and dogs, though frequently belittled, offer us a more emotionally sustaining and authentic form of communion with other animals than is to be won by shooting a pig with a high-powered rifle or slitting a frightened bird's throat.

Millions of people in the underdeveloped global South raise and keep animals; most do so, however, not out of romantic attachment to pastoral myths, but because animal husbandry remains one of the few sources of livelihood available to them within a cruel international division of labor. (Charities like Heifer International, which solicit donations to fund small-scale animal agriculture in the global South as the supposed solution to "ending hunger," falsify the origins of global inequality, while dooming millions of animals to brutalization and violence.) In the overdeveloped North, meanwhile, we long to recover what we never had but feel we've lost—a mythical Golden Age of harmony with nature. Our inability to mourn this loss has given rise to helpless rage, turned however not against the elites who bear responsibility for the disasters of society, but against the most vulnerable beings in our midst—the animals, whom we treat not only as our commodities but as our slaves.

5

FREEDOM IS SLAVERY

"Animals, whom we have made our slaves,
we do not like to consider our equal."
—Charles Darwin [1]

Freedom is constitutive of sentient life; it is what all conscious living beings seek, and even what they *are*. A moth or ant placed in a glass grows frantic trying to escape; a fish confined to a tank spends its waking life looking for the exit. Given the choice, every conscious being prefers liberty to captivity, and autonomy to servitude. And when an organism's will to freedom is thwarted, it suffers spiritual collapse. A dog chained in a yard, a pig confined to a crate, an orca forced to live inside a tiny pool at SeaWorld—all exhibit signs of depression and despair. Up to 80% of zoo animals exhibit some form of neurotic or stereotyped behavior, such as rocking back and forth, pacing or swimming in circles, pulling out their fur or feathers, or head-banging, in response to their confinement. Other behaviors may include "coprophagy (eating feces), regurgitation, self-biting and mutilation . . . and infanticide." To calm their captives, zoos prescribe antidepressants and anti-psychotics, including Prozac, Celexa, Haldol, and Valium.[2]

Despite such facts, it has become a token of faith among proponents of the new omnivory that, notwithstanding the lamentable excesses of factory farms, the billions of animals whose lives we perfunctorily summon into existence in order to violently extinguish again, mere weeks or months later, are benefited by this arrangement; that they consent to it; and that in some sense they arranged the whole thing.

On this view, the animals we exploit *prefer* confinement and even death to natural liberty. "To say of one of Joel Salatin's caged broilers, that 'the life of freedom is to be preferred' betrays an ignorance about chicken preferences," claims Michael Pollan.[3] When animal rights activists break open the cages of minks on a fur ranch, say, or free chickens from their battery cages, they are therefore acting not just irresponsibly, but against the interests and even wishes of the very animals they seek to rescue.

Our conviction that other beings are degraded inferiors intended for our use—"intended" here in the metaphysical sense, as an axiom of natural purpose independent of human culture—is the bedrock of our dominion, securing every form of animal exploitation. On this view, animals were "put here" for our purposes, either by a wise and loving God (the believer's version) or by a "providential" evolutionary order (the secularist's). Other animals are viewed not as thinking, experiencing, feeling subjects with needs, interests, or perspectives of their own, but as instruments of use. "This is the sort of farm machinery I like," hunter-farmer Wes Jackson remarks to Pollan, of a pig they sit watching together on Salatin's farm, because an animal "never needs its oil changed, appreciates over time, and when you're done with it you eat it."[4] Animal "machines" have the additional benefit of being reproducible. While a "pregnant mare at work is growing her replacement," Jackson notes elsewhere, one "does not come out in the morning and find a little baby tractor."[5] As Barbara Kingsolver writes, animals are our "four-legged tools"; they are "human property, not just legally but biologically."[6]

This notion, that animals are our natural property, is ancient in origin, and it long served as the basis of slavery, an institution that for thousands of years was the norm throughout much of the ancient world. Human slaves and domesticated animals shared a similar legal status under the Code of Hammurabi (1780 BCE), as property and an impressed labor force. The ancient Greek word for slave—*andrapodon*, for "man-footed creature"—appears to have been derived from *tetra-*

podon, "four-footed creature," suggesting that slaves and domesticated animals were once viewed nearly interchangeably.[7] As Aristotle observed, whereas a wealthy family might own human slaves, "oxen serve the poor in lieu of household slaves."[8] It was indeed a commonplace in the ancient world that slavery and animal husbandry were more or less the same practice. Most historians and anthropologists now believe that slavery grew out of and was modeled on animal domestication. As David Brion Davis, an authority on the Atlantic slave trade, observed: "To control such beasts . . . humans not only branded them but devised collars, chains, prods, and whips and also castrated and subjected certain animals to specific breeding patterns. . . . [T]he continual comparison of slaves to domestic animals suggests that as formal wars developed between more densely populated societies, similar techniques of control were used on captives."[9]

Slavery not only utilized the same tactics of coercion as animal husbandry, but adopted its view of natural hierarchy between inferior and superior beings. By about the sixth century BCE, some in Greece had criticized the practice of enslaving humans, prompting Aristotle to defend slavery as natural and just. Aristotle held that living beings—plants, animals, and humans alike—have a *telos* or end purpose which guides and organizes their development. Social inequality and hierarchy were therefore not products of culture, but aspects of nature, embedded in a Great Chain of Being. Dominating others, or being dominated, fulfilled one's natural purpose, according to the sort of being one was. Members of a subordinated and inferior class of beings therefore achieved their excellence only when made use of by their more perfect natural superiors. It was natural, then, for men to dominate women, for masters to dominate slaves, for stronger city-states to destroy or enslave weaker ones, and for humans to dominate other animals. Vestiges of this ancient view of natural hierarchy remain with us today in sex role stereotypy and the notion that women are not as capable as men—a view deriving in part from Aristotle's view of woman as an "incomplete" man who fulfilled her true being only when paired with a man in order to bear him children.[10] Racial, gender, and class inequalities are still justified in some conservative circles on grounds of natural roles or capacities.

Aristotle's arguments for slavery proved remarkably enduring, impeding the cause of social equality and freedom for millennia. More than twenty centuries after Aristotle's death, apologists for racial slavery in the Antebellum South would cite his *Politics* more than any text apart from the Bible in defending the slave system. In an Aristotelian vein, the anti-abolitionist George Fitzhugh described "slave society" as merely one of "a series of subordinations" in which "fathers, masters, husbands, wives, children, and slaves, not being equals, rivals, competitors, and antagonists, best promote each other's selfish interests when they do most for those above or beneath them."[11] Just as Aristotle had portrayed slavery as *good* for the slave too—because it helped the enslaved to fulfill his or her natural excellence as a slave—modern owners of enslaved persons argued that Blacks were improved by their enslaved condition. "A state of bondage, so far from doing violence to the law of nature, develops and perfects it . . . and in that state [the Negro] enjoys the greatest amount of happiness, and arrives at the greatest degree of perfection, of which his nature is capable."[12] Slave owners could even be seen as benevolent, helping the enslaved to become *what they are*, i.e., helping them to realize the purposes nature had intended for them.

Today, advocates for the "new" animal husbandry make the same arguments, echoing Aristotle's view that "as nature makes nothing purposeless or in vain, all animals must have been made by nature for the sake of men."[13] Domesticated animals are not hurt or damaged by us, but "completed" by the uses we make of them. Michael Pollan thus tells us that "the happiness of a working animal . . . consists precisely in serving as a means to human ends," while Jenna Woginrich, unwittingly recalling Aristotle's depiction of oxen as the poor man's slaves, calls working dogs "the poor man's pony," lamenting the fact that dogs are no longer as widely exploited as they once were.[14] Dogs "are seen less as a labor force and more as part of the family," whereas before they were "used on farms to haul carts to market, pull sleds, and carry supplies," like "horses and mules." (Why keep a dog solely as a companion when "with a properly fitted harness, a healthy Labrador retriever can pull 175 pounds, no sweat"?[15]) As the slaveowner William Harper argued in his defense of slavery in the nineteenth century: "He whose business is to labor, should be made to labor, and that with due diligence. . . . This is no less necessary to his happiness than to his usefulness."[16]

Race slavery differed greatly from earlier forms of enslavement in tying the slave's subordinate status to supposed unchanging heritable characteristics—a race "essence" said to establish the inferiority of people of African ancestry and to render them the "natural" and "animal-like" slaves of whites. Apologists for racial slavery often used animal domestication as "proof" of the naturalness of the slave system.[17] As Harper wrote in his *Memoir on Slavery* (1832):

> By what right is it that man exercises dominion over the beasts of the field; subdues them to painful labour, or deprives them of life for his sustenance or enjoyment? They are not rational beings. No, they are creatures of God, sentient beings, capable of suffering and enjoyment, and entitled to enjoy the measure of their capacities. . . . It is because the greater good is effected; not only to man but to the inferior animals themselves. . . .
>
> [W]ith the difference only of circumstances and degree, rests the right of the civilized and cultivated man, over the savage and ignorant. It is the order of nature and of God, that the being of superior faculties and knowledge, and therefore of superior power, should control and dispose of those who are inferior.

Enslaved persons had long been compared to animals in the ancient world; but the racialized system of slavery "animalized" specific human populations, based on phenotype and place of ancestral origin. Crucially, without the prior category of "the animal" as a degraded subject, race slavery would have lacked its metaphysical basis. Humans "naturally" made use of animals, and white Euro-Americans "naturally" made use of "animal-like" Africans. Just as the human intellect was meant to rule over mindless animal species, the white mind was meant to rule over more "weak-minded" Blacks. "It belongs to the being of superior faculties," Harper wrote, "to judge of the relations which shall subsist between himself and inferior animals, and the use he shall make of them; and he may justly consider himself, who has the greater capacity of enjoyment, in the first instance." However, the superior being must use the inferior one "conscientiously." Just as it was wrong to inflict pain on animals without the expectation of "adequate benefit" in return, it was likewise wrong to inflict "unnecessary" suffering on slaves.[18]

The notion that "superior" types had a natural right to exert absolute authority over their ostensible inferiors was thus the basis both of human dominion over animals and of white dominion over Blacks. While *de jure* human slavery was abolished in the nineteenth century, however, the ancient conception of other animals as our biological slaves, intended by nature to serve us, has remained intact. The same arguments once used to legitimate human slavery have been revived and put into play again, this time by apologists for the "new" meat economy.

According to Michael Pollan, to view animals as wanting liberty is "to misconstrue that whole relationship—to project a human idea of power onto what is in fact an example of mutualism or symbiosis between species."[19] But *power* is not merely an idea, it is a *relation*. And in their unguarded moments, even proponents of animal agriculture themselves acknowledge that their fundamental relation with animals is one of domination. Back-to-the-lander Alyssa Jumars thus recounts that, after she and her partner buy two mares to labor for them on their farm, "the horses began to test our authority in small ways." Distressed by "the sight and the jingling of harness," the horses would turn and stalk away when the women approached to halter them. "They'd take a step back to the side when we slid the harness over their backs, or raise their heads when we bridled them." At first, the women back down. But soon they become forceful. "What we unwittingly taught them was this: Throw a fit or act terrified of something and we will make it go away." The horses had gotten the mistaken impression that they had a say in the matter of harnesses and halters. "Our horses learned that we were pushovers and that they could get away with holding their own opinions and, ultimately, making their own decisions." So the women attach a "butt rope" to keep the mares together, so that they won't be able to "fan and turn inside out" to evade the women's control.[20]

The farmers' anger at the horses' attempt to exert their autonomy, to assert a literally *unbridled* will, recalls a passage in Plato's *Republic* when Socrates, evaluating the various forms of government, warns his friend Glaucon that, because the logic of democracy leads to complete equality and liberty, it threatens natural hierarchy. In a fully realized democracy, Socrates warns, children no longer fear or obey their parents, teachers are afraid of their pupils, masters and slaves are seen as equals, women exercise "complete freedom and equal rights" with men, and "even animals subject to man" have freedom. "Dogs behave like the proverbial masters—why, the very horses and mules stalk about in stately freedom and shoulder aside anyone who doesn't step out of their way, and everything else is bristling with freedom." Hearing this, Glaucon exclaims, "You're telling me my own nightmare."[21] End human dominion over animals, and you destroy the foundation of the state.

* * *

Slavery apologists rarely defended their practices on the straightforward grounds that they profited from slavery economically, psychologically, and even sexually. Nor did they admit that they *enjoyed* exerting power over the enslaved. Instead, they offered a host of metaphysical and "spiritual" rationales to justify their behavior. Racialized slavery wasn't a degradation of the human character, they maintained, but its *fulfillment*. The enslaved weren't damaged by the slave system; they were benefited by it. The owner of slaves wasn't acting selfishly, but out of selfless concern for the interests of his slave. Both in antiquity and in modern times, slavery was in fact often presented as a relationship between friends. "There is a community of interest, and a relation of friendship, between master and slave," Aristotle wrote, "when both of them naturally merit the position in which they stand."[22] Master and slave "have an identical interest," since the "slave is a part of the master, in the sense of being a living but separate part of his body."[23] This is why "slavery is the better and [more] just condition" for the master's natural inferiors.[24] White apologists for racial slavery in the nineteenth century later adopted these same views. The master watches over his slaves, Thomas Dew wrote in 1832, "with the kindest and most affectionate solicitude," winning "the kind treatment and generous sympathies of feeling hearts." The "slaves of a good master are his warmest, most constant, and most devoted friends."[25] Slave-owners had great natural affection for their slaves, and that feeling was reciprocated. Slavery was "all kindness on one side, and . . . affection and gratitude on the other."[26] "The relation of Master and Slave . . . is as the experience of all the world declares, naturally one of kindness."[27]

This same sentimental language has now been revived by meat apologists to defend our exploitation of animals. "Animals have been *good friends* to us throughout the millennia," Kathy Rudy writes in *Loving Animals*—a book which, notwithstanding its title, is a defense of exploiting and killing animals.[28] Lierre Keith similarly tells us that when she raises animals for slaughter, she's not harming them, but engaged in a "relationship . . . of mutuality and respect."[29] Keith describes the animals on her farm as "the joy of her days," as creatures who "accept you" and "come to you for help" and "cuddle sessions."[30] Later, she brings her cuddle partners to the butcher.

Real friendship, however, implies genuine mutuality and respect. That is why true friendship can be said to flourish only between equals, since inequalities of power undermine the reciprocal trust and mutual vulnerability that lie at the heart of the relation. Stockholm Syndrome, in which people abducted by terrorists develop warm feelings for their captors, identifying with their needs or interests in an unconscious bid for survival, is but an extreme example of the quotidian relations of inequality that stand in the way of genuine friendship. The greater the power differential in a relationship, the harder it is to preserve it from the corrupting taint of authority. This is why the relationship of "friendship" between the slave owner and the enslaved was anything but. Slavery was a relation of *unequals*, in which one side wielded literal powers of life and death over the other. And while we might well imagine, under some circumstances, the spontaneous upwelling of friendly *sentiments* between master and slave, we should be on our guard against attributing to such sentiments the qualities of true friendship. Nor should we imagine, in a case such as Jefferson's long-term relationship with Sally Hemings, that a "romantic" relation between dominated and dominator ever approached genuine reciprocity, as mutual awareness of the absolute vulnerability of the one party, and the absolute invulnerability of the other, would have thwarted the deeper communion that Aristotle, in his wiser moments, recognized as the true ground of love.

"Never listen when they tell you that Man and the animals have a common interest, that the prosperity of the one is the prosperity of the others. It is all lies. Man serves the interests of no creature except himself. . . . The life of an animal is misery and slavery." So declares Major, the prophetic elderly boar in George Orwell's satirical *Animal Farm*, to the other animals on Mr. Jones's farm. Major has gathered the animals together to reveal the terrible truth of their condition, which is that farmer Jones is not their friend, after all.[31] Few farmers, in truth, claim to maintain "friendships" with the animals they raise, both because most have no interest in such a relation and because they don't

have the time for it, being engaged in the practical business of reproducing and selling their animal properties. The burden of depicting
animal husbandry as "friendship" is therefore left, on the one hand, to
corporate agribusiness—whose bottom line depends upon convincing
consumers that their animal products are "ethical"—and, on the other,
to professional apologists of animal agriculture—journalists, farmers,
food writers, academics, filmmakers—who assure us that, in some
sense, animals *want* to be killed and eaten by us.

6

LOVE ME, BEAT ME, KILL ME, EAT ME

It is not enough for apologists of animal agriculture to suggest that farmed animals benefit from our "kindness" towards them; they must also be seen as *consenting* to their exploitation and death at our hands. Far from being the guileless victims of human cunning, the first animals we impressed to labor were the instigators of their own bondage. Long ago, they came to *us*, having sensibly determined that they would be *better off* with our help than left to their own sorry devices.[1] As animal behaviorist Stephen Budiansky writes, "the animals that we think of as domesticated chose us as much as we chose them." Thousands of years ago, they "entered into an alliance of mutual dependence" and "symbiosis" with us.[2] In this pleasing tale, the far-seeing and ingenious ancestors of modern turkeys, reindeer, cows, camels, pigs, chickens, aurochs, geese, sheep, etc., all had the same epiphany at once.[3] In a miracle of interspecies coordination, they decided to exchange the inconveniences of a "state of nature," in which all warred against all and none were safe, for the security and comfort of domestication by *Homo sapiens*.

In accepting this quid pro quo, the animals wonderfully anticipated the social contract theory of the seventeenth century English political theorist Thomas Hobbes, who described legitimate political rule as an arrangement in which a citizenry surrendered its rights of individual liberty to an absolute sovereign, in exchange for protection from foreign enemies and from one another. However, the clever animals proved even more "Hobbesian" than Hobbes himself. For they surrendered not only their own natural right to liberty, and that of their young, but also that of their future descendants. Without a backward glance, they cheerfully granted *Homo sapiens* the right to make use of every member of their kind for eternity, for any purpose whatsoever, so long as humans found it pleasing to themselves. As the political theorist John Locke observed in his later critique of Hobbes, however, a social contract between a people and a government can only be rightly held binding so long as the sovereign adheres to the agreed terms. What a free people can never do, Locke maintained, is to alienate its natural right to liberty once and for all time. Legitimate government is always provisional, subject to renewal and even to overthrow. Hence Thomas Jefferson's agriculturist-political dictum that "the tree of liberty must be refreshed from time to time with the blood of patriots & tyrants. It is its natural manure." If the animals chose human dominion, then, they did so illegitimately since, having surrendered the right to redraw the terms of the contract, they abandoned their liberty forever. And the proper name for one placed in permanent bondage to another is not "citizen" but "slave."

The distinction between these two roles could hardly be plainer. In legitimate forms of rule, there are well-defined limits to the power of the sovereign, and well-defined rights claimed by the citizen. In slavery, however, the situation is otherwise. The master claims a right to do whatsoever he likes to the slave, while the slave enjoys no reciprocal right to do what she likes to the master. In agriculture, similarly, the farmer castrates, suffocates, shoots, or stabs the animals who live under his absolute authority, claiming a *natural right* to engage in these acts. However, any animal who resists such treatment—who scratches, bucks, bites, or tries to run away—is subjected to harsh words and angry blows, when not dispatched to the nearest butcher. Slaves, too, who rebelled or tried to escape would be whipped, branded, castrated, chained, or hobbled, and their repeated insubordination meant death.

"It's a partnership," Keith nonetheless says of animal agriculture, echoing Joel Salatin's description of the animals on his farm as "partners in the land-healing ministry."[4] In this same egalitarian spirit, we saw, Whole Foods runs its "Global Animal Partnership" program depicting farmers, land animals, fish, and consumers as collaborators. In 2013, the chain launched an ad campaign featuring farmers, fishermen, and beekeepers holding aloft animals—including dead ones—under taglines that read, "*We Are Earthlings*," and "*Gopher and Farmer. One*." The message conveyed was one of mutual striving and common interest, notwithstanding the fact that while one party lived, the other died violently at the hands of the other. "We're all food," Jenna Woginrich writes pleasantly in *Barnheart*, her account of running a small animal farm. "Eating meat is what predators do," she says, "and human beings are nothing if not predators. I had no problem with a wolf eating me or my eating a deer. *We were all in this together*."[5]

The notion that "we're all in this together," once a common refrain, too, of slavery apologists, is reiterated with clockwork regularity by defenders of animal agriculture and hunting. Even the hunter and the hunted are depicted as working together in an equal partnership in which both are willing participants. "The hunter and the hunted deeply *affect* each other," writes Kathy Rudy. For both sides, "[b]eing part of a hunt means accepting vulnerability. In this world, the animal and the human exchange both risk and flesh as part of a sacred food chain."[6] However, Rudy does not explain in what sense a hunter armed with a high-powered rifle and infrared scope is "accepting vulnerability" or inviting "risk" in the same way as his unsuspecting victim downrange.

The idea that animals "want" to be captured or even killed has disturbing parallels with the myth in rape culture that a woman sexually victimized by a man must have been "asking for it."[7] Spanish writer José Ortega y Gassett justified hunting animals on grounds that it was "a relationship that certain animals impose on man, to the point where not trying to hunt them demands the intervention of our deliberate will. . . . The only adequate response to a being that lives obsessed with avoiding capture is to try to catch it."[8] But perpetrators of male sexual violence, too, often seek to justify their behavior by describing their victims as "seductresses" who brought the attack on themselves, even in cases where the woman fought back or struggled to get away.

English common law for centuries recognized the "conjugal right" of men within a marriage to make sexual use of their wives' bodies—a so-called marital rape exemption grounded in the principle of "implied consent."[9] Merely by entering into the marriage contract, the woman tacitly "agreed" to be made use of by her husband. The law expressed no opinion on the matter of whether a man should rape his wife; it only upheld his legal right to do so. Rape within marriage was indeed not seen as rape at all, but as a private matter, hence not of state interest. In a similar vein, our society treats the killing and eating of animals as a matter of private preference, not public concern: it is left to the individual's discretion whether, when, and how to exercise the presumed human "right" to kill other beings. An animal's mere existence is enough to imply consent to being slaughtered—meat advertisements often depict animals smiling and dancing on their way to the barbecue or butcher.

Celebrity locavore chef Jim Weaver describes cheese as "the oldest *cooperative effort* between animals and humans," averring that "we *still need each other* because it's impossible to make authentic, memorable cheese in a test tube."[10] Like other mammals, however, cows lactate for their young, not for members of other species; to make them produce milk for humans, farmers forcibly impregnate them, then sell the newborn calves into the veal industry. Enzymes are later torn from the slaughtered calves' stomachs for use in culturing cheese. While it is clear, then, why humans need cows to make dairy cheese, it is far less clear why cows, whose ancestors grazed the Earth long before humans arrived, should "need" us. One might as well say that the Romans and their slaves "needed one another," too, to build aqueducts and pave roads.

Since we are "all in this together," the animals must nonetheless be shown to benefit from the arrangement as much as we do. Thanks to domestication, Catherine Friend writes, "life got better for *both* humans and sheep."[11] "Sheep seem to appreciate what we're doing for them," she says.[12] Keith depicts the animals on her farm as so pampered that they come off as freeloaders—as when she complains that, during the winter, she has to dig through snow "so that my chickens would have something to drink." "I'm not exploiting them. They're happy, safe, warm, and fed. I'm the one who's miserable," she says. "Chickens won't even walk in snow, let alone haul supplies for me. . . . Chickens have gotten humans to work for them."[13] This sentiment, that the farmer "suffers" on behalf of her livestock and even sacrifices herself for their benefit, was a staple too of slavery apologia. The slave owner assumed the burden of "caring" for the enslaved individual, "worrying" about his or her health and safety, and "suffering" right along with the slave when the owner "had to" inflict corporal punishments on his human property. Having invested in a living commodity, the argument went then and goes now, the owner's natural interest in keeping that commodity healthy for market converges with the well-being and happiness of the enslaved.

What, then, of the countless documented cases of sadistic cruelty to animals in animal agriculture? Industry representatives and farmers dismiss such "abuses" as anomalies within an otherwise well-regulated and benign system. While acknowledging the evils of factory farms, they insist that there are nonetheless farmers who do "get it right by treating animals with love, care, and respect," as Rudy puts it.[14] The problem isn't animal agriculture, but how it's done. However, this line of argument, too, recalls nineteenth-century debates over slavery. When abolitionists publicized horrifying atrocities by the owners of slaves, slavery apologists accused them of cherry-picking their examples to exaggerate the slaves' suffering. Yes, the apologists would admit, an unscrupulous slave owner might sometimes abuse his property. But most slave owners were wiser. Reports of slaves being tortured or worked to death were exceptions within a system that otherwise functioned to the mutual benefit of the owner of slaves and the enslaved alike. Because "abuses" were rare, abolitionists therefore oughtn't besmirch the institution as a whole.

The situations of enslaved people, in fact, varied greatly from plantation to plantation. Even Rev. Benjamin Godwin, the British abolitionist firebrand, "admitted that the condition of the slaves may [vary] . . . by the views and dispositions of the owners . . . or of the overseers," and that "some masters and managers are more humane and considerate than others," exhibiting "more humanity, more calmness" than others. However, to focus on the "good" slave owners was to miss the point, Godwin said. The abolitionist position was not that "every slave suffers all the evils to which his condition exposes him," but rather that "he is subject to all these miseries, and . . . many [do] suffer them to the full, and all *may*."[15] This was as much to say that it wasn't the "abuses" inflicted by individual slave owners that was the problem; it was the institution of slavery. Though the treatment of the enslaved might vary from place to place and from owner to owner, his or her fate was always left to the caprices of the owner. Some owners of slaves treated their human property comparatively well—beating them "only" rarely, or keeping enslaved families intact—while others tortured, raped, or murdered their human property. Citing the abysmal treatment of farmed animals in Britain, Godwin observed:

> It is a man's interest, we know, to use his cattle well, and to take care that those who work them treat them properly; but, notwithstanding this, does not the brute creation groan under the cruelties of man? How many are injured through mere wantonness! How many through thoughtlessness! and how many a noble animal has been shamefully abused in a moment of passion! Besides, the owners of cattle are not always with them, and may even never see many of them; and men who have no interest in them may have the care and the working of them.

Violent abuse of animals in British agriculture was so much the norm, Godwin noted, that the Parliament had seen fit to pass legislation "to prevent cruelty to animals."[16] In the New World, we note, animals fared no better. After a visit to New England, the English author of *Animal Husbandry* (1775) declared that he knew of no country "in which animals are worse treated":

Horses are in general, even valuable ones, worked hard, and starved: they plough, cart, and ride them to death, at the same time they give very little heed to their food; after the hardest day's works, all the nourishment they are likely to have is to be turned into a wood, where the shoots and weeds form the chief of the pasture; unless it be after the hay is in, when they get a share of the after-grass. A New Englander (and it is the same quite to Pensylvania) will ride his horse full speed twenty or thirty miles; tye him to a tree, while he does his business, then remount, and gallop back again. This bad treatment extends to draft oxen; to their cows, sheep, and swine.[17]

To this day, animal farming remains a relation not of mutuality but of violent exploitation.[18] This is not to deny that some farmers feel affection for the animals they raise. But casual brutality is more common than compassionate care, and many farmworkers routinely curse, kick, beat, or administer electric shocks to force the compliance of their charges. Godwin maintained that, just as the interest of the farmer would always be at odds with the interests of his captive animals, "for similar reasons the interest of the slave-owner in his slaves is no sufficient security against ill-treatment."[19] The truth of the slave system was that "the interest of the master does not always run parallel with the slave's welfare. It may happen that circumstances may be such, that a degree of labor which is destructive to the slave may enrich his owner."[20] Today, thanks to undercover exposés by animal advocacy groups, the press periodically discovers some new shocking "abuse" in a system ordinarily viewed as harmless. But the distinction between "normal" violence in animal agriculture, on one side, and "abnormal" abuse, on the other, is untenable. A system built to effect the violent deaths of billions of unwilling subjects cannot help but produce extreme acts of cruelty, quite in excess of what is strictly speaking "necessary."

In 2001, a few hundred animals on small family farms in England, Scotland, and Wales were discovered to be infected with hoof and mouth disease. Though hoof and mouth disease is a non-fatal illness from which many animals recover, the British authorities ordered the mass killing of six million sheep, cows, and pigs. Soldiers were brought in to help with the shooting. To dispose of the corpses, authorities burned the bodies in giant pits, sending plumes of smoke across the English Channel. Peter Frost-Pennington, a semi-retired veterinarian who had joined the "front lines" (his words) of the massacre, killed animals for as much as twenty-three hours straight. He later told the BBC about an incident in which a boy, the son of a farmer, "had hand-reared a Highland calf" whom he was "trying to hide in his bedroom." "So I had to go in there and, as gently as possible, take it away from him. And then I had to kill it." Farmers who ordinarily would send their animals to be slaughtered had to kill them themselves, reportedly causing some of them great distress, if not trauma. Twenty years later, farmers who participated in the killings still found it difficult to speak about "the dark period."[21]

THE CASE OF THE ANIMALS VS. MAN

> "The Holy One, blessed be He, respects human dignity and knows our needs. He shut the mouths of beasts. For if they could speak it would have been impossible to put them in service to man or to stand up against them."
> —Midrash exposition of the Book of Numbers (Torah), eleventh-twelfth century[22]

Two thousand years ago, the Greek philosopher Plutarch noted that when "humans trap or trick animals into captivity . . . they reject food, resist thirst and choose to bring about and embrace death rather than accept enslavement."[23] Today, the animals we imprison in laboratories, slaughterhouses, zoos, and aquaria likewise resist our tyranny—they cry out, scratch or bite, try to escape, or mutely beg our mercy. If their protests go unheard, it is only because we choose not to listen, fearing the resonance of their cries for justice. Who, though, is to hold us accountable for our crimes against them, if not we ourselves?

This was the very question raised in *The Case of the Animals vs. Man Before the King of the Jinn*, a remarkable tenth-century work composed by a group of Islamic scholars known as the Brethren of Purity in what is now Basra, Iraq. In the story, the animals of the Earth give voice in court to their grievances against the human race. At a trial before the King of the Jinn, or genies (the supernatural beings of Arab folk myth), the representatives of the birds, fishes, insects, mammals, and other animals one by one give impassioned testimony against humans for their numberless crimes. Animals who had once "roamed the woodlands and wilds unhindered, in search of pasture, water, and all their needs," were "checked and trammeled." Gazelles and birds who had long "lived in peace and quietude in their ancestral lands" were forced to flee humans in terror, abandoning "the haunts of men for far-off wastes, forests, mountain peaks, and glens." Still the humans "set after them with all sorts of devices for hunting, trapping, and snaring, convinced that the animals were their runaway or rebellious slaves."[24] The animals describe "the exhausting toil and drudgery of hauling, ploughing, drawing water, turning mills, and being ridden," noting that they never consented to this usage but were "forced . . . to these tasks with beatings, bludgeonings, and every kind of duress, torture, and chastisement" throughout their lives. Furthermore, whosoever "fell into [humans'] hands was yoked, haltered, caged, and fettered." Then they were put to death. "They slaughtered and flayed him, ripped open his belly, cut off his limbs and broke his bones, tore out his sinews, plucked his feathers or sheared his hair or his fleece, and set him on the fire to cook, or to roast on a spit, or put him to even harsher tortures, torments ultimately beyond description." Without "weeping or complaining," the other animals watched as their comrades were "dismembered, disemboweled," "their heads, brains, and livers placed on butchers' blocks."[25]

Hearing all this, the humans merely scoff. "These cattle, beasts of prey, and wild creatures—all animals in fact—are our slaves," they tell the King. "We are their masters. Some have rebelled and escaped. Others obey grudgingly and scorn our service."[26] The relationship between human master and nonhuman slave, they say, is one of paternal solicitude:

> We buy and sell them, feed and water them. We clothe and shelter them from heat and cold, and protect them from predators that would tear them to pieces. When they fall ill, we treat their illness and take care for them. We train them when they're raw, bear with them when they're mad, put them out to pasture when they are spent—all in kindness and compassion for them. But these are things masters do for their servants and owners for their property.[27]

As the trial proceeds, however, the animals make the better arguments, demolishing the excuses offered by the humans in defense of their dominion, from an upright posture and fairer form to intelligence and superiority of senses. The animals establish the beauty of animal forms, the inferiority of the human senses, and the cleverness of many species, observing that while a human will often become lost even when traveling down a familiar road, animals are able to navigate unerringly over great distances. The humans, meanwhile, worried that the judge might want to see the deed or bill of sale proving the animals to be their property, scheme to deceive the court: "We'll say we had these documents, but they were lost in the Flood."

In the end, the humans establish that they differ from other animals in one crucial respect—the presence of saintly persons among them. As such, only humans are potentially capable of spiritual enlightenment. But the trial ends without judgment. As the Brethren explain in their introduction, their aim has been "to touch on man's overreaching, oppression, and injustice against the creatures that serve him." Though the Brethren fail to offer an alternative to our uses of other species, they provide an unflinching account of the suffering animals endure at human hands, while showcasing human perfidy, vanity, arrogance, and sadism.

The only thing that has changed in the interim between ancient Basra and today is the scale of our abuses. That the animals we imprison and violate still have the status of our slaves is confirmed in periodic news reports of animals "escaping" from zoos, farms, and even aquariums. If the escapee should be recaptured and returned to captivity, the episode is reported in a humorous way. If, however, the animal is shot to death by the police, then the episode is represented in a "tragic" light, as the "sad" outcome of an "escape." In either case, it is taken for granted that humans have the natural right to keep other beings in captivity for their uses, and to thwart their manifest desire for freedom. Some philosophers still maintain that animals, lacking reason, cannot be said to be capable of freedom. Yet the fact that animals attempt to resist or escape our control shows that they fully comprehend the distinction between liberty and forced confinement.

Chickens frantically try to hide their eggs from the humans who come each morning to collect them. Oxen refuse to plow if their team partner should become injured. Sheep guess which way the farmer is going to lunge at them, then coolly bolt in the opposite direction. At the National Aquarium in New Zealand, an octopus named Inky waited for everyone to leave the building one night, then shoved aside the lid of his tank, pushed himself through the opening, slid across the floor, and escaped by squeezing "through a narrow pipe leading to open waters."[28] In 2018, the BBC reported that a cow being led to a slaughterhouse in southern Poland "sought sanctuary on the islands of Lake Nyskie" after overpowering the men who were leading her, breaking through a metal barrier, and swimming across a reservoir.[29] Here in Massachusetts, a sixteen-hundred-pound cow leaped a five foot high fence to escape a slaughterhouse in Hopkinton, then evaded capture for forty days and forty nights, despite unusually heavy snowfalls. Emily, as the cow became known, was eventually adopted by Meg and Lewis Randa, directors of the Peace Abbey in Sherborne, where she lived for another eight years before dying of uterine cancer, surrounded by the loving humans who cared for her. There are hundreds of similar examples of what the animal industry and news media alike call "runaways," the same term once used to designate fugitive slaves.

Sometimes animals resist our attempts to harm them with counterforce. In *Moby-Dick*, Melville relates a true incident in which a sperm whale, enraged at the violence being done to her comrades, made precise headlong dashes at the bow of a whaling ship to amplify the force of her attack, sinking it. One scholarly analysis of the behavior of sperm whales during the nineteenth century concluded that whales not only engaged in strategies of resistance, but taught one another how best to evade and attack the humans hunting them: their defensive maneuvers and attacks proved so successful that they caused a nearly 60% decline in whalers' successful strikes.[30] In 1994, an abused and traumatized circus elephant named Tyke suddenly snapped in the middle of a performance in Honolulu, murdered her abusive trainer in front of the crowd, and bolted out of the circus tent, running through heavy traffic and dodging cars. She was shot at least twenty times by angry men wielding rifles and pistols, until she finally collapsed in the street. In the heartbreaking video of her death, she can be seen struggling to stand, her eyes filled with indescribable suffering as she looks about, in vain, for safety or the comfort of a friend, as men and women in the street can be heard screaming, "Fucking animal!" and the men fire more rounds into her bleeding head.[31]

Such incidents, including documented cases of once-captive domesticated animals adapting well to a free life, are ignored by those who prefer to see farms, circuses, zoos, and other institutions of captivity as beneficent institutions intended for the "safety" of the animals held captive within them. "If farm animals have civil rights," Barbara Kingsolver asks sarcastically, "what aspect of their bondage to humans shall they overcome? Most wouldn't last two days without it."[32] But slave owners once made the same arguments. Abolition "would be extreme cruelty to the African savages," one eighteenth-century apologist said, because slavery "saves [them] from massacre, or intolerable bondage in their own country, and introduces them into a much happier state of life."[33] Compare Thomas Dew's remark in 1832, that "Liberty has been the heaviest curse to the slave, when given too soon,"[34] to Michael Pollan's contention, more than two centuries later, that "Liberation is the last thing such a creature wants."[35]

Slave apologists wrote a great deal, and not inaccurately, about the suffering of "wage slaves" in Europe and the northern states—of adults and children made to labor up to sixteen hours a day in filthy, dangerous factories and mines during the early waves of industrialization. Freed slaves were even "less free after emancipation than before," since, once freed, their "obligation to labor was increased; for they were compelled to labor more than before to obtain a livelihood, else their free labor would not have been cheaper than their labor as slaves." Freed slaves thus "lost something in liberty, and everything in rights—for emancipation liberated or released the masters from all their burdens, cares and liabilities, whilst it increased both the labors and the cares of the liberated serf." In contrast to wage laborers, among slaves one found "no starvation, no begging, no want of employment."[36] Once "elevated" above their natural condition of privation, slaves were "happy, content." Slavery supported the slave "in comfort and peace," while "restraining" his vices. Furthermore, slaves were "utterly incapable, from intellectual weakness, ever to give us any trouble by their aspirations."[37]

Owners of enslaved people were not wrong about the brutalities of the wage labor system (socialists had drawn attention to such brutalities for years). But their "concern" for the suffering of freed slaves was bad faith, rooted not in empathy but in race hatred and pecuniary self-interest. Today, much as slave apologists once cited statistics on the brutal and degrading conditions suffered by children working in factories to justify slavery, apologists for animal agriculture invoke the horrific conditions of industrialized animal agriculture—and the hazards of natural liberty—to justify the violence and degradation of animals on smaller, ostensibly "humane" farms. Pollan thus defends animal agriculture on grounds that "the life expectancy of a farm animal would be considerably briefer in the world beyond the pasture fence or chicken coop." Joel Salatin similarly maintains that the chickens on his farm "have an easier life than they would in nature," because "[w]e protect our animals from predators and weather. We give them good food and care of them, and in return, they are more prolific."[38]

While it is true, however, that escaped farmed animals, genetically tailored by capital to serve human interests, find themselves at a disadvantage when suddenly confronted with freedom in an unknown and hostile environment, they stand a better chance of survival outside the bounds of the farmer's property than within them. Even a commercially bred hen with a weak heart stands better odds of survival by escaping Salatin's clutches than by remaining within them, since every one of the animals at Polyface are killed while still juveniles. (Pigs, who can live up to twenty years, are generally killed at six months; chickens, who in nature can live up to fifteen years, at six to seven weeks.) Colonies of feral chickens—domesticated birds who managed to escape human captivity to live and squabble another day—have been found thriving years later, long after the compatriots they left behind have been served for dinner or been ground up as fertilizer after dying from the trauma of confinement. On the Hawaiian island of Kauai, escaped chickens were found living in a free colony, "evolving into something quite different from their wild predecessors, gaining some traits that reflect that past, but maintaining others that had been selected by humans." Similar cases have been documented of "other populations of animals, including dogs, pigs and sheep, that have broken free of captivity and flourished."[39] So powerful is the myth that animals "benefit" from our exploitation, however, that hunters and locavore proponents often argue that even wild animals are *better off dead* than to be exposed to the hazards of freedom in nature. "Being instantly beheaded sure beats being ripped apart by a fox or run over by a truck," quips farmer Jenna Woginrich.[40]

In locavore farming accounts, the narrative veers boozily between "sentimental" concern for the animals, on one side, and schadenfreude at their misfortunes, on the other. In *The Dirty Life: A Memoir of Farming, Food, and Love*, her account of buying and running an animal farm on Lake Champlain, Kristin Kimball describes a newborn calf as "an intimate, practically a member of the family." Yet in other passages, her descriptions of the calf are callous and mocking, as when she notes that the calf one day will be "in her mother's place, tenderly licking clean a new baby"—and "she would not get to keep hers, either."[41] After snatching the calf from her mother to sell for veal, Kimball describes how the mother "lingered around that spot for days, searching, lowing. I think that in her wordless way she blamed us for her loss."[42] Far from sympathizing with the cow's panic and grief, Kimball makes fun of the "molassesslike thought" that supposedly kept her from intervening in time to save her calf. "We expected Delia to follow, but she couldn't understand where her calf had gone. She nosed the grass where she had given birth, wondering if it was still there but invisible. She bawled urgently and would not move from the spot." Eventually, Delia "stopped bawling for her calf. From then on, it was as though there had never been a calf, or she had willed herself to forget."[43]

It is impossible to read such passages without being reminded of Thomas Jefferson's similar view of enslaved Black women after their children were ripped from their sides and sold to a new white owner. "Their griefs are transient," Jefferson wrote in *Notes on the State of Virginia*. "Those numberless afflictions . . . are less felt, and sooner forgotten with them. In general, their existence appears to participate more of sensation than reflection."[44] Like humans, cows in fact have excellent memories, and they recognize their offspring years later if given the opportunity to reunite with them.[45] Psychologists and biologists have furthermore established that mammals and other animals exhibit PTSD in the wake of emotional trauma. Some cows have been discovered to have given birth to their calves in secret, then hidden them in the bushes to keep the farmer from taking them again, much as the enslaved mother of Moses hid him in the bullrushes.

KILL BILL—AND LOU TOO

Even in cases where farmers do develop affectionate bonds with the animals they exploit, the "friendship" between oppressor and oppressed lasts only so long as the latter remains of profitable use to the former. Then the relationship takes on a decidedly less friendly aspect. Such proved the case concerning Bill and Lou, two draft oxen at Green Mountain College in Rutland, Vermont, before the college went out of business in 2019.

Nestled alongside the meandering Poultney River amid majestic white pines, tamaracks, and sugar maples, the college long prided itself on its sustainability curriculum, which included a working farm where students were taught to plant crops and to raise cows, chickens, and pigs for milk, eggs, and meat. Year after year, Bill and Lou toiled on behalf of their human overseers, pulling plows and other heavy loads in snow, rain, and sun. Beloved on campus and in town, the gentle oxen responded affectionately to the hugs and caresses people came to give them. One day in 2012, however, Lou sustained an injury to the joint of one of his rear legs, making it impossible for him to pull. In response, Bill, Lou's close companion of eleven years, went on "strike," refusing to labor without him. College administrators then convened a campus-wide meeting to determine the oxen's fate. Should Bill and Lou be put to pasture, allowed to live out the rest of their lives in peace? Or might there not be some better use for them?

Students, staff, and faculty were invited to weigh in on the matter. Some argued that after many years of faithful service, Bill and Lou had earned a retirement. But others saw things differently. Bill and Lou were "meant" to labor. Now that they couldn't or wouldn't work, they had stopped contributing to the farm and had become merely a drain on the Earth's resources. To spare the oxen's lives would thus go against the college's ecological mission. And so, after the public airing of views, college administrators announced their verdict: both animals would be put to death. Bill and Lou would be taken to a butcher, shot in the head, and bled to death. Then their bodies would be made into hamburgers and served to students in the cafeteria. It would be a teachable moment in the meaning of "sustainability."

As news of Bill and Lou's fate spread online, ten thousand people signed an online petition urging the college not to kill the oxen. Protestors held vigils at the entrance of the college, where they were met with angry jeers by Green Mountain's students. The *New York Times*, National Public Radio, and other media reported on the controversy. VINE, a nearby animal sanctuary in Vermont, offered to take the oxen and care for them for the rest of their lives, at its own expense.[46] But Green Mountain refused. "If sent to a sanctuary," the college explained in a statement, "Bill and Lou would continue to consume resources at a significant rate. As a sustainable farm, we can't just consider the responsible stewardship of the resources within our boundaries, but of all the earth's resources." What the college did not say, however, is that Green Mountain's students and faculty themselves would be allowed to "continue to consume resources," and at rates far exceeding those of the two oxen, driving their Chevy pickups and BMWs, shopping online, and jetting overseas for vacations and conferences.

In the end, Aristotle's ancient view of animals as mere living tools won the day. Bill and Lou had a *telos*, and that was to serve human purposes. And now that they were no longer of use, they had lost their right to exist. As the controversy swirled, Steven Fesmire, a philosophy professor at the school, chastised Green Mountain's critics, claiming they had no right to question the college's decision since the community had engaged in an "inclusive deliberation" that had met the demands of procedural justice. "We strive to be a community that listens to, responds to, and thoughtfully incorporates different voices," Fesmire wrote. "Yes, Bill and Lou's voices too."[47]

But Bill's and Lou's voices hadn't been included in the discussion that decided their fate. Had the two oxen been brought to the public hearing, perhaps their guileless affection and curiosity would have served as eloquent testimony of their desire and right to live. Had members of the community listened, they might have "heard," in Bill's refusal to leave the side of his long-time companion, the voice of a kind spirit. Instead, however, the community chose to privilege the voices of the teamsters who had driven the oxen, coercing their labor each day. Fesmire claimed that it was they, Bill and Lou's overseers, not those who were distant from on-the-ground considerations, who were "obviously the best-positioned proxies to speak for the oxen's interests."

This notion, that morality—like politics—is local, was also common in slavery apologia. White Southerners used the claim of "states' rights" to circumvent the federal government's attempts to regulate the spread of slavery, essentially arguing that each state was entitled to its own principles of right and wrong. Slave apologists told Northern abolitionists to butt out of their affairs, saying they had no moral authority to criticize Southern institutions, being too remote from the "on-the-ground" realities of plantation life. In a bitter rebuke of abolitionists, slavery proponent Harper wrote that it was "extraordinary" that "those who complain and clamor, are not those who are supposed to feel the oppression, but persons at a distance from them, and who can hardly at all appreciate the good or evil of their situation."[48] "We who have the best opportunity of judging" the situation, he wrote, stood accused of being "incompetent to do so, and to be blinded by our interests and prejudices." Skeptics of slavery were being told "to distrust or disbelieve that which we daily observe, and familiarly know," by people who had never owned a slave or even visited a plantation.[49]

After weeks of controversy, Green Mountain College cancelled its plan, citing alleged death threats made to the owners of the slaughterhouse where Bill and Lou were to have been taken and killed. A few months later, after the controversy had died down, the college quietly had Lou "euthanized," ostensibly for health reasons. Some time later, under circumstances that still remain a mystery, Bill disappeared.

PART III
LIES OF KILLING

7

MURDER, SHE WROTE

The HeliBacon company in Houston, Texas, offers helicopter rides over forested lands to massacre wild pigs using automatic weapons. Patrons, virtually all men, choose from among dozens of different weapons, from shotguns, carbines, and Glocks to a belt-driven Browning M2 .50 caliber machine gun—a massive anti-aircraft weapon that has been used by the US military in dozens of conflicts, including Vietnam and Iraq. The kinetic energy of a single .50 round on a body is enough to turn organs into pulp and bones into splinters. (The US military has long used live goats and pigs as experimental subjects to study the physiological effects of high-velocity rounds, partly to provide surgeons with experience in treating battlefield trauma.) As the copters swoop down over the terrified animals, HeliBacon's guides indicate desirable targets like "sounders"—groups of mother pigs and their piglets. Pigs not killed outright lapse into shock, dying slowly from their wounds and staggering in agony with their shattered intestines or other organs hanging out, as the men hoot with delight.[1]

Aristotle described hunting as war against animals, and war as the hunting of humans, and the two practices have always been the province of men. Nothing indeed more defines the masculine as soldiering and hunting. As ecofeminist Marti Kheel observed, the hunter's "intimacy with death," his ritual of "oneness" with nature, serves to confirm "his masculine self-identity."[2] The same holds true of warfare, the ultimate proving ground of masculine prowess. Four out of five hunters and nine out of ten recreational fishers in the US are men; about the same percentage of men occupy combat roles in the US military. Soldiers refer to combat as "hunting" enemy soldiers; sports hunters meanwhile invoke the language of war and its sadistic violence. A cover story in *Hunting Magazine*, entitled "Calling All Killers," features a photograph of a rugged white man in military camouflage and face paint on its cover, holding a rifle with a scope in one hand and a dead fox in the other. In *Elk Hunter*, *Marlin*, and hundreds of other magazines catering to fetishes for killing particular species, advertisers hawk military-grade weapons and accessories—night vision goggles, sniper scopes, hollow-point bullets, combat knives, range finders. HeliBacon boasts that its Bell 212 helicopter has been adapted by many countries "for national defense forces." The company's high-end promotional video depicts a helicopter flying against a red sun—an homage to a scene in the film *Apocalypse Now* of a fleet of Bell UH-1 Hueys on their way to mow down civilians in a Vietnamese village.

The multi-billion-dollar industry in hunting and fishing, like the animal economy generally, is so obviously a patriarchal enterprise that it seems almost redundant to point it out. The "double helix" of human supremacism and capitalism, described in an earlier chapter, is rooted in masculinist violence, and the same is true of the animal economy through which the two systems find their confluence. It was white men from Europe who invaded the Americas and used cattle, horses, and dogs to subjugate the Native human inhabitants, whom they raped, enslaved, and exterminated—a historical trauma whose faint imprint still lingers in ranching culture, with its iconic trope of the cowboy rounding up sheep or cows on horseback, wielding a whip. As Carol Adams shows in *The Sexual Politics of Meat*, meat-eating and the killing of animals have in fact been associated with masculinity and the domination of women for thousands of years.[3] It is still men who take over the barbecue pit and "fire up the grill," and men who are supposed to need and crave animal flesh more than women. In 2006, Burger King rewrote the lyrics to Helen Reddy's famous 1970s feminist anthem, "I Am Woman," linking masculinity and meat consumption to promote its Texas Double Whopper burger. The ad depicted angry men streaming into the streets to protest against "feminine," emasculating foods, shouting, "I will eat this meat!" "I am man, hear me roar / In numbers too big to ignore / And I'm way too hungry to settle for chick food! / Oh, yes, I'm a guy! / I'll admit I've been fed quiche! / Wave tofu bye-bye! / Now it's for Whopper beef I reach."[4] Hungry-Man Dinners, the popular meat-based frozen meals, are still advertised today with the slogan, "Eat like a man."

Today, the more the animal system comes into doubt as a result of its ecological contradictions and pandemic risks, the more it has become necessary to shore up the gendered nature of *meat* as a source not only of nutrition, but of masculine virtue. TV shows like *Duck Dynasty* and *Deadliest Catch* reinforce our association of masculinity with meat and the killing of animals; sexist pundits like psychologist Jordan Peterson and talk-show host Joe Rogan meanwhile promote bestselling books like *The Carnivore Diet*, which recommends a meat-only diet. Meat has even become a flashpoint in the culture wars, with Republicans in dozens of US states pushing legislation to ban vegan foods and cellular meats—a defense not merely of their states' economies, but of white rural masculinity. Since compassion is viewed as a weakness in boys and men, veganism is associated with effeminacy. To impugn the masculinity of liberal men, therefore, the political right has taken to deriding liberal men as "soy boys"—much as white Europeans in the nineteenth century ridiculed the "effeminate rice eaters" of Asian peoples to justify colonialism.[5] (Tofu has been eaten by Japanese, Chinese, and Korean peoples for millennia; the animus in American media culture against tofu is partly rooted in anti-Asian racism.[6])

Even as the effort to anchor masculinity in violence against animals intensifies, however, we are paradoxically seeing an effort to involve more women in the domination of animals.[7] While it is still overwhelmingly men who run the cattle, dairy, and meat industries, and who hunt, fish, and trap animals for sport, we are seeing a cultural shift in the way society represents men, women, and animals. One of the most striking things about the new carnivory, in fact, is that it is often being promoted with the greatest enthusiasm and moxie not by men, as one might expect, but by women. In thousands of news stories, magazine articles, books, films, and blogs, women are being celebrated for taking up new roles as pig farmers, cattle ranchers, butchers, and hunters. Killing animals is no longer exclusively men's work, the stories tell us, but the very horizon of women's empowerment. As Lily McCaulou writes in *The Call of the Mild: Learning to Hunt My Own Dinner*, an account of her transition from urban journalist to big-game hunter, "hunting is the final frontier of feminism."[8]

Such a notion, that dominating and hurting animals is a path to women's liberation, would have startled feminists of earlier generations. "Scarcely a human being in the course of history has fallen to a woman's rifle," Virginia Woolf pointedly observed in *Three Guineas*, "the vast majority of birds and beasts have been killed by you, not by us."[9] From the vegetarian Amazonian women in Charlotte Perkins Gilman's utopian sci-fi novel *Herland* (1915) to Frida Kahlo's self-portrait as a wounded deer pierced with arrows, feminists have long emphasized the parallels between male domination of women and masculine cruelty towards nonhuman animals. But no longer.

In 2010, journalist Peggy Orenstein wrote an influential article for *The New York Times*, "The Femivore's Dilemma: Can Chickens Save the Desperate Housewife?," describing scores of women who had flocked to farming, hunting, and butchery as a form of self-empowerment. Since then, thousands of other women have joined in. For these women, nothing could be more repugnant than the musty feminism of their predecessors, with its specter of an angry activist clutching her dog-eared vegetarian *Moosewood Cookbook* as tightly as she clung to her millenarian fervor.[10] These post-feminists don't want to unseat patriarchy, they want a seat at the table; they want to lean in, and they want their grass-fed steaks lean, too. More than a cultural curiosity, the "femivore" phenomenon has become central to society's efforts to legitimate the failing meat economy. By depicting violence against animals as a form of women's empowerment and maternal care, femivorism is providing patriarchal society with a novel set of rationales for maintaining its boundless cruelties.

THE NEW FEMININE MYSTIQUE

Until recently, the literary expositors of husbandry and hunting were nearly all men, writers like hunter-rancher Wes Jackson and organic agriculture expert J. I. Rodale. Today, however, more and more women are leading the charge. Dozens of women have written memoirs about dominating animals as a way to achieve a purpose-driven life. Women have written books about designing "humane" slaughterhouses (*Humane Livestock Handling*) or becoming taxidermists (*Still Life*), about becoming cattle ranchers (*My Ranch, Too: A Wyoming Memoir*) or marrying them (*Righteous Porkchop*), becoming butchers (*Killing It: An Education*) or marrying them (*Cleaving: A Story of Marriage, Meat, and Obsession*). By far the most common books in the genre, though, are memoirs by novice women farmers. With dozens of such books in print, sporting titles like *Hit by a Farm, Confessions of a Counterfeit Farm Girl, Country Grit: A Farmoir of Finding Purpose and Love*, and *Barnheart: The Incurable Longing for a Farm of One's Own*, the women's farming memoir has become a leading genre in contemporary women's nonfiction. Many of the books are bestsellers that have been lavished with praise by critics.

The memoirs take the form of the bildungsroman, the coming-of-age novel popular in the nineteenth century depicting the moral and psychological maturation of its youthful protagonist. In the classic bildungsroman, the (male) protagonist feels restless or lost, and casts about for some purpose adequate to his ambitions and passions. The hero struggles with self-doubt, lost love, or personal setbacks. By the end, however, he has triumphed over adversity and forged a more authentic self. The "femivore" bildungsroman traces a similar narrative arc, recounting its author's painful path to self-discovery and self-reliance. Unlike the hero of the traditional bildungsroman, however, the memoirists are able to achieve authenticity only by dominating animals.

In *The Feminine Mystique* (1963), Betty Friedan famously addressed the tedium and alienation of the suburban housewife. Women who'd benefited most from the economic boom of the 1950s, and for whom life was supposed to be good, felt instead "a strange stirring, a dissatisfaction, a yearning" for something more. In interviews, women from all walks of life, though mostly middle-class white women, told Friedan of a "problem that has no name." "Sometimes," Friedan wrote, "a woman would say 'I feel empty somehow . . . incomplete.' Or she would say, 'I feel as if I don't exist.'" As one woman tells her: "I've tried everything women are supposed to do—hobbies, gardening, pickling, canning, being very social with my neighbors, joining committees, running PTA teas," but nothing works.[11]

The authors of the women's farming memoirs, nearly all of them white and comfortably middle-class or affluent, sound a lot like the women profiled by Friedan, expressing similar feelings of dislocation or alienation. As the books begin, the women are reeling from romantic or professional blows, or both. A former food reporter for the *Chicago Tribune* takes up animal farming when she finds herself "without income, heartbroken, and terrified" after being left by her husband and fired from her job. In *Killing It: An Education*, Camas Davis's chronicle of her transformation from magazine editor to celebrity butcher, the author begins her story walking away from her personal ground zero, having recently lost a ten-year relationship and been fired from her job at the foodie magazine *Saveur*. "I broke my own heart. I wrecked my career," Davis writes. "Who was I? Where was I?"[12] Like many restless American writers before her, she flees the wreckage of her life for the relative safety of Europe. Ernest Hemingway went to Spain to drink and watch bullfights; Davis travels to the French countryside to be tutored in the fine arts of butchery and *charcuterie*.

For most of the memoirists, though, the problem isn't losing a job—it's having one. Alienated from corporate life and feeling "burned out, apathetic, and bored" with what they term their "sheltered" and "spoiled" urban lives, the women walk away from lucrative positions as journalists, editors, food critics, and marketing directors. Though there are many ways to address feelings of alienation, from therapy to volunteering in a soup kitchen, for these women only the farming cure will do. Feminists once dreamed of changing the world; all these memoirists want is a Farm of Their Own.

Or, rather, an *animal* farm of their own. Though many of the women grow vegetables and fruit, too, it is no part of their vision to lord it over an apple orchard or petunia patch. Forty acres, yes, but the mule's the thing. Driving the women from their urban lives is what Jenna Woginrich, the author of two farming memoirs, calls "barnheart," a condition suffered by "those . . . who wish to God we were outside with our flocks, feed bags, or harnesses instead of sitting in front of the computer screen," women who "are overcome with the desire to be tagging cattle ears or feeding pigs."[13] As she observes in *One-Woman Farm*, farming is a way to prove that "as a single woman I can manage an entire flock."[14] For women grown tired of having to please their boss one minute, then rush home to begin the Second Shift the next, controlling animals is a way to escape feeling controlled themselves. "I'm damn sure a ewe trying to deliver a lamb doesn't care about meeting a spreadsheet deadline," Woginrich writes.[15] Tired of being tethered to the corporate machine, now *she'll* do the tethering.

Bereft of community and a sense of deeper purpose, the women flee metropolises like New York, San Francisco, and Seattle to homestead in rural townships in Michigan or Wisconsin, alone or with a lover or spouse or (more rarely) a family in tow. For Susan McCorkindale, a senior marketing director at *Family Circle*, not even $400 sea-salt pedicures and a $30,000 year-end bonus can relieve the stressful tedium of her privileged life: she and her husband buy a five-hundred-acre beef farm in Virginia. Jessie Knadler, a senior editor with a woman's magazine, exchanges her life in Manhattan, where she "splurged on

Miu Mius, partied hard, and lived for Kundalini yoga," for down-home life on a farm in "the badlands of Montana."[16]

No sooner are the women ensconced in their farmhouses, however, than their troubles begin. The novice farmers make blunders, struggle with doubt, and contend with early frosts and broken farm equipment. The flint against which the women strike their souls, though, are the animals they raise for slaughter. In *Chickens in the Road*, Suzanne McMinn's "coming-of-age story of a woman in her forties," a chronicle of her transformation "from publishing diva to reluctant pasture princess," raising animals satisfies the author's "deep-seated need to test myself"—"[m]ilking a cow made me prove myself every single day."[17] For Kristin Kimball, an Ivy Leaguer from an aristocratic East Coast family, dominating animals effects her metamorphosis from party girl who "stays out until four, wears heels, and carries a handbag" to cowgirl who can "shoot a gun, dispatch a chicken, dodge a charging bull, and ride out a runaway [animal] behind panicked horses."[18]

Scenes in which the author exerts mastery over a large animal feature prominently in many of the books, signposts along the road to self-sufficiency. Seeing another woman controlling a horse named Steele for the first time, Woginrich admires how she "converses with Steele through the black leather lines, her voice, and her carriage whip." Woginrich soon learns this "language" herself, "the way a child learns it, by holding up things and repeating what they are out loud: *Carriage whip. Blinders. Singletree. Lines.*"[19] When Merlin, a horse she's riding, balks at carrying her up a hill, Woginrich digs him sharply with her heel, then gives him the taste of rawhide—a piquant reminder to Merlin of the true terms of their "conversation." The mastery the women achieve is real, not notional—the mental and physical domination of another being. As Kimball writes in *The Dirty Life*, controlling a horse means "you're on top, a position of power."[20] For the first time in their lives, the women feel in control. "I rise up on the big pasture from the back of a horse," Suzanne McMinn reflects in the closing pages of her memoir. "And in my hands, I hold the reins."[21] In mastering the animal, she has mastered herself.

Though each memoir ostensibly relates an original story of self-discovery, the sameness of the books complicates their authors' claims of existential authenticity. The title of memoirist Ellen Stimson's best-selling book, *Mud Season: How One Woman's Dream of Moving to Vermont, Raising Children, Chickens and Sheep, and Running the Old Country Store Pretty Much Led To One Calamity After Another*, is representative of the themes and literary sensibilities of memoirs across the genre. The women poke fun at their "greenhorn" farming ways, marvel at their new Carhartt mud boots, and crack wise about goat and sheep penises. Several recount identical "comical" showdowns with "mean" roosters, whom they vanquish at the chopping block. "Bats and Bears and Skunks. Oh My," reads one chapter title; "Calves' Heads and Black Snakes and Groundhogs, Oh My!" reads another, in a different book by a different author. Even as the women depict themselves as roughing it, enacting pastoral rituals that "people have been doing for thousands of years,"[22] they surf the internet, play *FarmVille* on their iPhones, and curl up at night to a Netflix movie and a fine Chablis after a hard day wrangling sheep, milking cows, and cutting off the heads of the sensitive creatures they lovingly depict as their infants and children.

MOTHERING "BABIES"—THEN KILLING THEM

There have been any number of farming memoirs written by men, including the bestselling *The Bucolic Plague* by Josh Kilmer-Purcell, about a gay couple who leave their jobs in Manhattan to set up an animal farm on an old estate in the country.[23] As in the women's memoirs, the gentlemen farmers portray themselves in a self-deprecating and comedic light, as smug city slickers who get their comeuppance wading in cow dung. Like their female counterparts, too, the men portray their rural experiments as a way to achieve a sense of authenticity and connection to nature. However, there are far fewer farming memoirs by men and, unlike the memoirs by women, the male authors don't couch their farming adventures as cure-alls for depression, romantic disappointment, or career crisis. Nor do they depict animal husbandry as a revelatory exercise in parental caregiving.

The first book to popularize the gentlewoman farmer narrative was Barbara Kingsolver's bestseller, *Animal, Vegetable, Miracle*, a critique of corporate agribusiness wrapped in a personal account of the Kingsolver family's experiences running a small organic animal farm. Published in 2007, *Animal, Vegetable, Miracle* was the first bestseller to center maternal and natalist themes in the new discourses of animal husbandry. "April 23, my babies due!" Kingsolver scrawls in her calendar, marking the day the chicks she's ordered are to arrive from the hatchery. "Our turkeys would be pampered as children," she explains, saying that she has ordered the birds to instruct her daughter in the responsibilities of mothering. "Some parents would worry about a daughter taking on maternal responsibility so early in life, but Lily was already experienced," having helped care for chickens at the family's previous home.[24]

Kingsolver's approach would subsequently inspire scores of similar farming memoirs by women (Orenstein's "The Femivore's Dilemma" would appear in the *Times* just three years later).[25] Maternal themes appear in these books too—signaled in the books' cover photographs of the authors smiling in mud boots, clutching chickens, lambs, or baby pigs, infant-like, to their gingham-clad chests. "We would make babies," Catherine Friend writes in *Hit By a Farm*, after she and her partner buy a farm in Minnesota to raise sheep.[26] Another author puts a "basket of gear and supplies" by her back door, like "a hospital suitcase for a mother-in-waiting" or "a midwife . . . preparing for a midnight delivery."[27] For memoirist Ellen Stimson, the decision "to foster a little girl and a little boy"—a pair of lambs—fills the author with trepidation because "it had been a long time since I had had a baby."[28] As the pregnant animals approach their due dates, the women anxiously take their temperatures and check their cervixes. When the babies are born, the women are over the moon. "Ohmygodohmygodohmy-god," Friend enthuses on birthing day. "We'd made a baby boy."[29] Cra-dling the "sturdy little wool-baby" in her arms, Suzanne McMinn feels "starry-eyed."[30] Pastures in birthing season are described as "nurser-ies" and "out-of-control daycare" centers, while herding lambs is said to resemble a "fire drill in a kindergarten."[31]

By controlling the bodies of other animals, the women are able to demonstrate superhuman maternal powers. One author writes of her joy in having "a baby on my lap," while boasting that her "skills prog-ress to the point I can feed five babies at once."[32] Slipping out of bed in the small hours of the morning after breast-feeding their own new-borns, the women go out and milk cows and goats, yielding brimming vats of milk that would make La Leche League green—or white—with envy. Ordinarily, a nursing mother can produce only a few pints of milk each day; Jenna Woginrich however is soon producing "more than 45 gallons of fresh milk" each month. "Holy cow!" she writes. "Strike that. Holy goat! *I'm doing it!*"[33] In a fantasy of limitless fertility, the women "produce" thousands of eggs and help birth llamas, sheep, cows, alpacas, rabbits, and goats. For memoirists who are single and have longed for children of their own, rearing farmed animals becomes a way to achieve an elusive motherhood. "I had become a single parent raising a goat," Woginrich writes, recounting how she learned to let down a goat's milk by massaging her teats.[34]

The traditional human dependent is of course not the domesticated pig, chicken, or llama, but the human infant. However, that kind of dependent, the sort demanding unwavering parental attention and care, has long been sign and symptom of woman's subordinate social status. So long as women remain solely responsible for bearing and raising children, they remain socially disadvantaged. Having a child is not merely to *have* a dependent, it is to *be* dependent. Hence the importance placed by earlier feminists on universal free childcare, as a way of freeing women to pursue careers. Today's "femivores," however, have gravitated to a new kind of dependent, one that allows them to engage in the pageantry of maternalism, but without the risk of being tied down. These are babies who can be "loved" and "cared for," but also gotten rid of once their company grows tedious. Most of the memoirists want only ersatz children, ones requiring only a simulation of maternal love and responsibility. Casual indifference to the fates of their "babies" is the norm in the memoirs. When the women aren't killing the animals outright, hence, they're killing them through malign neglect.

Animals die left and right on the women's farms, with such frequency that the reader needs a scorecard to keep up. Sheep get crushed to death between bales of hay. Chickens fall between slats of pallets, or get "mashed between the side of the feeder box and the wall of the chicken house," or have their necks broken when the women accidentally crush them with heavy objects.[35] One rabbit gets her leg caught in the steel mesh floor and tries to gnaw it off, dislocating her vertebra and paralyzing her "from the waist down."[36] Snowstorms on the McCorkindale farm leave behind what the author jokingly calls "a very nice dusting of dead chickens" when the suffering birds freeze to death.[37] Cows give birth alongside electric fences, incinerating their newborn calves. "Bad things happen," Catherine Friend observes blandly after one ewe gives birth along an electric fence, killing two lambs.[38] (When she and her partner accidentally get their flock of sheep pregnant out of season, they correct the error by selling them all for slaughter.) As more than one memoirist remarks: "There's a saying in farming, if you're going to have livestock, you're going to have deadstock."[39]

Such pearls are meant to distract the reader from the fact that it is the authors themselves who've placed their vulnerable charges at mortal risk. It is they who will betray their "babies" in the end, ensuring that not one escapes a violent death. When Kingsolver's chicks arrive from the hatchery, the author at first finds them "adorable," recounting how "they imprinted on me as Mama and rushed happily to greet me wherever I appeared." Kingsolver confesses to feeling like "Cruella de Ville" for having deceived the young turkeys into thinking that she's their mother (their real one having already been killed) and taken them under her wing for the sole purpose of killing and eating them. Once the chicks mature into young adults and begin exerting their own agency and will, however, Kingsolver no longer wants them around. "Many of us were relieved that year at harvest time," she confesses.

Up to the very moment of slaughter, Kingsolver compares her relationship to the birds to that between a mother and her children—a tacit acknowledgment that the violence she is to inflict constitutes an act of betrayal. Moments before delivering the coup de grace using a "kill pipe"—she has placed the bird's body inside a tube to immobilize her, so that she can then cut her throat—Kingsolver registers the "downy softness and a vulnerable heartbeat" of the animal whose life she is about to extinguish. "I felt maternal, while at the same time looking straight down the pipe toward the purpose of this enterprise."[40] In Shakespeare's *Macbeth*, after Lord and Lady Macbeth determine to murder King Duncan and his men, guests under their roof, Lady Macbeth privately begs the "spirits" to "unsex" her by "damming up the access and passage to remorse." Only by tamping down any "compunctious visitings of nature"—compassion—can she proceed with her "fell purpose." The memoirists similarly suppress any natural stirrings of empathy in order to destroy their young charges, producing scenes in which maternal affection suddenly gives way to violence and unfeeling cruelty.

"I stroked his warm, warty head. . . . I could feel his heart beating, slowly," writes Novella Carpenter in *Farm City: The Education of an Urban Farmer* of Harold, the loving turkey she has raised, seconds before cutting off his head.[41] Catherine Friend, meanwhile, describes how she "clung fiercely to this tender animal in my arms, wanting to protect her from whatever dangers lay ahead"—except for herself. When an affectionate lamb becomes smitten with Friend, following her around and demanding to be patted on the head, she names him "Mr. Playful," gushing to her partner, "I feel like kissing him right on his nose." Weeks later, Friend sits in her pickup outside a slaughter-house, weeping, as "Mr. Playful" is killed. By suppertime, though, she's right as rain again, sitting down eagerly to dine on the lamb's body. Eating Mr. Playful's "savory and incredibly tender" flesh is her way of "honoring the lamb *that died*" (my italics).[42]

Novella Carpenter, ruminating about killing the pigs she's raised, wonders whether the animals are "really as intelligent as everyone" says they are. Would she "end up keeping the beasts as seven-hundred-pound pets," or instead melt them down into fat? "Of course it would be the latter," she writes. "I knew myself well enough by then. A prag-matic farmer, not a soft sentimentalist."[43] Ironically, though Car-penter and other femivores accuse vegans of "sentimentality," it is they who engage in sentimental depictions of the animals they kill, treating them not as individuals worthy of respect, but as platforms for their own narcissistic displays of affect. In a conversation with another farmer about killing chickens, Carpenter remarks, "It's sol-emn," recounting how "we both touched our hearts."[44] These sorts of empty sentimental gestures, like Friend crying in her pickup, or the *de rigueur* ritual of "thanking" the animal corpse before a meal, recur throughout the memoirs. Sentimentality, a form of thinly disguised bad faith, is not to be confused with genuine *sentiment* or feeling. As James Baldwin observed in his critique of the white liberal sensibility of *Uncle Tom's Cabin*:

> Sentimentality, the ostentatious parading of excessive and spurious emotion, is the mark of dishonesty, the inability to feel; the wet eyes of the sentimentalist betray his aversion to experience, his fear of life, his arid heart; and it is always, therefore, the signal of secret and violent inhumanity, the mark of cruelty.[45]

Baldwin's observation explains how the sentimentality in these accounts bleeds so easily into sadism. A dark undertow of violence runs beneath the memoirists' narratives, as caring and killing get woven into a lethal maternalism, and infant care dissolves into bloody spectacles of death.

In *Blood, Bones & Butter*, Gabrielle Hamilton's memoir about becoming a chef, the author confesses that each time she changes diapers on a "noncompliant child" she's reminded of trussing chickens and wrangling eels. Hamilton wistfully describes her family's spring lamb roasts during her childhood, when the lambs "with their little crooked sets of teeth and milky eyes" were slaughtered by a local butcher, then skewered "onto ten-foot poles made of ash," as her family "roasted four or five of the whole little guys." In a macabre parody of maternal watchfulness, the author writes: "The lambs were arranged over the coals head to toe and head to toe, the way you'd put a bunch of kids having a sleepover to bed." The lullaby for the sleepover is the sound of the lambs' blood as it drips "down into the coals with a hypnotic and rhythmic bliss. . . . Hiss. Hiss. Hiss."[46]

Many of the memoirists speak of "getting their hands dirty," a euphemism for enacting violence. "I had daily intimacy not just with *dirt* dirt, but with blood, manure, milk, pus . . . the grease of engines and the grease of animals, with innards," writes Kimball in *The Dirty Life*.[47] Another memoirist observes that "most of my story" was "written in sweat, tears, and even a little blood."[48] And there will be blood. Buckets and buckets of it. Blood pouring out of the torn tracheas of cows, blood gushing out of the throats of thrashing pigs, caught in giant buckets. Perhaps, confesses Catherine Friend, even "more blood than I was comfortable with."[49] With despotic fury, the women stab rabbits, dismember deer, and roam the barnyard lopping off heads. Farms become abattoirs, cemeteries, killing fields. One memoirist traps a raccoon, then shoots him with a rifle as he cowers in a cage. "Wow," she writes. "I felt strange. I'd just killed an animal. I felt good and bad all at the same time."[50] But the truth is, she feels very good. Though the women wonder whether they'll be "tough enough" when the moment of truth comes, they prove eager and even impatient to kill.

When journalist-cum-hunter Lily McCaulou kills her first animal with a well-placed "head shot"—"a clean, perfect kill" of a pheasant in a canned hunt (the animals are raised in captivity, then released before the hunters in a confined space to be shot)—she experiences "euphoria." Driving home, she recounts, "I roll down the windows, crank up the radio, and sing at the top of my lungs." Like a man boasting of having deflowered his first virgin, the author writes that "no other kill . . . evokes such pure elation as my first." McCaulou—who compares herself to a modern-day Diana the Huntress—soon graduates from killing birds and small mammals to slaying larger animals. Her moment of arrival comes the day she finds herself "kneeling before a bull elk, up to my shoulders in blood," "drenched in blood and laughing" at her "earlier squeamishness."[51] For McCaulou and the other memoirists, shedding the blood of animals becomes a way to reenact earlier rituals of maturation, loss of childlike innocence with the "adult knowledge" that "death is the substance of life."[52] In a kind of reverse transubstantiation, real blood gets transformed into something metaphysical—an aesthetic of the sublime and an "authentic" self. In *Farm City*—named one of the Top 10 Books of 2009 by Dwight Gardner, daily book critic for the *New York Times*—Novella Carpenter invokes the rite of menses when, renouncing her former vegetarianism, she throws out her *Moosewood Cookbook* and replaces it with *The Encyclopedia of Country Living*, an instruction manual on DIY slaughter. After her first kill, Carpenter reports, the book becomes "marked with blood."[53]

A leading force in locavore politics in the San Francisco Bay area, Carpenter is an especially avid killer, someone who enjoys seeing animals die. Of the first pigs she has raised, Carpenter writes, "I was going to have to kill one of Simon's babies." "Yeah I gotta find someone to execute those fuckers." She hires a female butcher named Sheila to do the deed, telling her, "I really want to see the pigs die." Later, when she learns in a phone call that Sheila has gone ahead and killed the animals without her being there, Carpenter is so infuriated that she slams down the receiver and screams, "*Cunt!*" Seeing the dead pigs' bodies for the first time, she impulsively reaches over to a pig's severed head and scoops its raw brains into her mouth, pronouncing them "delicious."[54] In another passage, Carpenter boasts of the "bloody revenge" she enacts on a possum who's made his way into the poultry enclosure one night. Recalling "the cuteness of my ducks, and the goose who would rest her head in my lap," Carpenter takes a shovel and brings it "down on the opossum's neck," thrusting repeatedly until his head rolls off. "Caught up in protecting my babies," she quips, "I had become a savage."[55] Her fierce determination to protect her "babies" is nowhere in evidence weeks later, though, when she carries a trusting white duck into her house, places him in the bathtub, and decapitates him with a pruner. "He quacked and swam around for a few minutes. . . . I merely squeezed the loppers shut. The duck went from being a happy camper to being a headless camper. I plucked and eviscerated him outside on a table."[56]

Flippant passages like these, in which the memoirists mock their victims, give the lie to the authors' claims to love and "respect" animals. Catherine Friend finds it amusing when a lamb strays against an electric fence and receives an 8,000-volt shock (a voltage so high that it burns a hole in a leather glove), causing him to shoot "straight up in the air" and to run crying to his mother as the other lambs "scatter in panic."[57] When a new lamb is born on Friend's farm, she and her partner "steal it from its mother" in order "to do things to it." "We sneak up to a pair of sleeping twins and each pick one up. The ewe no longer sees her babies on the ground and panics."[58] Similar heartbreaking scenes, of traumatized sheep and cows returning day after day to the place where they last saw their baby, sniffing the ground and lowing in distress, can be found in many of the memoirs, their authors betraying not the least sympathy for their victims, let alone remorse for their cruelty. The women joke about the impending doom of their victims, finding humor in their very guilelessness and vulnerability. Woginrich, observing that the pig she has raised will soon "die in the same place where she has spent the last three months sleeping and eating," remarks: "It will surprise the hell out of her." And it does. On the fateful morning, as Woginrich reaches down to scratch the pig's ear, the pig turns and looks at her "curiously," wagging her "little curled tail" and making "gentle" noises. "I'm proud of this Pig," Woginrich writes. Soon, three men arrive in a truck, seize the trusting animal, slash her throat, and carve her body up into slabs. Woginrich sticks around to watch. It's her way of taking "responsibility," she writes. "I *need* to be there," she says, to bear witness to the "whole process, from holding a piglet in a dog crate, squealing in my arms, to the day its head lies on a snowbank."[59]

ROMANCING THE KNIFE

Food is often tied to sex in human culture, and a number of the memoirists find ways to link the killing or eating of animals to eroticism. "This gravy makes my nipples hard," murmurs the young wife of a Navy officer after sampling a gravy made from a turkey; Novella Carpenter meanwhile describes herself as "dizzy with desire" at the sight of a stack of bacon, confessing to the sin of "pork lust."[60] For many of the women, pleasure in killing animals gets bound up with their romantic attachments to men. "Don't you have to tie off the anus and penis first?" Lily McCaulou's husband lovingly reminds her as the couple kneel together before the warm body of an elk. Moments before this pillow talk, the couple have been crawling together through the muck of a damp forest, chasing down the mortally wounded elk McCaulou has shot through the heart. Later, over dinner, the lovers raise glasses of wine in "a simple toast, loaded with thanks: To our elk."[61] One elk, one kill, one heart.

For many memoirists, the best way to win over a man is to strike down an animal. Suzanne McMinn describes "killing chickens [as] the last new thing" she and her lover did before breaking up—a "kind of fitting punctuation to our life together."[62] For Kristin Kimball, killing and eviscerating a pig is the first activity she shares with Mark, a handsome young farmer she interviews for an article. Kimball finds that she is "not disgusted, but enlivened" by the experience of killing, so much so that the next morning she finds herself padding barefoot around Mark's kitchen, eating his organic sausages, after sleeping with him the night before.[63] The couple grows closer with every assassination. "Mark and I moved through the steps of slaughter gracefully . . . a co-ordinated team of two," Kimball writes. "Mark handed me the gun, I handed him the knife." Together, the couple sneak up on a cow they've named Kathleen, whom they find "grazing quietly" in a field. They put a bullet in her head, then slash open her throat so that her "hot blood poured out on the grass."[64]

All of this violence suggests nothing so much as a wish on the part of the women to be accepted as co-equals in the death cult of patriarchy. In male-dominated societies, sexual desire is sometimes blurred with a desire to inflict suffering (an impulse seen, for example, in violent pornography). "For each aspect of eros," observes feminist theorist Nancy Hartsock, "the centrality of hostility, the wish to do harm, marks a fascination with death—the death of the other as a separate being, the denial of one's own body in order to deny one's mortality, and the recasting even of reproduction as death."[65] These impulses, deeply rooted in masculine culture, have only been amplified under conditions of advanced capitalism where, Herbert Marcuse once noted, "constructive and destructive achievements, work for life and work for death, procreating and killing" get blurred together.[66] George Orwell observed that false reconciliation of opposites—freedom as slavery, war as peace, etc.—is a characteristic of totalitarianism; today we find similar attempts to reconcile opposites in the new omnivorism, as killing animals gets conflated with caring for them, and death is blurred with life.

Conflation of death and life sometimes even takes the form of the authors' own fantasies of self-destruction. In her bestselling book, *The Ethical Meat Handbook*, Meredith Leigh, a prominent carno-locavore in North Carolina who runs do-it-yourself slaughter workshops, goes so far as to imagine her own murder. After a pleasurable day spent slaying animals on her farm, Leigh writes:

> We separate hearts and heads, we roll fleeces for later washing and tanning. We slaughter two more lambs, Maybelle and Whiteface. We share silence and sadness each time. Each time, I feel my breathing, and I feel gratitude, for precious life as well as for suffering. . . . I think, I could stand to die here. Here, in this pasture, under these mountains, this sky. If, when my time comes, someone lays me down in green grass and soothes my body, and someone I love then lovingly cuts my throat, and my blood runs into the grass and fertilizes the soil, and my body is used for food and necessity, I could handle that.[67]

Leigh offers this dissociative fantasy as a sign of her supposed connection to animals and nature. In reality, it signifies contempt for animals and renunciation of the life principle. Of the hundreds of animals Leigh kills, none will be given the opportunity to choose the place, the time, or the means of their deaths. The author's supposed gesture of solidarity with her victims collapses into grotesque sentimentalism, a defense against her own aggression.

HUNGER GAMES

In 1974, a young chef at a feminist food collective in Ithaca named Moosewood published a new book of vegetarian recipes. The *Moosewood Cookbook* soon became one of the most popular cookbooks of all time, and the name of its author, Mollie Katzen, became synonymous with vegetarianism. In 2017, however, Katzen announced that she had started eating meat again. "For about 30 years I didn't eat meat at all, just a bite of fish every once in a while, and always some dairy," Katzen told an interviewer with *Food and Wine* magazine. "Lately, I've been eating a little meat. People say, 'Ha, ha, Mollie Katzen is eating steak.' But now that cleaner, naturally fed meat is available, it's a great option for anyone who's looking to complete his diet." Katzen now claimed to have been misunderstood all those years. She'd never said that she didn't "want people to eat meat"; she'd only "wanted to supply possibilities that were low on the food chain." The heroine of vegetarians everywhere now mocked them. "For people who are against eating meat because it's wrong or offensive to eat animals," Katzen said, "even the cleanest grass-fed beef won't be good enough."[68] Katzen's about-face represented more than a change in diet—it was the repudiation of a movement and a moment when many Americans, particularly women, had become open to a new way of relating to food and to animals. How had the nation gone from the feminist-vegetarian *Moosewood* to the spectacle of women hunting moose in the woods?

While women have been drawn to animal husbandry for many of the same reasons that men have, such as a longing for a more "authentic" relation to nature and to the sources of our food, femivorism has specific features all its own, as a cultural response to the contradictory demands on women in the twenty-first century.

We have seen that some femivores explicitly describe their domination of animals as feminist. Whether one agrees with that characterization, however, will depend on how one construes the history and meaning of feminism, and whether one finds oneself satisfied with a conception of women's progress that emphasizes their formal rather than substantive equality with men. In the late 1960s and early 1970s, radical feminists sought not merely formal parity with men but a broader transformation of patriarchal norms and institutions, including an end to militarism, imperialism, racism, and rape culture. As the feminist poet and essayist Adrienne Rich wrote in "Toward a Woman-Centered University" (1973–1974), the question facing women wasn't merely whether they should be equal participants in society alongside men, but "whether this male-created, male-dominated structure is really capable of serving the humanism and freedom it professes." Rich and other radical feminists argued that it was not, and that patriarchal society's "suicidal obsession with power and technology" was incom-

patible with general liberation and a just society. True women's liberation thus implied the creation of a new society, based on principles of
universal freedom and nonviolence.[69]

It was this same vision of a just world that ecofeminists like Marti
Kheel and Ynestra King would later lay claim to in their work, highlighting human oppression of animals as one of the most destructive
features of patriarchal society. The high-water mark of these efforts
was Carol Adams's book, *The Sexual Politics of Meat*. By the time Adams's book appeared in 1990, however, the women's movement had
been in decline for years, and feminist interest in vegetarianism had
waned along with it. With the election of President Ronald Reagan
in 1980, a period of broad political reaction had set in, transforming
the political and cultural landscape and leading to a retrenchment of
traditional gender norms. Liberal feminism, oriented around winning formal parity with men, now came into ascendancy. More radical
figures in the movement, those who had questioned the underlying
values of the patriarchal system, including speciesism, were eclipsed.
Over time, mainstream feminism moved ever further away from environmentalism, vegetarianism, and animal rights.

By the 1990s, women had gained entry into previously closed pro-
fessions and had won important legal victories for reproductive rights
and against discrimination in the workplace. However, despite these
and other advances, women remained socially subordinate to men.
Women remained responsible for the bulk of domestic labor and
child-rearing, they were still paid less than their male counterparts,
and they remained as susceptible as before to male sexual assault. For
white middle-class and upper-class women in particular, the group
that had arguably gained the most from post-70s feminist reform,
equality had come to seem tantalizingly close, but also agonizingly
out of reach. As Susan Faludi observed in *Backlash: The Undeclared
War Against American Women* (1991), "[b]ehind this celebration of the
American woman's victory, behind the news, cheerfully and endlessly
repeated, that the struggle for women's rights is won, another message

flashes. You may be free and equal now, it says to women, but you have never been more miserable."[70]

This contradiction, between the promise of gender equality, on the one hand, and women's continuing status as the social subordinates of men, on the other, created the cultural opening for femivorism, a regressive project in which some middle-class white women, partly under the mantle of liberal feminism, have channeled their frustration and rage over the unfinished business of sexual equality into animal husbandry and other forms of animal harm. It is no accident that the phenomenon arose during a period of patriarchal retrenchment and neoliberal austerity—during the rollback of women's rights and a cultural retreat into various "localisms" that came at the expense of broader civic engagement. The influx of women into animal pastoralism siphoned off some women's energies into a depoliticized movement, one that substituted rural domesticity for a more robust conception of feminist struggle. Before she began running an animal farm, Kristin Kimball confesses, "the word *home* could make me cry," because "I wanted one. With a man. A house. The smell of cut grass, sheets on a line, a child running through a sprinkler."[71] After forsaking professional lives in the city, she and other post-feminist pioneers set furiously to work canning, preserving, pickling, gardening, knitting, sewing, quilting, baking, and making homemade jerky, transforming themselves into "domestic superheroes" (as more than one memoirist describes herself) in a ferocious return to stereotypically "feminine" activities, now improbably re-cast as tactics of empowerment.[72]

Few women today, however, welcome the idea of a complete return to domestic life. Some countervailing demonstration of women's power within the domestic sphere is therefore needed to paper over the contradiction between the femivores' avowed quests for authenticity and independence, on the one hand, and their socially prescribed longings to fulfill traditional gender roles, on the other.[73] And domination over animals has provided it. In the femivore memoirs, violence against animals serves as a kind of psychic ballast, keeping the women from sinking entirely under what would otherwise be merely another form of conventional domesticity. By "mothering" animals, then killing them, the women have found a way to square the circle of a new femininity that demands that women be both vulnerable *and* strong, domesticated *and* self-sufficient. By raising pigs and sheep—then bearing eager witness to their deaths—the women are able to exhibit traditional caring behavior while also demonstrating the "toughness" and ruthlessness we stereotypically associate with men. Having spent their lives in a world centered around men and their brutal deeds, women can now claim a piece of the action for themselves. Hence the "swagger," as Jessica Applestone, co-owner of Fleisher's Grass-fed and Organic Meats, calls it, among women taking her butchering class for the first time. "There's a macho performal [sic] nature that some of these people crave," she says. "And what better a performance than the blood and guts of butchery?"[74]

Tellingly, many of the memoirists seek out male approbation rather than meaningful connections with other women.[75] Many recount the ritual of learning to wield a gun, a potent symbol of masculine power that allows them to claim a "transgressive" status, while nonetheless engaging in a practice that keeps them safely within the bounds of existing patriarchal norms. "I ran my hand over the smooth, dark wood of the stock and shivered," Kimball writes, caressing her first rifle. "Hand me a bow and arrow or a rifle and *it makes sense*," Woginrich confesses. Fielding a gun for the first time, Catherine Friend thinks: "Gosh, this is fun. Hand me more bullets." After considering different weapons, Friend settles on an air pistol, for killing groundhogs and other "pests" on her farm. ("We're going to shoot those SOBs," a woman staying with her remarks.) "I yearned for more space, more breathing room," Friend writes.[76] And how better to carve out a little *Lebensraum* in the wilderness than with a blazing firearm? Soon the hills around the memoirists' farms are alive with the sounds of gunfire, as the farms and their surrounds get transformed into free-fire zones for killing deer, possums, pigeons, squirrels, and any other living being hapless enough to wander across the women's defense perimeter in search of food, shelter, or a mate. Memoirists who have described themselves as liberals suddenly reveal a patriotic fascination with all things military. "I've always fantasized about being one of those Navy SEALs, Special Forces, or Delta Force dudes, I think it would be a blast," McCorkindale writes.[77] "I begin to understand why hunting is often compared to war," McCaulou confesses. Like soldiers victorious in battle, she and the other women keep tokens of their victims' bodies—feathers, tails, teeth, etc. Suzanne McMinn nails the tail of the raccoon she's killed to her front porch as a warning to other "pests"— much as colonial officials once impaled the heads of defeated Native warriors on poles at the town gate.

Even the memoirists' insatiable hunger for meat and blood as "enlivening" foods—a recurring theme in many of the accounts—suggests nothing so much as a sublimated desire to participate in society as the true equals of men. Many memoirists describe themselves as former vegetarians or vegans whose cravings for flesh supposedly overwhelmed them. Of her time as a vegetarian, Kristin Kimball writes, "there was something about it, something more primal, a kind of craving, my body yelling, EAT THAT, I NEED IT."[78] McCaulou confesses, "when I don't eat meat for a few weeks, I start to crave a hamburger as a vampire does blood."[79] There is poignancy to such accounts, unfolding as they do against the backdrop of a culture obsessed with food and with women's relationship to it. Vegans are familiar with the "pathological vegan," usually a woman, who throws herself into veganism to force herself into being thinner; the "converted" femivores appear to have exchanged one pathological relationship to food for another.

TEMPLE OF THE ABATTOIR

The myth that animals can be raised and killed humanely and with "compassion" has today been adopted not only by organic farmers and locavores but also by the world's largest meatpackers. Smithfield, owned by the WH Group in China—the world's largest killer of pigs—advertises itself as the "World's Leader in Animal Care," while Tyson Foods, the world's biggest killer of chickens, boasts that its "Animal Well-Being" program "promotes the health, safety and well-being of the animals."[80] In this context, "femivorism," with its rhetoric of womanly care, has come to serve as a strategic bridge between smaller-scale animal agriculture and factory farming.

Judith Capper, a self-proclaimed "livestock sustainability consultant" to the US cattle industry, invokes her femininity to legitimate factory farming. In a blog entry entitled, "Do Moms Have Instant Beef Credibility?," Capper links stories of women as nurturing mothers and domestic providers to the "caring" work of industrialized animal agriculture. Noting that women "who have children are trusted by female consumers more than the traditional scientific image of an older man in a white lab coat," Capper urges male ranchers to ask their "wife, girlfriend, daughter, mother, granddaughter, or niece to . . . let the female consumer know why . . . beef is a great choice for our families, and why we spend time caring for baby calves almost as if they are our own children." Only women can make "that female-female connection that, like it or not, does promote an instant degree of trust." At a meeting of the International Livestock Conference, one prominent male cattle lobbyist praised Capper for helping "to improve the image of beef sustainability," noting that "Jude Capper is credible because she is female" and suggesting that Capper would soon become "even more credible when she has children" of her own. Recounting the lobbyist's praise later on her blog, Capper revealed that she was seven months pregnant. "I am gaining credibility by the day . . . pound by pound . . . literally." With her new "baby bump," she would have even "more opportunities for conversations about the importance of beef in pregnancy nutrition."[81]

While Capper is not widely known outside the beef industry, the same cannot be said of animal behaviorist and meat industry consultant Temple Grandin, the most consequential figure in the "feminine-washing" of mass violence against animals. Grandin first rose to celebrity in the 1990s, on the basis of her unsubstantiated claim that her autism has imbued her with a mystical ability to "know" what other animals are thinking and feeling. Leveraging these supposed powers of insight, Grandin has built a lucrative career helping meat companies slaughter animals more efficiently and "humanely" by eliminating sensorial clues that might otherwise tip off cows, sheep, and pigs that they are facing imminent death. That Grandin should be universally praised for "caring" about animals tells us everything we might care to know about society's need to justify its murderous impulses. In a rational order, an obsession with designing means to effect mass killing would be seen as perverse, if not as anathema to the proper values of society. Against the backdrop of a pathological society, however, a woman who professes "to care" so for much for animals that she has devoted her life to helping millions of them go uncomplainingly to their doom is held up instead as an exemplary figure. In 2009, Encyclopedia Britannica published an article entitled, "We Salute Temple Grandin, A Hero for Animals," and in 2010, *Time* magazine named Grandin one of the 100 Most Influential People of the Year. The same year, NPR ran a story entitled, "Temple Grandin: A Life Devoted to Animals," and HBO aired a hagiographic biopic, *Temple Grandin*, starring the glamorous actress Claire Danes. In 2013, the Museum of Modern Art in New York preposterously described Grandin as "an animal rights activist," while praising one of Grandin's "design concepts"—a kill-chute designed to pacify and reassure animals as they approached their deaths at the slaughterhouse.[82] If Grandin hadn't existed, the culture would have had to create her—but in a sense it did.

Only with the waning of a more substantive feminist politics could causing harm to animals come to be mistaken for genuine women's liberation. Waging war on animals is the continuation of post-feminist politics by other means—a way for some women to work through the conflictual nature of twenty-first century femininity, without however challenging the prerogatives or values of men. Today's real-life Dianas and Katnisses may not be able to shatter the corporate glass ceiling or to send conservative state legislators scattering for cover before they can close another abortion clinic, but they can make some deer or pig *pay*. But sticking pigs is not the same as sticking it to the Man. With its false pieties of "respect" for animals, and its love of guns, knives, and blood, femivorism signifies a maladaptive response to women's subordination, a reactionary stance allied with some of the most destructive features of our patriarchal culture.

THEIR KINDNESS TOWARD EACH OTHER

Reading these disturbing memoirs, it is easy to forget that most vegans are women, as are many leading figures in animal advocacy—women like Brenda Sanders, whose Afro-Vegan Society is doing extraordinary community organizing about racism, veganism, and health in the Black neighborhoods of Baltimore; or pattrice jones, the director of VINE Sanctuary, who tried to save Bill and Lou, the Green Mountain College oxen; or Jenny Brown, co-founder of Woodstock Animal Sanctuary, who drew on her own experiences as a disabled woman to develop prosthetics for rescued animals maimed and crippled in the industrialized agriculture system, restoring them to mobility and an active life.[83] These and many other courageous women I might name have modeled genuine care and respect for animals by rescuing them from slaughterhouses, running sanctuaries, and educating the public about the true nature of animal agriculture.[84] There are many caring men, too, who have dedicated their lives to animal advocacy—men like Robert Grillo, director of Free from Harm, and the British animal advocate Kim Stallwood. However, it isn't these men and women being profiled by the media or being awarded handsome book contracts with the top presses. Only those who exploit and kill animals are deemed worthy of public interest.

It was not so very long ago, however, that more justice-oriented perspectives on animals could still be found in the media. In 1990, on the twentieth anniversary of Kate Millett's pathbreaking book, *Sexual Politics*, Simon & Schuster published Millett's memoir, *The Loony-Bin Trip*, about her struggle with a bipolar disorder while living in a women's collective on a former working farm in New York. Millett's account of visiting a rural horse auction reminds us that there are more ethical, and more meaningfully feminist, ways for us to think about our relationship with other animals, besides doing violence to them.

Millett arrives at the auction expecting the pleasant atmosphere of a country fair. Instead she finds herself confronted by a spectacle of ritualized humiliation and violence. Everyone at the auction, except for Millett and the friend she has gone with, are men. It turns out that the horses and ponies are there not to be sold as pets, as Millett had thought, but to be auctioned off by the pound to be killed for dog food. A "tangible climate of fear" pervades the arena, as the animals sense death in the air—the horses are neighing in fright and a tiny pony is "crying out in small cries." As the auction gets underway, men poke and prod the terrified animals, forcing them around the viewing ring. "It is not anger they feel, any more than deportees in boxcars or behind barbed wire—it's gone way beyond anger," Millett writes. "Their situation is too desperate, too inferiorized for anger, that implies some peer relationship, a testing of forces that are matched. They are no match for Luther's Auction, not even hundreds of them." The shocking thought comes to her that "these creatures are like slaves—bought and sold to whomever and wherever, without control over any part of their destiny."[85]

Seized by pity and emboldened by a sudden upswing in her mood disorder, Millett throws herself into the bidding, determined to save as many animals as she can. She succeeds in saving three—a small pony and two horses. The larger horse, a discard from a summer children's riding camp, she names Big Jim. "You don't condescend to this animal," she writes. "The pony is like a kid; this is an adult male; awesome, proud, powerful."[86] After the auction, Millett returns to the farm to await the animals' arrival. When the transport truck finally arrives, she helps each one down the ramp. Finally, it's Big Jim's turn. After leading him down, Millett begins walking him slowly towards the stalls, away from the field where the other horses are.

Suddenly, "the other horses whinny from the field," and Big Jim whinnies back. "The calls are imperious, urgent, powerful," Millett writes. "They obliterate people as they call from kind to kind. How eager they are to claim him and how entirely the need of them takes over the big horse." Big Jim begins irresistibly pulling Millett towards the other horses, slowly at first, then with increasing urgency. Now Millett has to run to keep up with him. "Then I am only something impeding him," she says. "Take it easy, you're scaring me, I say to him, and he actually slows down a bit. But he cannot contain himself, cannot resist, and we take the road to the gate of the field in far too much of a hurry for me." As Millett throws open the gate of the corral, Big Jim rushes past her:

> It is a passion, what they have toward each other, the urgency of that neighing. It must be more than they feel for humans except in rare cases. And these refugees must have everything to tell each other, to heal each other of death, having nearly died in the auction barns and escaped here. . . . But the remarkable thing is their kindness toward each other, the courtesy, one almost wants to say, of their society. The way they have paired off, pony with pony, and the gray horse with the palomino, and now Jim with Big Molly, the mare who is boarding with us, a neurotic who chews on wood and is forced to wear a restraining band. Jim has gallantly taken on this difficult personality and they are from the first inseparable. . . . I think, going back to the pond, what a very nice fellow he is, this horse, and how charitable they are toward each other as beings.

At the moment when Big Jim begins to pull away from her, Millett realizes what she "feared but already knew," which is that Big Jim "is mysterious and of himself and will not always do what I want: thank me for keeping his life, and hold me in gratitude."[87] The epiphany comes to her that Big Jim is a being with his own needs and interests, separate from hers, and that "there will always be this distance of awe between us, the unknown across species." Rather than fight this uncomfortable realization, Millett allows herself to be humbled by it. Surrendering her need to control Big Jim, she finds herself existentially lighter, relieved of the burden of her dominion.

It is a remarkable passage. One of the outstanding feminist theorists of the twentieth century, Millett models a quite different way of relating to animals than we have seen elsewhere in this chapter and in this book, where malignant narcissism, sentimentality, and bad faith in men and women alike destroy any possibility of genuine communion with other beings, and where animals assume the form only of remote figures, glimpsed callously from an unbridgeable distance.

8

HARRY LIME DISEASE

In the film *The Third Man*, starring Joseph Cotten and Orson Welles, an American named Holly Martins (Cotten) travels to occupied Vienna at the end of the Second World War to take a job working with his friend, Harry Lime (Welles), only to learn that his friend is dead, having been killed by a car the day before. In a plot twist—spoiler alert—Martins learns that Lime has staged his own death to avoid responsibility for a crime: during the war, he knowingly sold contaminated penicillin to a hospital, causing the agonizing deaths of many children. The two men agree to meet at an amusement park, atop a giant Ferris wheel. As their gondola lifts them high into the air, Martins confronts his friend over his terrible crime. However, Lime only smiles. Gesturing matter-of-factly at the tiny figures on the ground far beneath them, he says genially, "Look down there. Would you really feel any pity if one of those—*dots*—stopped moving forever?"

Gazing on a pasture of grazing cows on a ranch in South Dakota, Michael Pollan similarly describes seeing not individual beings, but "perambulating black dots."[1] From this "black sea of bovinity," as he terms it, Pollan selects one "dot"—an Angus steer labelled 534—and arranges to have him transported to a feedlot in Kansas. Later, once fattened, the cow will be killed and carved up into meat. Pollan travels to South Dakota and Kansas to make these elaborate arrangements so that he can later write about his experiences in print. The cow he buys is merely an object to be manipulated and destroyed for his literary purposes.

Glimpsed remotely or from a great height, every individual appears insignificant, a speck among other specks. The result is a total collapse of moral perspective. We succumb to "Harry Lime Disease," so to say, when we lose sight of others as unique, vulnerable "someones" worthy of our solicitude and compassion, seeing them only as interchangeable objects to be manipulated or even destroyed at our caprice. In its symptomology, the condition most resembles the set of character traits we associate with antisocial personality disorders like psychopathy.[2] Psychopathy is characterized by shallow emotions, an inability to empathize with others, and a lack of remorse or guilt after inflicting harm on others. Psychopaths are often intelligent and socially at ease, even charming, owing to their fearlessness and supreme lack of self-doubt. Though psychopaths are unable to feel many emotions, they are often adept at observing and mirroring the feelings of others, making them master manipulators. Psychopaths don't feel they should be constrained by the moral realm. Rather, they treat the world as a completely open field of action, but for themselves alone. Ethical constraints, in short, are for "little people." Though few psychopaths become murderers, the inability of psychopaths to empathize with others, coupled with their manipulative outlook and utter lack of moral inhibitions, make them potentially dangerous. While psychopaths don't generally go out of their way to harm others, neither do they respond the way ordinary people do when encountering others in distress. And when they do choose to harm others, they are incapable of feeling remorse or taking responsibility for their actions. Hence Harry Lime's reaction when Martins confronts him on the Ferris wheel—bemused indifference.

Though we think of psychopathy as something exotic or rare, the stuff of horror films and frightening headlines, researchers have discovered the disorder to be more widespread than once thought. Furthermore, every quality that researchers identify with psychopathy, including "impaired empathy, sympathy, guilt, remorse, shame, and love," can readily be observed in our own collective behavior towards other animals.[3] While most people are able to empathize with some animals, that empathy is selective and typically doesn't extend to the animals we exploit. Violence against nonhumans is not only sanctioned by society, but encouraged and monetized. We kill hundreds of billions of sea and land animals each year without feeling remorse or guilt; we even believe that we have a *right* to our violence, so much so that should an "angry vegan" question the desirability of these arrangements, we feel indignant. The animals we exploit are merely "perambulating dots," *things* whose lives, interests, and needs have no significance beyond the uses we might make of them. Ours is a society of Harry Limes.

EMPATHY AS A WAY OF KNOWING OTHERS

The most characteristic feature of Harry Lime Disease is an absence of empathy. Empathy is not so much a "feeling" as a mode of perception and *knowing*—a "sixth" sense rooted in our bodies that provides us access to the internal states, feelings, and perspectives of others. Embracing a distraught friend after the sudden death of her spouse, we find ourselves shedding tears, too; when our child forgets his lines in the school play, we feel his embarrassment, as though it were us up on stage. It is empathy that enables us to know when our baby's diaper needs changing, and whether our friend is really "doing fine," or is only saying so. Used in conjunction with reason and our moral imaginations, empathy enables us to "feel" our way into the experiences even of those distant from us, such as strangers from another culture or historical era—as when we see a news story about a family of refugees drowned at sea, or read a historical account of an enslaved mother's grief as her children are taken from her at an auction.[4]

Empathy can also provide us access to the subjective experiences of other animals. To illustrate this point, I would ask you to go to my author's website (www.JohnSanbonmatsu.com), where I have posted videos in cognitive ethology, or the study of animal minds. Look for the footage of a group of donkeys at the Ezelshoeve sanctuary in Baarle-Nassau, in the Netherlands. In the short video (two minutes long), we see seven or eight donkeys approach the body of a dead donkey lying on a blue plastic tarp. The donkeys crowd around their dead friend, braying and wailing as they investigate his body, before suddenly lapsing into silence. One lets out a high-pitched cry, while another tugs at his face with his teeth, and others paw at their friend with their hooves, trying to revive him. On the periphery of the tarp, the sanctuary staff look on in grief, weeping. We, too, though watching this scene from a temporal and spatial distance, find ourselves deeply affected by the donkeys' grief. Though "being-a-human" and "being-a-donkey" are very different ways of being-in-the-world, we and donkeys participate in a shared *lifeworld*, or structure of experience. Feelings and moods are contagious, even across the boundary of species.

When I show this video in class, my students often express surprise that donkeys are capable of "human-like" feelings. However, the donkeys are no more "human-like" in their expressions of grief than we are "donkey-like" in ours. The limbic system, the part of our brains responsible for our emotions and behavior, consisting chiefly of the amygdala and hippocampus, is among the oldest regions of the proto-mammalian brain, dating back some 150 million years. Long before the earliest hominids, other species were living emotionally vivid lives. We are thus latecomers to empathy. So fundamental is empathy to human social life that the philosopher and psychoanalyst Edith Stein believed it to be the "glue" that makes possible our relations with one another. Our ability to empathize with others may even be a precondition for society itself—for the experiences of community, belonging, mutuality, and love that make life worth living. It follows that the suppression of this capacity is likely to be injurious to social and moral life. For if I cannot *feel* my way into your experiences, then I may also feel no emotional disinhibition against manipulating or harming you.[5]

In Philip K. Dick's science fiction novel *Do Androids Dream of Electric Sheep?*, fugitive "replicants," intelligent beings bioengineered to serve as slaves for humans on colonized planets, are hunted down by a policeman named Deckard. Replicants are human in every way but one: they lack empathy. The only way for an investigator to identify a replicant, therefore, is to administer a "Voight-Kampff test" to register their emotional responses to signs of distress in others. In *Blade Runner*, the film version of the novel, a suspected replicant is presented with the hypothetical scenario of encountering a tortoise lying on its back, "its belly baking in the hot sun, beating its legs trying to turn itself over." The replicant, though, has no idea what is expected of him. Having nothing to gain personally from helping the tortoise, it doesn't occur to him to turn him over. Realizing that he isn't going to pass the test, he murders his interviewer.

Most of us would pass the Voight-Kampff test without difficulty. When we see a vulnerable "someone" in danger or distress, like a struggling bird tangled in a fishing line or a child running into traffic, we feel spontaneous concern for their well-being. That emotional response can then become the basis of moral deliberation and action.[6] After emotionally registering the *need* of the other, that is, we can then use reason to decide what, if anything, is the appropriate thing to do about it. Psychopaths, though, respond quite differently to the distress of others. The philosopher Emmanuel Levinas described the "face of the other" as the basis of moral life: seeing the vulnerability of the other's naked face before us, we feel responsible for the other's well-being. But the situation is quite otherwise for the antisocial personality. Nothing indeed more sharply sets the psychopath or sociopath apart from ordinary people as their response to *vulnerability*. For them, weakness and vulnerability elicit contempt or aggression, not sympathy.

In one interview, a woman diagnosed with psychopathy recounts an episode in which she came across a tiny baby possum drowning in a pool where she was to give a swimming lesson. The possum was "struggling, struggling to try to get out of the pool, and I thought, 'Oh! Baby opossum must have fallen in the pool in the night or in the early morning.'" But the animal's desperation elicits no emotional response in her. So after concluding that there is no advantage to be gained in rescuing the possum, she drowns him with a hose. "I never have really felt anything for animals," she remarks with a smile. "I've never had a pet or felt, like, a connection to animals," she tells the interviewer.[7] Psychopaths are perfectly able to recognize their distress and vulnerability of others; they are just indifferent to it.

People with antisocial personality disorders treat distressed humans and nonhumans with equal callousness. Not only do many serial killers compare the butchering of humans to the butchering of animals, sometimes the behaviors even overlap—as in the case of Canadian pig farmer Robert Pickton, who tortured, killed, and cannibalized at least twenty-six women, burying their remains on his hog farm, where he also killed thousands of pigs. Most serial killers torture and kill nonhuman animals while children, before growing up to murder humans. So normalized is violence against animals in our culture, however, that it isn't always easy to distinguish a child's "ordinary" cruelty towards animals from the kind of behavior indicative of a budding psychopath.

When I myself was a boy, it pains me to say, I killed insects with wanton abandon. I swatted flies, sprayed RAID on wasps, and crushed spiders underfoot. For the colonies of ants who lived in our front lawn, meanwhile, I cultivated special malice. The ants were merely living their own lives, fulfilling their own purposes, and they posed no threat to anyone, least of all to me. Yet I killed them by the hundreds, and I did so in a way calculated to cause them suffering. I killed them not in passion or anger, but with the cool detachment of a behaviorist. I knew that after the ants had withered under my blows, scrambling back inside their burrow to safety, they would eventually venture out again, slowly and cautiously. Having observed their psychology, I would win back their trust in order to betray them again. Forensic psychologist Gwen Adshead observes that individuals with psychopathy are often not merely "indifferent to others' distress" but "have a positive emotional response to it."[8] Vulnerability, in short, can be a goad to violence. This sadly was true in my case—it was the ants' very vulnerability that attracted me. Simply, I had singled out the ants because they were even more vulnerable than I was. Only years later did I come to understand that my violence towards the ants was displaced aggression, a way of dealing with the bullying and trauma I experienced as a child. My mode of address to the ants was unmistakably antisocial, though I had great affection for other animals and would never have harmed them.

Adshead compares the mentality of psychopaths to that of hunters—in both cases, the perpetrators "seek out . . . and target those that will not be protected or cannot protect themselves, those who are weaker and more vulnerable."[9] Both "take pleasure in hurting others and exerting control" over weaker beings.[10] Like psychopaths, hunters are often skilled at reading the behavior of their victims. They may have a sense of what their prey is thinking, which avenues of escape they may revert to, and so on, while nonetheless being incapable of *feeling* their way into their experiences. Hunters can thus kill again and again, causing terror and agony to their victims, without experiencing anything but satisfaction. In *The Omnivore's Dilemma*, Michael Pollan recounts joining a group of friends to ambush a community of mother pigs quietly foraging together with their babies in the woods. Pollan shoots one of the pigs as she tries to flee, shattering her skull and leaving her piglets to starve. Afterwards, he describes feeling "pride," "relief," and "gratitude." The "one emotion," though, that he "expected to feel but did not" feel, he confesses, "was remorse, or even ambivalence." Instead, he "felt absolutely terrific—unambiguously happy." Pollan describes a photo taken of him at the time, "kneeling on the ground behind a pig the side of whose head has erupted in blood that is spreading like a river delta. . . . The hunter's rifle is angled just so across his chest. . . . One proprietary hand rests on the dead animal's broad flank." Meanwhile, the author himself is "looking into the camera with an expression of unbounded pride, wearing a big shit-eating grin."[11]

Had Pollan instead stalked and killed a Labrador retriever, then boasted in print about his "unbounded pride" posing beside the dog's still-warm body, the blood "spreading like a river delta" from her exploded head, readers would have been repulsed and likely seen the author as a moral monster. Owing to our society's unjustified contempt for pigs, however, Pollan's pleasure in killing only lent him credibility in the eyes of his readers—even though there is no ethical difference between killing a pig in the woods and shooting a dog in one's neighborhood (leaving aside the harm done indirectly to the dog's human companion). Only social convention and prejudice lead us to hold the one act admirable and the other repugnant. Occasionally, hunters kill dogs by accident, mistaking them for some other "killable" canine species. In such moments, the moral incoherence of hunting culture breaks into the open—as happened when a woman in Montana shot and skinned a Siberian husky, claiming to have mistaken him for a wolf pup. The public was outraged, though millions of other equally intelligent and emotionally complex animals—foxes, rabbits, deer, bears, etc.—are routinely killed each year for "sport."

Sociopaths and psychopaths are astute observers of the *external* behavior and intentions of others. As one psychopath told an interviewer, "it's like being on the outside looking in." He or she knows "the words but not the music," as researchers studying psychopathic military offenders put it.[12] The sadist observes the victim's suffering as through the wrong end of a telescope, at a remote emotional distance. "If they knew they were going to die you'd see much more agitated behavior," Temple Grandin assures Michael Pollan, about animals killed at the slaughterhouse.[13] Grandin sees animals only from the "outside," as a set of external signs. Though her efforts to "reduce" the suffering of animals in slaughter are widely seen as evidence of her "compassion" for animals, her behavior demonstrates the opposite—indifference to the vulnerability of her victims. Grandin can stand and watch thousands of animals being shot, stabbed, or gassed to death, without emotion. Witnessing an animal at his or her moment of greatest vulnerability, Grandin evidently feels no fellow feeling, only detached curiosity and a professional interest in the "process." Some people with autism may find it challenging to empathize with or recognize the distress of others; it is therefore possible that Grandin's emotional detachment while seeing animals being killed has a neurological basis. However, others with autism are able to form close empathetic bonds with other animals, and some (like my friend Emily Moran Barwick, who runs the Bite-Size Vegan website) are outspoken advocates for animal rights. In any event, Grandin's callousness towards animals is indistinguishable from the callousness of non-autistic people in the animal industry. It is also important to distinguish Grandin's inability to empathize with animals, whatever its origins, from the frank sadism and toxic masculinity exhibited by Michael Pollan in his account of his pig hunt.

Researcher Kerrin A. Jacobs observes that many psychopaths "act in a way that dramatically exceeds common, socially set thresholds of aggressiveness, manipulation, cruelty, cold-bloodedness, and so forth," exhibiting little patience for "the restricted moral realm."[14] The case of Richard Kuklinksi, a serial killer and hit man for the top Mafia families in New York and New Jersey, is indicative. Kuklinski, who murdered as many as 200 people, took pleasure in looking his victims in the eye as their lives melted away. "I'd be looking in her eyes, I would see the blankness come over it, I'd watch 'em die, I wouldn't just shoot them and walk away. I saw the surprise, the shock"—then the blankness. After stalking one stranger, a man whom he felt had slighted him, Kuklinski strangled him outside a bar using a nearby clothesline, swinging him over his shoulder like a bag of laundry so that he could *feel* him die. The man's body, he recounted, "was twitching and kicking. . . . I kept him a while, after he stopped, I kept him a while, just to make sure. . . . I actually felt him die. . . . I felt him go limp."[15]

Similar descriptions, of taking pleasure while watching others die, are common in accounts of killing by hunters, ranchers, and locavore slaughterers. Recounting her killing of the cow she has named Kathleen (described in the previous chapter), Kristin Kimball writes: "She bled and kicked, parody of flight, her eyes blank. . . . I wrapped a chain around one of her hind legs, and then she kicked again. . . . I held the leg for a moment, felt the strength seep from the big muscles. It takes time to drain all the life from a living thing, as though life were a substance. . . ."[16] Tommy Lynn Sells, who murdered as many as eighty people, including children and infants, recounted similar feelings while killing. "It's the sensation of the blood. It's the sensation tying that scarf around your neck and just watching your eyes. . . . It's the sensation of seeing that skin pull apart."[17]

As criminologist Scott Bonn observes, psychopathic killers "view their innocent victims as inhuman objects to be tormented and exterminated for their own amusement."[18] Many people take similar delight in inflicting suffering on nonhuman animals. After cutting an animal's throat, they enjoy watching them thrash about in their blood while their eyes go blank. Such individuals would likely score highly on Hare's Psychopathy Checklist—a kind of Voight-Kampff test used to identify people with antisocial personality disorders. Some of the "femivore" memoirists exhibit such psychopathic traits as extreme cruelty, impulsiveness, and lack of self-control. Whether they are psychopaths in the clinical sense, however, is less salient than the fact that society grants vicious individuals the "right" to wield such total power over vulnerable beings, without any accountability or sanction for their sadistic behavior.

Millions of ordinary people seek out opportunities either to inflict violence on animals or merely to watch others inflict it. In Spain, bulls are ritually tortured and stabbed to death in stadiums, or are set on fire and chased and beaten through the streets, until they die, moaning in agony. Organizers of the live pigeon shoot in Hegins, Pennsylvania, abduct the birds from the streets of New York and other cities, shove them into crates, and transport them to a fairground in Hegins to be killed. The pigeons are then released before a cheering crowd and shot to death. After each "round," small children are sent into the field to tear the heads off birds who were wounded but not killed outright, amidst raucous cheers from the crowd. Other towns across the US invite similar public slaughters of squirrels, turkeys, and other species. In 2023, when officials in New York City announced a new campaign to exterminate millions of rats, the mainstream news media ran dozens of columns and editorials joking about the impending slaughter, with journalists gleefully offering creative ways to kill them—even though rats are as emotionally sensitive and intelligent as our own companion animals.

Pathological indifference to suffering is on the menu, too, of *Shark's Fin and Sichuan Pepper*, a foodie memoir by Fuchsia Dunlop that finds its author traipsing up and down China on a quest to eat as many exotic animals as possible. The book, one reviewer observed, "reads like a bill of lading for dismembered occupants of Noah's Ark: rabbits' heads and turtles' feet, duck tongues and ox throat cartilage, goose intestines and pigs' brains."[19] Even the most extreme forms of cruelty leave the author unmoved. "There isn't a sense there that you're killing an animal," Dunlop writes, "it's simply that you are preparing an ingredient for the table. . . . No one thinks anything of skinning frogs and rabbits while they're still alive."[20] On a panel at the Sydney Writer's Festival in 2011, meanwhile, celebrity chef Anthony Bourdain joined British journalist A. A. Gill in mocking animal rights and defending the exploitation of geese for *foie gras*. "I think it's a bullshit issue," Bourdain said. Gill agreed, saying, "I . . . don't really care if animals suffer. If I'm perfectly honest, I don't give a shit."[21] The audience laughed at both quips.[22]

In recent decades, the media have shown special interest in men and women who seek out opportunities to kill and butcher animals with their own hands. Killing animals oneself, rather than buying meat neatly packaged at the supermarket, is seen as a sign of moral virtue, a demonstration of one's commitment to a more "authentic" and "honest" relation to animals and the food system. However, the opposite is true. The desire not to harm others, and not to see others harmed, is an attribute of a healthy psyche. There is therefore no more "virtue" in killing an animal with one's own hands, instead of buying meat at the store, than there is in filming oneself abusing children in one's own basement, instead of "merely" consuming child porn produced by others. Levi Cole, a critical care nurse in Oregon, says he took up animal slaughter because it "gives you a whole different reverence for what you're doing." "Who wants to be a hypocrite?" Cole asks. "So I could become a vegetarian, or I could kill my own animal."[23] But there are worse things than hypocrisy, and deliberately inflicting harm on others is one of them.

We are all susceptible, to some degree and at various times, to aggression and even to the rare sadistic impulse. Virtue, however, lies in resisting our antisocial tendencies, and in cultivating our better characters. That our society encourages the disinhibition of our worst impulses by celebrating violence towards animals in no way authorizes us to participate in such evil ourselves. Nor does it excuse our indifference to harms committed by others. "It is very tempting to take the side of the perpetrator," Judith Herman observes in *Trauma and Recovery*. "All the perpetrator asks is that the bystander do nothing." By contrast, the victim asks us "to share the burden of the pain," demanding our "action, engagement, and remembering."[24]

EMPATHY IN OTHER ANIMALS

Many of Charles Darwin's fellow naturalists believed that other animals exhibited only two emotions, rage or fear. However, Darwin showed that, like us, other species experience joy, jealousy, terror, astonishment, impatience, and other emotions. Darwin cited one observer who witnessed an elephant "captured and bound in Ceylon" who, after being "overpowered and made fast," exhibited a "grief . . . most affecting," lying on the ground and "uttering choking cries." Animals also exhibit compassion and empathy for one another: "The mother calls incessantly for her lost young ones; for instance, a cow for her calf; and the young of many animals call for their mothers."[25]

Empathy has since been observed in many other species. Young female chimps have been observed carrying water in their mouths and taking it to an older female who had difficulty walking, then emptying it into her mouth.[26] Capuchins will go out of their way to provide monkeys in adjacent enclosures with food, if they see that they don't have any.[27] In India, rhesus monkeys were observed tending to a baby monkey after he was hit by a car. The "monkeys encircled the injured infant, whose hind legs were crushed and who lay in the road unable to move." "Some of them massaged its legs. Finally, they left the scene carrying the injured baby with them." ("It was very emotional," a shopkeeper at the scene reported.[28]) At a train station in the Indian city of Kanpur, a macaque was observed reviving another monkey after he had been shocked into unconsciousness by an electrified rail. The macaque spent an hour biting, pushing, and even dunking his friend repeatedly in a puddle of water, in an effort to revive him. Eventually, he succeeded.[29] (You can find this video on my website.)

But it isn't just primates who exhibit empathy. Scientists in the Netherlands have shown that pigs are highly sensitive to the feelings and emotional states of others, feeling happy when other pigs experience something pleasant, but becoming distraught when seeing other pigs suffer.[30] A dolphin stunned into unconsciousness by a dynamite charge was observed being rescued by two fellow dolphins, who held him above water with their bodies (holding their own breaths in order to do it).[31] Younger elephants have been seen bringing food to an older bull who was too sick to forage for himself;[32] in one case, an elephant whose trunk had been brutally amputated by a poacher was seen being fed by another elephant, though a stranger to herself. Should a baby elephant fall into a pond or river, adult elephants become frantic and work together to save the youngster from drowning. Rats, too, are empathic. In one cruel experiment, researchers put a rat in a water tank without means of escape, then released another rat in an adjacent, dry compartment to watch.[33] Seeing the other rat about to drown, the dry rat worked frantically to free her fellow. Subsequent experiments have shown that rats will sacrifice their own interests—even a favorite reward like chocolate—in order to save a drowning stranger. (Ironically, even as such experiments establish empathy in rats, they also establish lack of empathy in human scientists socialized to accept animal experimentation: the latter continue to repeat this experiment, inflicting trauma on their sensitive captives, again and again.)

Birds and reptiles, too, are highly sensitive to the well-being and suffering of others. Scientists have observed crows conducting funerary rites for their dead; I myself once saw a distraught sparrow frantically trying to revive a friend lying in the road after being struck by a car. The naturalist Konrad Lorenz, who observed greylag geese closely for most of his life, concluded that geese who experience the loss of a life-partner feel terrible grief: they fall into deep despondency and even seem to lose interest in life.[34] Even reptiles appear to have empathy. Turtles and tortoises have been observed coming to the rescue of their fellow creatures when found flailing on their backs: in a real-life version of the Voight-Kampff test, the animals can be seen working singly or with others to set their desperate comrades right again.

We are raised to think of the natural world only in terms of competition, violence, and suffering. But while predation and competition are indeed fixtures of nature, so too are symbiosis, mutuality, empathy, and altruism between members of different species. At the Basel Zoo, chimpanzees were seen rescuing an injured bird who had fallen into their enclosure—after handing the bird around, they gently set the creature outside their cage.[35] In another case, an orangutan attempted to rescue a drowning baby bird, initially by trying to coax it onto a leaf, and then, when that failed, by removing the bird and placing her on the ground. In 1996, after a three-year-old boy fell into the gorilla enclosure at the Brookfield Zoo in Illinois, a western lowland gorilla named Binti-Jua cradled him in her arms, then "laid him gingerly at the feet of waiting paramedics."[36] A similar incident occurred ten years earlier at a zoo in the UK. After a five-year-old boy fell into the gorilla enclosure, a male gorilla named Jambo went to the unconscious boy and gently stroked his back, interposing himself between the child and the other gorillas in a protective gesture, until the boy was rescued.

Since ancient times, mariners have reported dolphins coming to the aid of drowning people, and dolphins have been seen rescuing drowning dogs, as well. Elephants have been observed coming to the rescue of rhinos drowning or becoming stuck in the mud.[37] There are many documented cases of dogs seeking help for injured or incapacitated human companions, dragging them to safety from fires, saving them from drowning, or going to seek help from other humans. Dogs have also been seen rescuing deer, birds, and other dogs from danger. On YouTube—an extraordinary repository of ethological films—hundreds of videos can be found of nonhuman animals engaged in similar acts of altruism: a bear gently rescuing a drowning bird from a pool of water; an elk pulling a drowning marmot out of his water tank; a horse feeding another horse through the bars of a stall; a pig who, seeing his goat friend flailing in a stream, leaps into the water to push him out; a dog frantically attempting to revive several suffocating fishes lying on a concrete floor by pushing water into their mouths.

The ethologist Frans de Waal suggested that empathy is one of two great "pillars" of moral behavior in animals, the other being reciprocity or a sense of fairness. Far from being a uniquely human trait, then, empathy is an adaptive way of "knowing" that is widely distributed throughout the animal realm. If, as Edith Stein maintained, empathy is the precondition for human social existence, it may also be a precondition for the interspecies relations necessary for a thriving biotic community. Though some scientists have attributed empathy to a neurophysiological mechanism—mirror neurons that fire in our brains when we witness an emotional state in another—empathy is much more complex than this, requiring a consciousness capable of judgment. Animals don't merely "act from instinct," but respond in often creative and intelligent ways to the urgent situations presented by others in distress. The very existence of such a capacity is evidence of highly sophisticated cognition in other species, suggesting an ability to grasp meaning, context, and the perspectives and needs of others.

TREATING HARRY LIME DISEASE

We share a natural capacity for empathy, then, with many other animals. However, in our species that capacity can become blunted by culture. Prejudice, habit, and structures of power and inequality can distort our ability to perceive the vulnerability of others or to respond in a morally appropriate way to their suffering. As we saw, Thomas Jefferson, observing the behavior of enslaved mothers after their children were taken away and sold, wrongly concluded that they experienced only "transient" grief. Jefferson's immersion in slave culture, and his own white supremacist beliefs, dulled his moral insight and senses, preventing him from empathizing with his supposed racial inferiors. We likewise find it hard to empathize with the beings we exploit, having been raised to view them as degraded inferiors and "tools."

In *The Omnivore's Dilemma*, Pollan makes an elaborate show of "getting to know" the "perambulating black dot" he has purchased, visiting the cow in person at a distance in a supposed effort to become acquainted with "my boy," as he calls him, before returning home.[38] The cow is then transported to a feedlot in Kansas, where, Pollan jokes, he will pay "for his room and board (all the corn he could eat) and meds."[39] Pollan pays the animal one more brief visit, at a feedlot, to see how well he has fattened. For the occasion, he has worn "the same carrot-colored sweater" he'd worn months earlier at a ranch in South Dakota—ostensibly to help the steer recognize him. Instead, however, author and animal stare "dumbly at one another," without any feeling of connection. "Glint of recognition?" Pollan writes. "None, none whatsoever." He adds, "I told myself not to take it personally; 534 and his pen mates have been bred for their marbling, after all, not their ability to form attachments."[40]

It is an urban myth, however, that animals bred for food are not as emotionally complex or intelligent as other animals. Nor are they in any way less capable of forming bonds of friendship. I know many observant people who have lived alongside rescued cows, pigs, chickens, sheep, and other exploited animals, and they reliably report them to be just as expressive, curious, and affectionate as any cat or dog. My friend Harold Brown grew up in Michigan in a family that had raised animals for generations. As a boy, he worked on his grandfather's ranch, where he milked cows, helped deliver calves, and dehorned, castrated, and butchered animals. Later, Harold worked on a dairy farm. Although he had always had affection for the animals he raised, it wasn't until he suffered a heart attack—ironically, due in part to his consumption of beef and dairy—that he began to question the system he had been a part of, and his role in it. Eventually, Harold decided to leave the dairy business. A man who had spent his life exploiting and sometimes killing cows now became a vegan and even adopted a rescued steer named Snickers at an animal sanctuary.

One day, Harold stopped by the sanctuary to see if Snickers, whom he'd visited only briefly a few times before, would still remember him months later. Arriving at the sanctuary, he found all the cows but Snickers being lavished with attention by visitors. On a whim, Harold opened his arms wide and called out, "Hi Snickers!" To his amazement, Snickers came running across the barnyard to him, then pushed his massive head against Harold's chest. Harold, who'd been raised in a conservative rural community where boys were taught to repress their feelings, broke down. "I had this immediate mental image of a light switch right over my heart," he later recalled. He had turned off this "compassion switch" his whole life when he needed to disconnect himself "mentally, emotionally, and even spiritually" from the animals he butchered and ate.[41] Now, Harold leaves the switch on, and is a full-time advocate for abolishing animal agriculture.

The reason Michael Pollan, by contrast, doesn't feel a personal connection to steer 534 at the feedlot is not because of a cognitive deficit in the cow, but because of an empathy deficit in Pollan. It does not occur to him that a being who has been brutalized and treated with violent indifference throughout his young life—from the time he was torn from his mother's side at birth to his experiences of being castrated and branded with an iron without painkillers, then being prodded and shoved onto a crowded truck and driven hundreds of miles to a feedlot—might understandably be wary of the man in the sweater standing beside the feedlot's staff veterinarian. Pollan feels no "glimmer of recognition" between himself and his "boy" because he himself has closed the door to such a possibility. He sees only what he is prepared to see—an animate dot in a "black sea of bovinity."

As Harold's experience shows, though, just as we have learned dissociative behavior towards animals, we can also unlearn it. As children, we have to be taught not to pull our sibling's hair or shove other children off the monkey bars. We then internalize this parental authority as moral authority, associating our feelings of empathy and compassion—and, concomitantly, feelings of moral censure (shame and guilt)—with abstract notions of right and wrong. Culture and upbringing therefore play a key role in our ability to engage in empathic connection. Unlike true psychopaths, whose lack of empathy and inability to feel remorse are now thought by some researchers to be genetically based and "hard-wired" into their neurology, most of us can be cured of our moral indifference towards others—if we are only willing to rethink our prejudices and assumptions.

A FLY DROWNING IN A GLASS OF WATER

"The animal . . . is certainly another existence, and this existence is perceived by everybody," observed the philosopher Maurice Merleau-Ponty. If an animal weren't such an existence, then the seventeenth-century philosopher Baruch Spinoza "would not have spent so much time considering a drowning fly," as Spinoza did. Even a drowning fly has an existential significance, corresponding to a *situation* in which a distressed consciousness finds itself. And we can perceive this existential significance if we open ourselves to it.

Mahayana Buddhists have argued for centuries that we can be taught *karuṇā*, or compassion, for all suffering beings. Even insects, they hold, are deserving of our respect and solicitude. When we see a fly on our leg, our first response may be to kill it. But as Pema Chödrön explains, summarizing the views of Tibetan monk Trungpa Rinpoche, by giving in to our violent impulse we only "sow more seeds of aggression and insensitivity," hindering any "awakening" of our heart. Instead, we might "try having a friendly response to the fly." "You could just look at it in a kind way and either let it be there or gently put your hand near it so it will fly away. This transforms the fly's visit from an annoying event into an opportunity for sowing seeds of kindness and tolerance and appreciating the sacredness of life. It turns into a small way of becoming more open-hearted and open-minded—in order words, of freeing yourself."[42]

Today, I no longer kill insects and spiders. Sometimes, ant scouts find their way onto my kitchen counter. Instead of killing them, I mist them lightly with a water bottle, to encourage them to explore elsewhere. The ants eventually get the message and disappear from my kitchen. Occasionally, some other tiny consciousness will stray into my domicile—a moth or fly, a spider or wasp. I have no desire to harm them, either. Instead, I gently take them outside, using a butterfly net I keep in my hall closet for that purpose. I do these things not to assuage my guilt over my past injustices to the invertebrate world, nor out of a Kantian sense of objective moral duty, but simply out of concern for my visitors' well-being. It pleases me to set them outside, and they are pleased to be free again.

9

BLOOD AND SOIL

"New snow has all but covered the blood.
A farm exhales."
—Jenna Woginrich, *One-Woman Farm*

"All people are Nazis; for the animals, it is an
eternal Treblinka."
—Isaac Bashevis Singer

During the 2010 Winter Olympics in British Columbia, a company
called Whistler Outdoor Adventures offered tourists the chance to run
their own Iditarod by renting sled dogs to drive across the ice.[1] When
the games concluded, however, and demand for the dogs slackened,
Whistler's parent company ordered the staff to reduce its "stock" of
dogs. The task fell to an employee who'd previously been responsible
for the animals' care. A reporter for the *New York Times* described
what happened next:

> The killing went on for two days, and several of the deaths were
> grisly. . . . When an initial shot failed to kill a dog that was the mother
> of the employee's family pet, she ran around with her "cheek blown off
> and her eye hanging out" until she was felled by a rifle with a scope,
> according to the report. The bullet also penetrated another dog, which
> was not supposed to be part of the kill and which suffered for about 15
> minutes before dying.
>
> Another dog, left for dead for 20 minutes, emerged [crawling] from
> a mass grave only to be shot again, the report said. The employee said

he eventually wrapped his arms in foam padding after the frightened dogs began attacking him.[2]

Some of the dogs were killed "execution style." In other cases, the worker "wrestled the dogs to the ground and stood on them with one foot to shoot them."[3] One hundred dogs were shot or stabbed to death.

After news of the massacre leaked to the Canadian press, causing an uproar, Whistler released a statement assuring the public that it had only instructed its employee "to euthanize" the dogs in "a proper, legal and humane manner."[4] For some, however, reports of the massacre, with their descriptions of dying victims crawling out of mass graves after being shot, conjured up images not of "euthanasia," from the Latin for a "good death," but of atrocities and war crimes. Despite the public's revulsion at the killings, however, the Canadian Parliament passed no new legislation to prevent similar massacres from occurring in future, whether of dogs or of other animals. "Under Canadian criminal law," the reporter noted, "it is not illegal to kill dogs using a gun, provided it is done without undue suffering."

In a sense, the entirety of our treatment of other beings revolves around this one belief: that we are permitted to kill animals for our purposes so long as we don't cause them to suffer "unduly." There is a scene in the science fiction film *Independence Day*, depicting an alien invasion of the Earth, in which the US President finds himself in the grip of a telepathic exchange with one of the invaders. "What do you want us to do?" he asks his enemy, to which the alien replies, "Die." We ourselves ask as little of the other beings with whom we share our world: we don't want the animals we exploit to suffer "unnecessarily," only as much as is necessary for them to die. And animals deserve to die, we think, because they do not deserve to live.

This was the view, we saw, of farmer Jay Bost in his winning essay for the "Defending Your Dinner" contest in the *New York Times*. "Am I willing," Bost asked, "to divide the world into that which I have deemed is worthy of being spared the inevitable and that which is not worthy?" And Bost said that he was. All conscious beings can be separated into one of two categories—those deserving of continued life, and those undeserving of it. And only human beings make it into the first group. This idea, that some beings are simply *unworthy of life*, and that as a consequence of their worthlessness it is permissible to kill them en masse, so long however as it is done "humanely," is not without historical precedent. A century ago, the same idea appeared in Europe—only, the beings deemed unworthy and "killable" happened to be human.

In 1920, Karl Binding, a professor of law at Freiburg University, and Alfred Hoche, a physician, published *Authorization for the Destruction of Life Unworthy of Life*, arguing that the vitality of the German nation was being sapped by the growing ranks of individuals they termed *lebensunwertes Leben*, or "life unworthy of life." Those unworthy of life fell into one of two categories: the physically disabled and chronically ill, whose lives were compromised by suffering; and the mentally ill and mentally enfeebled ("imbeciles") whose "degenerate" natures made them useless to society. The authors argued that the humane thing to do was to allow the German state to kill them. Written at the height of the eugenics movement, Binding and Hoche's manifesto presented state euthanasia as a mercy not only to society, but to the "unworthy" individuals themselves. It was well known that physicians sometimes overdosed terminal patients with morphine to relieve their suffering at the end, and few doubted that allowing such patients to die painlessly was humane and just. Why, then, shouldn't physicians also be permitted to euthanize the chronically ill, the disabled, and the cognitively impaired? Such defective individuals would be relieved of the "suffering" caused by the worthlessness of their lives, while society would in turn be relieved of a drain on its finite resources by "idiots."

Though Binding and Hoche couched their arguments in humanitarian terms, their "concern" for suffering could not disguise their violent contempt for the persons they deemed expendable. As Saul Friedlander observes, the authors "used the argument that the terminally ill deserved the right to a relatively painless death to justify the murder of those considered inferior."[5] Apart from *Mein Kampf*, no other book proved as influential in shaping later Nazi attitudes towards mass killing as Binding and Hoche's slender work. Two decades later, Adolf Hitler operationalized Binding and Hoche's proposal, ordering his personal physician and the chief of the Reich Chancellery to arrange the killing of so-called *Ballastexistenzen*, "subpersons" whose existence was unnecessary "ballast" weighing on society. Though the killings were conducted in secret, the Nazis had prepared the German public for the slaughter with eugenicist charts showing "alarming" year to year growth in the mentally disabled population, warning that "imbeciles" would soon outnumber healthy Germans, destroying the nation. Thousands of mentally and physically disabled adults and children, war veterans, epileptic and autistic children, and chronically ill patients were subsequently murdered by the German state.

The three ideas that served as the basis of this grotesque state crime—that some beings are unworthy of life; that mass killing of such beings can be conducted "humanely"; and that enacting such violence is simply part of "the cycle of life"—have been put into circulation again today, this time by "enlightened" omnivores in defense of the animal food economy. Disturbingly, we find more than a passing resemblance between the system of animal agriculture and the totalitarian state.

LIFE UNWORTHY OF LIFE

Initially, the victims of Hitler's euthanasia program were killed through starvation or poison injection. Soon, however, the Chancellery hit upon the idea of gassing victims using carbon monoxide. Secret gas chambers were hastily constructed in several cities in Germany and Austria beginning in 1940. By the end of the war, Hitler's Aktion T4 program (named for Tiergartenstrasse 4, the street address of the Chancellery) had "euthanized" as many as 200,000 people.

Significantly, the program served as a trial project for the much larger extermination of European Jewry, Roma, and other "enemies" of the Third Reich.

Throughout this period of state criminality, Binding and Hoche's perverse language of "humane" and "painless" mass killing found its way into the Nazis' own self-justifications for their genocidal policies. Even as the Nazis sought out opportunities to humiliate, torment, and kill their Jewish and Roma victims—working them to death as slaves in labor camps and factories, conducting scientific experiments on them, forcing mothers to watch the murder of their children—they reverted time and again to the rhetoric of *care* in eliminating their victims. Genocide was internally legitimated in Nazi documents as a "good death" for those who did not "deserve" to live. Killings were supposed to occur as instantaneously and impersonally as possible, ostensibly without "suffering."

The SS embraced gassing as the most efficient and "compassionate" way to liquidate enemies en masse, with the Aktion T4 program serving as the inspiration for more industrial-scale facilities at Auschwitz and other death camps. The Nazis settled upon Zyklon B, a cyanide-based pesticide already in wide use for exterminating insects and small mammals, as the preferred means. It took but a minor technical adjustment to switch the targeted population from nonhuman parasites to supposed human ones.[6] The *sonderwagen*, or gas trucks, were a second means of killing in quantity, employed by the *Einsatzgruppen*, the mobile killing units of the SS, initially against members of the Polish intelligentsia. As the Wehrmacht drove further east, Reinhard Heydrich, Hitler's deputy, who directed the *Einsatzgruppen*, repurposed them to murder the thousands of Jews now under Nazi control. After members of the *Einsatzgruppen* complained about the "stress" of shooting Jewish women and children at close range, the SS began experimenting with mobile gas chambers. Victims would be herded into vans, then driven to mass graves. The truck exhaust was diverted into the back, and the victims would be killed during the short journey to their destination.

Rudolf Höss, Commandant of Auschwitz, described "the Zyklon-B method . . . as . . . more 'humane'" than other methods.[7] August Becker, the SS officer and chemist who helped design the *sonderwagen*, saw his method in the same light, complaining that van drivers sometimes failed to press down enough on the accelerator, leading victims to lose consciousness but not to die. "It has proved that if my instructions are followed and the levers are properly adjusted death comes faster and the prisoners fall asleep peacefully," he wrote his superiors. "Distorted faces and excretions, such as were observed before, no longer occur."[8] In reality, the women, men, and children who were gassed died horrific deaths. The victims of the *sonderwagen* realized that they were being slowly smothered, and parents died trying to shield dying children from the carbon monoxide. Becker, however, unable to empathize with his victims, could perceive their death agonies only from a vast, uncomprehending distance, as external "behaviors."

The suffering of Jews and others at Treblinka and other camps— transported by train in the same cars used to ferry cattle to their doom—was even more horrific. The victims, deceived into thinking they were to be given showers, were made to strip naked, then beaten and marched at gunpoint into a large room. Then the doors were slammed shut and the lights suddenly went out. As the terrified people screamed and struggled to open the door, realizing the trap, an operator on the roof dropped canisters of Zyklon B into a chute. The poison landed in a grate-covered hearth, spreading the gas quickly throughout the chamber. Minutes later, when the doors were opened again, the victims were found in a pile near the door, the weaker ones on the bottom, crushed by the stronger ones in their desperate struggle to escape. A Jewish *Sonderkommando* (work crew) then removed the bodies and cleaned the chamber so that the next batch of victims could be brought in.[9]

RETURN OF THE GAS CHAMBER

In a kind of return of the repressed animal origins of the Holocaust, the meat industry has lately embraced gas chambers as the final solution to the problem of "animal welfare"—as the "humane" way to liquidate animals in the millions. Even the *sonderwagen* have made a comeback. Organic farmers can now pay to have a mobile gas chamber called a Mobile Poultry-Processing Unit (MPPU) driven directly to their farm, to save them the trouble of having to transport their victims to a slaughterhouse, or to kill them themselves. State wildlife officials, too, have borrowed from the SS toolkit. Because Canada geese and ducks are now flourishing in urban areas due to climate change, wildlife officials in New York, Colorado, and other states have been herding them, too, into mobile gas chambers. The birds are corralled into the vans, the doors are quickly shut, and the truck exhaust is pumped into the sealed compartment, where the birds slowly suffocate to death on their way to the incinerator.

Temple Grandin is the leading proponent of using gas chambers to exterminate animals. "Gas chambers are better than having slaughter plant workers capture and shackle thousands of distressed, flapping birds each day—a practice that causes a high percentage of broken wings," Grandin told the Canadian Cattlemen Association (in a reporter's paraphrase). "Birds don't like to be hung upside down," Grandin said. "If you go to a chamber system, you get rid of the stressful situation. People are not going to torture dead chickens." An added benefit, the reporter noted, is that "gas chambers also make workers' lives easier."[10] Grandin's enthusiasm for gas chambers also extends to mammals. "Gas chambers have also been adopted by hog operations to make the task of disposing of surplus or runt piglets easier for barn workers, especially the new recruits."[11]

There is nothing "humane," however, about being gassed, whether the victims are human or nonhuman. An undercover investigation at Black Eagle Farm, an organic, "sustainable" animal operation in

Virginia, documented the excruciating suffering of chickens during the farm's "depopulation" process. After turning off the lights to the henhouse to disorient the birds, workers grabbed the hens by their legs and violently pulled them from their perches, then took them outside and shoved them into coffin-like metal boxes five feet long and three feet wide, 200–500 individuals at once. After slamming the door to the chamber shut, they then pumped freezing cold CO_2 into the tank through a hose. The terrified birds inside struggled to escape, injuring themselves and others in the process. Investigators found that while "birds on top burn and suffocate to death," those lower in the chamber were often found alive and suffering an hour later.[12] Workers would then seize the injured birds and smash their heads in with boards.

Grandin, we have seen, earns her livelihood by making adjustments to corrals and kill chutes, so that doomed animals are given the illusion of safety. The SS, too, went to elaborate lengths to deceive their victims about what was about to happen to them, installing fake shower heads in the gas chambers and disguising the walled corridors leading to shooting pits with branches from pine trees. When victims arrived at Treblinka, they were given haircuts and delousing to make them think they weren't in imminent danger. Then they were killed. The Nazis did these things not out of kindness, but to prevent their victims from rebelling, hence impeding the efficient functioning of the apparatus. Similar attention to the psychology of the victims is evident in animal husbandry and in blood sports—as when hunters deploy duck decoys or artificial calls to fool animals into thinking they are safely among comrades. Some slaughterhouses still employ a Judas goat or sheep—an animal raised on the premises and hence accustomed to the smell of blood and brains and death—to lead their victims calmly to their deaths. The owner of Dalla Terra Ranch, a "grass fed organic lamb operation" in Iowa, has credited Grandin for getting the lambs to go their deaths "quietly and without agitation or fear," with "no fighting to turn back, no bawling, no injured animals." The owner thanked

Grandin for her "wonderful advice and insight into how to improve what was previously an *unpleasant* event for the livestock."[13]

Sardonic irony and euphemism to describe violence against animals is a staple of many farming narratives—as when Barbara Kingsolver describes killing animals as "a lot less fun than spending an autumn day picking apples off trees," or when chef Jim Weaver describes force-feeding birds for *foie gras* as "probably not as fun as paddling in a pond." With a wink and smile, organic farmers meanwhile quip that the animals they raise have a nice life and "only one bad day." Ironic understatement was a staple too of internal Nazi communications. "This is not a pretty business," Harald Turner, Chief of Staff of the Military Government under the Third Reich, remarked of the mass shooting of thousands of Jews in Serbia.[14] In a letter dated July 16, 1941, Heinz Höppner, the Higher SS and Police Leader of Warthegau, similarly warned Adolph Eichmann that, as winter came, Jews captured and imprisoned by advancing German forces would not have adequate food. "One might weigh honestly," Höppner wrote, "if the most humane solution might not be to finish off those of the Jews who are not employable by means of some quick-working device. At any rate, that would be more pleasant than to let them starve to death."[15]

It would be a grave insult to the victims who died at the hands of the Nazis to credit such monsters as Höppner, Himmler, or Höss with having genuinely "cared" about the suffering of their victims. However, we do not need to accept the Nazis' own lies about their behavior to recognize the value that a rhetoric of "humane" murder might have for the perpetrators themselves. Even as the Nazis justified their deception of their victims on grounds that doing so helped make "for a less stressful and therefore more 'humane' dying experience," as one scholar puts it, their "concern" was utterly cynical, a way to distance themselves from their crimes. In his book *Ordinary Men*, his account of the men of Polish Reserve Police Battalion 101, who massacred thousands of Jews, scholar Christopher Browning exclaims, "a quick death without agony of anticipation was considered an example of human compassion!"[16] In reality, Nazi policy had nothing to do with compassion, and the Nazis' "humane" methods caused unspeakable suffering in their victims, whether the latter were gassed in darkness in a chamber or shot in a field in the sunny countryside.

Some researchers have suggested that Hitler instructed Heinrich Himmler, architect of the Holocaust, to implement the genocide "as 'humanely' as possible."[17] But as Robert Payne notes, Hitler on the contrary "told Himmler that it was not enough for the Jews simply to die; they must die in agony." Himmler then "turned the problem over to his advisers, who concluded that a slow, agonizing death could be brought about by placing Jewish prisoners in freight cars in which the floors were coated with . . . quicklime . . . which produced excruciating burns. The advisers estimated that it would take four days for the prisoners to die, and for that whole time the freight cars could be left standing on some forgotten siding."[18] Overt sadism aside, however, the suffering of the Nazis' victims was merely the byproduct of the policy of extermination. Once the decision to kill had been made, everything else was to be permitted. Nazi quips about "pleasant" deaths and "humane" murder only served to demonstrate the vast differential in power between perpetrators and victims, those authorized to kill and those authorized to die.

Today's apologists for the meat economy similarly make use of understatement and irony to emphasize their total supremacy over their animal victims. Notwithstanding their claims to "care about" the animals they kill, even the most "conscientious" of meat apologists can't help mocking the vulnerability of their victims. It is more than coincidence that the slaughterhouse ramp designed by Temple Grandin is known in the meat industry as "the Stairway to Paradise," while the funnel at Treblinka, through which prisoners were herded to their deaths, was called *Himmelweg*, or "Road to Heaven," by the SS.[19] Sadistic mockery of victims has long been a feature of modern animal agriculture. More than a century ago, the ramp leading to the killing floor at the Chicago Yards was called the "Bridge of Sighs," after the

Ponte dei Sospiri, or Bridge of Sighs, in Venice. The latter, constructed in the early seventeenth century, conveyed the condemned to a prison from which there would be no return, a one-way trip to sorrow.

"SHOULD THE BABY LIVE?"

Surprisingly, Binding and Hoche's discourse of "humane" killing has been revived today not only by apologists for the "new" animal economy, but also by Peter Singer—the utilitarian philosopher credited with having inspired the modern animal rights movement.

Utilitarianism, again, is the moral theory that tells us we should act in such a way as to maximize the greatest happiness for the greatest number of people—or, in Singer's version, of all sentient beings—while minimizing their pain and suffering. The trouble with the theory, critics have long contended, is that because utilitarians tend to value individuals only as "vessels" or carriers of happiness, they fail to recognize the dignity of the individual. This can make it hard for them to explain why killing someone is wrong, particularly in cases when the life of that "someone" tends to yield more unhappiness than happiness overall. There is thus a tendency in utilitarianism to view the lives of persons as fungible or interchangeable, which in turn can potentially render those unable to defend themselves vulnerable to grave harms. This has led Singer to maintain that causing animals to suffer is worse than killing them—and also that killing disabled human infants ought to be legally permissible.

In 1985, Singer published a book with bioethicist Helga Kuhse called *Should the Baby Live? The Problem with Handicapped Infants*, suggesting that it should be legally permissible to kill babies born with severe disabilities. Recycling a line of argument first developed by Binding and Hoche, the authors noted that physicians already exercise discretion in allowing terminally ill patients and severely disabled newborns to die. Why, then, not permit more "active" interventions? The authors rejected the idea that human life has any "irreducible value" in itself, and they denied that all lives could be considered of equal value.[20] The fact is, they wrote, that "some lives are not worth living."[21] It would therefore be "the very best for all concerned" in cases of severe disability that children be killed—provided that it be done "swiftly and painlessly."[22] The authors gave the example of a baby born with Down Syndrome: if the mother doesn't want the child, they maintained, it should be legally permissible to kill it.

Let us grant the authors' contention that in cases of extreme suffering, an individual may well prefer death to life. In such cases, killing may reasonably be held permissible—as when an individual in extreme pain is dying and wishes to be relieved of their suffering. However, Singer has been too quick to devalue the lives and experiences of disabled people—"defectives," as he has sometimes called them—and his views on when, and under what conditions, intellectually disabled individuals may be legitimately put to death have rightly been described by critics as "troublingly imprecise."[23] More disturbingly, like Binding and Hoche, Singer and Kuhse defended infanticide in *Should the Baby Live?* not merely as a way to prevent future suffering, but also on grounds that it would minimize the costs to society of caring for the disabled. Pointing to the "alarming increase" in the number of "children enrolled in some form of special education"—a 15% increase between 1977 and 1982, "from 3.5 million to 4 million"—Singer and Kuhse warned that society might be fast approaching "a limit to the burden of dependence," observing that if "we attempt to keep all handicapped infants alive, irrespective of their future prospects, we will have to give up other things which we may well regard as at least equally important." As more and more disabled people end up in state care, "already stretched resources will have to be stretched even further."[24] It would therefore be reasonable for a community to "decide that its resources are more urgently spent on other tasks than caring for handicapped new-born infants" rejected by their parents.[25] The authors proposed lethal injection to deal with the problem.

In defending this position, Singer and Kuhse criticized as incoherent the view that while all humans have inherent value, all nonhuman animals have none. Since some animals in fact exhibit equal or greater cognitive functions than so-called "marginal" cases of mentally disabled humans, they pointed out, arguments for the sanctity or unique dignity of human life are insupportable. Rather than extend the notion of inherent dignity to all sentient beings, however, the authors instead used evidence of complex cognition in other species to deny inviolable rights to *all* individuals, of whatever species—including humans.

At a conference in the Dutch city of Utrecht some years back, Singer spoke on a welfarist panel entitled, "Animals and the Harm of Death." The broad take-away from the panel was that killing animals does not harm them, because death can only harm beings with a sense of self through time and therefore with an ability to anticipate and plan for the future. Earlier that morning, at the same conference, a panel of Dutch scientists had proceeded on the basis of this same view, in a discussion of the most "humane" ways to kill farmed animals. The researchers had displayed graphs plotting the time, from seconds to many minutes, that it took the brain activity of victims to cease after being subjected to various "treatments." Was it better to shoot them or to gas them? To suffocate or electrocute them?

I happened to be at this conference, and I attended both panels. When Singer's panel ended, I approached him and asked him how, as a "preference" utilitarian who'd staked his career on the principle that we ought to maximize the preferences of other animals, he could deny that the one preference that animals have above all others is *to live*. Singer curtly replied that I hadn't shown that animals in fact have such a preference. I responded that an animal will endure even great pain and abuse if she or he believes it will help them live longer. So great is the desire to *live* that a fox caught in a hunter's trap may even gnaw off his own limb, to free himself. I cannot recall what Singer said in reply. But my feeling at the time, and since, is that there is something wrong with a moral philosophy that purports to care about the "happiness" of a class of beings, whether farmed animals or disabled children, while remaining indifferent to their violent deaths.

The ancient philosopher Epicurus held that death does not harm us—only the fear of death does.[26] Few people, however, have agreed with Epicurus through the ages. The reason we hold murder to be the most serious of crimes, worse than torture, is because death is the only truly irreparable harm an individual can suffer. The individual loses everything by death—all possibility, all hope, all qualities. "If death is not a bad thing," the philosopher Adam Beresford asks rhetorically, paraphrasing Aristotle's view, "why is it wrong to bring it upon someone else?" As Beresford notes, "Aristotle is the only Greek philosopher who doesn't need to answer that profoundly silly question, because he is the only one to hold on to the common-sense view that death is a very bad thing indeed."[27]

BLUT UND BODEN: THE CYCLE OF LIFE AND DECAY

In Orwell's *1984*, the totalitarian state of Oceania uses language to render opposite ideas falsely equivalent to one another, in order to prevent the citizenry from thinking outside the terms of the given order. (If freedom is slavery, then to resist slavery is pointless, since it amounts to resisting freedom.) In the Newspeak of today, the enlightened omnivore similarly equates the freedom of animals with their enslavement, equates killing animals with caring for them, and even collapses the existential distinction between life and death—all to prevent us from thinking outside the terms of the animal system.

"Life and death are the same moment," thus writes Lierre Keith in her attack on vegetarianism. "It is a profound spiritual truth that you cannot have life without death," echoes Joel Salatin. "Life requires death," Derrick Jensen says, affirming that "all eating requires death." "Everything has to die sometime," a woman rancher agrees. "Through the commonality of death," intones Jason Mark, the chief editor of *Sierra* magazine, "we reaffirm our kinship with the other animals on Earth." Do such authors mean that, as we and other suffering beings share a similar existential condition, a similar vulnerability to death, we ought to show animals compassion, as a way to affirm our creaturely solidarity with them? They do not. Rather, they mean that the best way to "reaffirm our kinship" with other animals is *to kill them*.[28] As Jason Mark elaborates in his *Sierra* editorial on "The Moral Case for Meat":

> I would argue that while every creature deserves the respect of a humane death, no animal has the right to live forever. Humans included. We, too, will end up as worm food, the cycle of life and death turning once more. I can't imagine a better end than having my ashes dumped in the compost pile, so that my bones might feed the soil that helps feed my family.[29]

The reader searches in vain, however, to learn how the author wishes to die, or to be killed, so that he can be composted. While locavores sermonize endlessly about "the cycle of life and death," they hold their own lives, and those of the ones they love, infinitely dear. It's only the lives of other animals they hold cheap. In their view, the latter ought to be grateful for our condescension in granting them life—however briefly conferred and however violently snatched away again.[30]

The omnivore's equivocal contention that life "requires" death is meanwhile true only in the banal sense that a world in which organisms literally lived forever would eventually run out of resources. That is a far cry from Keith's assertion, though, that "for someone to live, someone else does indeed have to die," by which she means *to be killed*. All forms of agriculture, it is true, take an ecological toll on other beings. Growing crops leads to the deaths of millions of insects, mice, and other small animals, who get caught up in harvesters and other farm equipment. However, we could minimize such collateral damage by utilizing new technologies and methods, if we chose to. Furthermore, since most crops are fed not to humans but to nonhuman animals raised for slaughter, switching to a plant-based diet would radically reduce the number of animals killed by mechanized agriculture.

For the enlightened omnivore, though, violence and death are not to be feared or minimized, but welcomed as beautiful, life-giving, metaphysical truths. Killing insects in her garden one day, Keith has the epiphany that "life isn't possible without death," and that the soil "wanted" death—"Blood meal, bone meal, dead animals." So Keith begins "feeding" her soil "blood and bones." "I've learned to kill," she writes, "And I've learned to say my own grace."[31] But Keith's aesthetic unity between blood, soil, and violence has troubling historical antecedents: similar ideas in the early organic foods movement were championed by British fascists, then later also taken up by the Nazis. For the latter, metaphysical qualities of blood and soil were inseparable from a wider conception of cyclical nature and of the cleansing violence that made its harmony possible. As Fritz Wirz, a Nazi professor of medicine, maintained: "Blood and Soil is [critical to] . . . the metabolic cycle of humans, animals, and nature."[32] Goebbels himself commissioned at least seven feature-length films on the subject of blood and soil, among them *Ewiger Wald* ("The Eternal Forest"), depicting "a Master Race whose roots lie in the sacred soil fertilized for centuries by the richness of their blood."[33] Such films evoked not merely connection to the land, but rituals of violent blood-sacrifice; as Kiernan observes, "only advanced industrial killing could give Germany back its primeval past."[34]

Appeals to the supposed eternal verities of nature to legitimate violence have always been dangerous, but never more so than in the case of Nazism. For fascists in Italy and Germany alike, violence was a way to achieve a higher spiritual state of national being.[35] "Nature knows no political boundaries," Hitler wrote. "She places life forms on this globe and then sets them free in a play for power." The Nazi jurist Carl Schmitt elaborated on this concept, maintaining that, in Tim Snyder's words, "racial enemies were chosen by nature" and the "superior" race had the responsibility "to struggle and kill and die."[36] Mass killing of more vulnerable beings was seen not as an ethical problem, but as an instantiation of "natural" facts—life, death, violence, suffering—which must lie forever beyond the reach of moral judgment.

Rudolf Höss, before joining the Nazis and rising in their ranks to become SS commandant of Auschwitz, had been part of the proto-fascist, back-to-the-land agrarian movement known as the Artaman League.[37] In his autobiography (published after his execution for crimes against humanity), Höss describes the killing at the Auschwitz death camp in pastoral terms: "In the spring of 1942, hundreds of blossoming people walked beneath the blossoming fruit trees of the farmstead, most of them never guessing they were on their way to the gas chambers, and to death. I can still see this image of *growth and decay* quite clearly" (emphasis added).[38] In her book *Eichmann Before Jerusalem*, scholar Bettina Stangneth remarks of this passage: "Thinking about the eternal cycle of growth and decay made the extermination of millions of people into a natural occurrence, and the murderers into a force of nature, the right hand of natural law."[39] Höss aestheticized mass killing, passing off a deliberate policy to murder millions of innocent people as a thing of beauty, merely part of the natural cycle of life.

Today we find a similar aestheticization of mass killing in omnivorist discourse, as when Michael Pollan praises Salatin's farm for offering a view of "the whole cycle of birth, growth, death, and decay." Eager to participate in Salatin's death-dealing—both because he is "curious," he writes, and because he wants to know "if I could bring myself to do it"—Pollan personally slits the throats of dozens of chickens, blankly watching their violent spasms as they die. Absorbed in "the rhythm of the work," Pollan finds that he's able to "kill without a thought to anything but my technique," to the point where he "got fairly good at it."[40] In a rare moment of self-awareness, he acknowledges that "the most morally troubling thing about killing . . . is that after a while it is no longer morally troubling." (Such "psychic numbing," as psychologist Robert Jay Lifton termed it, is also well-documented among perpetrators of war crimes.) Pollan wonders idly if the chickens he's killing can "smell the blood" or "recognize the knife" in the hands of their killers. But he shrugs off the question, saying, "I have no idea."[41]

My late friend Karen Davis, however, who spent more than three decades living with and caring for chickens, believed that chickens are well aware of what is being done to them and others. "Lest anyone think that chickens don't mind hearing and seeing other chickens die violently in front of them, nothing could be further from the truth."[42] Pollan, though, is too immersed in killing the animals to have "much time for these reflections, because you're working on an assembly (or, really, disassembly) line," which "has a rhythm of its own that soon overpowers your mind as well as your body." Occasionally, the sinister nature of the workings of Polyface Farm intrudes upon Pollan's pastoral idyll, when a "death smell" rises up from the "rotting flesh" of the compost piles. But the pleasure Pollan takes at mealtime smothers any faint stirrings of conscience. "Thankfully, all of that, the killing cones, too, had retreated to the mental background for me, chased by the smoky-sweet aromas of the meal, which I found myself thoroughly able to enjoy." Only when the birds are dead do they truly come "alive" in Pollan's prose, in aestheticized descriptions of their corpses—"viscera [as] unexpectedly beautiful, glistening in a whole palette of slightly electric colors, from the steely blue striations of the heart muscle to the sleek milk chocolate liver to the dull mustard of the gallbladder."[43]

"HITLER WAS A VEGETARIAN"

"We shall never be rough and heartless when it is not necessary," declared Heinrich Himmler, the head of the Gestapo and the overseer of the concentration camps. "We Germans, who are the only people in the world who have a decent attitude towards animals, will also assume a decent attitude towards these human animals." As Nestar Russell sardonically observes: "When the sensitive Himmler instructed that 'human animals' be killed—much like with other animals—it was preferable these acts be undertaken without cruelty—all were gently to go to sleep."[44]

Apologists for the meat economy sometimes bring up Hitler's vegetarianism, and the Nazis' "love of animals," as evidence of a supposed affinity between animal rights and Hitlerism. In reality, the Nazi view of "humane" mass murder coincided with their view of the "humane" killing of animals, and the two views reinforced one another. Many Nazi and SS officials had personal backgrounds in animal breeding and husbandry before the war, and once in power they applied this same "skill set" to implement Hitler's eugenics program. Himmler had himself studied animal agriculture at university, and had once been a chicken farmer: as one SS newspaper boasted, Himmler merely "enlarged on [these practices] subsequently with regard to breeding, selection, and perhaps even what he understood by extermination of vermin."[45]

In 1944, the Nazis passed the strongest animal welfare law in Germany's history. Like other Nazi laws, it was framed in antisemitic terms—as a way to contrast supposed Nazi "sensitivity" towards animals with the "cruelty" of the Jewish people, whose kosher laws specified that animals be conscious when butchered. "The animals protection movement," the law read, "strongly promoted by the National Socialist government, has long demanded that animals be given anesthesia before being killed. The overwhelming majority of the German people have long condemned killing without anesthesia, a practice universal among Jews . . . as against the cultivated sensitivities of our society."[46] However, just as the Nazis' "decent" attitude toward their human victims failed to spare those victims the least suffering, their "decent" animal welfare laws failed to end the exploitation, killing, or suffering of animals under the Third Reich, either.

The Nazis were obsessed with health, fitness, and eating "natural" foods; the latter, particularly whole grains and plant-foods, were seen as important for staving off food scarcity and preserving Aryan racial supremacy. However, the Nazis saw themselves as enlightened omnivores, not ethical vegetarians, and they believed that the "natural diet for Germans was a 'mixed diet' containing both meat and plant food."[47] Meat production in fact increased under the Third Reich, as Hitler's generals struggled to get animal flesh to the frontlines—in the belief that meat was integral to the strength of the German fighting man. (In occupied Poland in 1940, Aryans received an allotment of nine ounces of meat each week, while Jews were allotted less than two ounces.[48]) The Nazis meanwhile banned vegetarian societies in Germany and in the lands they occupied, and persecuted their leaders. They also conducted horrific scientific experiments on nonhuman animals—as well as on Jews, Roma, and prisoners of war.

Hitler followed a largely vegetarian diet, not out of concern for animals, but as "a model of dietary virtue" (publicly) and "to control his weight, digestive troubles, insomnia, nerves, and muscle tremors" (privately).[49] He was not fastidious about his diet, however—a "flexitarian" until the end, Hitler continued to indulge now and then in his favorite liver dumplings and Bavarian sausages. As for Hitler's vaunted love of dogs, that too has been exaggerated. As Charles Patterson observes, "Hitler often carried a dog-whip and sometimes used it to beat his dog in the vicious way he had seen his father beat his own dog."[50] Though Hitler was fond of Blondi, his German Shepherd, what he seemed most pleased by was Blondi's adoration and obedience. And in his final days, Hitler showed no more respect for Blondi's life than he had for any of the lives of his millions of other victims. Worried that the cyanide he'd been given might not be potent enough, he instructed an SS physician to test it on Blondi first.[51] It worked. Hitler decided to use a different method, anyway, and shot himself the next day. The following afternoon, Goebbels and his wife Magda asked an SS dentist to administer morphine to their six children. After being sedated, the children were administered ampules of cyanide. Hitler's regime thus ended as it began—in the "compassionate" murder of children.

THE ANIMAL OF BAD FAITH

In his book *Anti-Semite and Jew*, published after the war, the philosopher Jean-Paul Sartre sought to explain how an ideology as plainly irrational and dangerous as antisemitism should have continued to thrive in France even after the Nazis' murder of European Jewry. Antisemitism was not merely a "belief" or "opinion," Sartre held, but a "passion" or existential project around which the antisemite organizes his or her identity and sense of life purpose. In *choosing* to hate Jews, the antisemite adopts "a comprehensive attitude . . . not only toward Jews" but towards society and history, as well. For the antisemite, hatred of the "other" serves to lend meaning and order to an otherwise confusing and threatening world. Without the figure of the Jew, the antisemite would be nothing, for it is only "vis-á-vis the Jew and the Jew alone that the [antisemite] realizes he has rights." There is nothing the antisemite has to do to merit his superiority, as it is bestowed at birth. Merely in "treating the Jew as an inferior and pernicious being," he or she affirms membership in "an elite."[52]

A similar psychological structure subtends our dominion over nonhuman animals. My *worth* as a human being derives from the *worthlessness* of all other beings of the Earth.[53] Just as a bank creates money by putting a mark in its ledger to record a new asset, I open the ledger of nature and scrawl down the compound word, "*not*-animal," creating at a stroke a value for myself that hadn't existed before. Even if I commit murder, I retain an inherent dignity lacking in every "mere beast," simply because I am human. I may know nothing of literature or physics, but I can take pride in the accomplishments of Shakespeare or Einstein, as if I myself had penned *Hamlet* or invented the general theory of relativity. Yet it would never occur to me to take responsibility for Pol Pot or Hitler, too.

If our contempt for other beings was a matter of simple ignorance, then we might be easily "cured" of it through education. However, the meat-eater doesn't arrive on the scene a *tabula rasa* open to better arguments, but comes armed with a glittering array of ready-made arguments, whetted against his appetites, to defend against every inconvenient truth. As Sartre observes, antisemitism isn't ignorance, but an existential orientation towards the world. With its "slender scientific coating," antisemitism always "precedes the facts that are supposed to call it forth." This makes the antisemite "impervious to reason and to experience."[54] The speciesist, likewise, "knows" in advance of every fact that all animals are "the same," i.e., inferior. If it is shown that animals use language, it will then be claimed that they can't use syntax. If it is shown they can use syntax, it will be claimed they lack domain general intelligence. And so on. We move the goal posts to justify our prejudices. And at some level we know it.

The term for this habit of self-deceit is what Sartre called "bad faith." Ordinarily, when we accuse someone of acting in "bad faith" we mean that he or she has acted duplicitously towards another. Someone who makes a promise without intending to keep it is said to have acted in bad faith. However, in Sartre's usage, bad faith is a lie in which we are both the deceiver and the deceived. We know the truth, but we hide that truth from ourselves. In this way we seek to avoid responsibility for our choices and values.

In Aesop's fable of the fox and grapes, a fox repeatedly leaps at ripe grapes just outside her reach. Finally she turns away, muttering bitterly that they were probably sour, anyway. The fox finds it easier to blame the grapes, and to tell herself she never "really" wanted them, than to admit her own limitations. That is bad faith. We engage in bad faith either by avoiding some "displeasing truth" or, contrarily, by clinging to some "pleasing *un*truth."[55] To put it differently, I can pretend to myself that I am something that I am not, or I can pretend to myself that I am *not* what I in fact am. Consider a man who cheats on his partner and lies to her about it, telling himself, "After all, I don't want to hurt her—it's best if she doesn't know." He represents himself to himself as being *what he is not*—a faithful, loving partner—while denying what he in fact *is*—a person unable to keep his commitments.

By presenting his lies to his partner as altruism, the man tries to escape responsibility for his actions. But whatever he chooses to tell himself, he has behaved badly.

Our relations with other animals are suffused with this psychological structure. Scientists describe "sacrificing" animals in their experiments—rather than killing them. Wildlife officials speak of "managing" animal "resources"—instead of shooting, gassing, or stomping to death millions of animals, often at the behest of cattle ranchers. Hunters portray the animals they terrorize and kill as "equal" participants in a "sport," claiming to hunt in order to promote "conservation"—when in truth they hunt because they take pleasure in exerting violent power over other beings. These and other perpetrators of animal harm rely on euphemism less to deceive the public than to hide the truth from themselves. Few people, likewise, know the true nature of the meat industry, but most also would prefer not to know. Hence the bad faith arguments deployed by meat-eaters when confronted with veganism. Vegans are told that "plants are alive too" (though plants aren't conscious and don't suffer); that "lions eat gazelles" (though, unlike lions, we aren't obligate carnivores); that "we need protein" (though animal protein is no higher in quality than protein from plants: there is more protein in two slices of whole bread, or two tablespoons of peanut butter, or half a cup of cooked lentils, than in two slices of bacon).[56] Such arguments are offered not in earnest, but to fend off genuine moral reflection.

Vegans are meanwhile mocked in our society not because their positions are ridiculous, but because they pose a threat to the violence of the established order. "What he wishes, what he prepares, is the death of the Jew," Sartre observed of the antisemite. Though "not all the enemies of the Jew demand his death openly," still "the measures they propose—all of which aim at his abasement, at his humiliation, at his banishment" amount to the same thing, which is a desire for the Jew's death. We have likewise organized our material and psychic lives around the death of the animal. The degradation of nonhuman animals in our culture, in children's books poking fun of farting dogs and stinking pigs, in the humiliated captives we put on display at zoos and aquaria, or brutalize or kill in public spectacles like rodeos, bull fights, and sport fishing shows, are invocations of the pogrom.

It is no accident that George Orwell should have chosen a small family farm as the basis of his allegory about totalitarianism in *Animal Farm*: both animal agriculture and totalitarianism take as their basis the annihilation of the individual.[57] "The State is everything, the individual nothing," as Benito Mussolini put it. Primo Levi, in his survivor's account of Auschwitz, observes that the SS exterminated the Jews twice—first psychologically, by stripping them of their humanity as individuals, then physically, by murdering them. The one was the prelude to the other. When Jewish work details were marched outside the gates of Auschwitz through the bitter winter cold, Polish villagers mistook their wretched condition for moral debasement:

> They think . . . that as we have been condemned to this life of ours, reduced to our condition, we must be tainted by some mysterious, grave sin. They hear us speak in many different languages, which they do not understand and which sound to them as grotesque as animal noises; they see us reduced to ignoble slavery, without hair, without honour and without names, beaten every day, more abject every day, and they never see in our eyes a light of rebellion, or of peace, or of faith. . . . [M]uddy, ragged and starving, and mistaking the effect for the cause, they judge us worthy of our abasement. Who could tell one of our faces from another?[58]

If, as the Jewish philosopher Emmanuel Levinas maintained, the "face of the other" calls out to us in its very vulnerability, requiring a moral response from us, then the erasure of the face is the essence of totalitarianism.[59] "If you want a picture of the future," the state functionary O'Brien tells George Winston at the end of Orwell's *1984*, "imagine a boot stamping on a human face—for ever."

But other animals, too, have faces. And just as the Nazis tattooed their prisoners with numbers, we brand farmed animals and staple numbered tags to their ears, not merely to control them, but to efface their individuality. In 1940, Joseph Goebbels, the German Minister of Propaganda, commissioned a film entitled, *Der ewige Jude,* "The Eternal Jew," the most notorious of the many films made by the Nazis depicting Jewish people as worthless "vermin." To depict Jews as parasites living off the body of the German *Volk,* the Nazis resorted to cinematic tautology, employing film footage taken inside the very ghettos that the Nazis themselves had created and forced the Jews into. Images of starving Jews reduced to ghostly, abject figures suffering from disease, terror, and despair were then used by the Nazis to make the case for the Jews' own elimination. "The Jew" was not old or young, fat or thin, man or woman, farmer or student, but an eternal type— the "Jewish bacillus," as Goebbels termed Jews in his personal diary. Like the Nazis, who crowded their victims into ghettos and concentration camps, we crowd animals into filthy, airless warehouses, zoos, and Concentrated Animal Feeding Operations, then use their misery as proof of their abjection.[60] At the zoo, capuchin monkeys chase one another on concrete perches and fake trees, covered in their own feces and driven half-mad by the relentless gaze of thousands of gawking human primates. Penguins, crowded onto plastic ice at the aquarium, are ridiculed by children for their stink. Confronted with undercover video footage of pigs lying prostrate in their own urine and excrement on the killing floor, moaning, we may turn away in disgust at *their* filth. Mistaking the effect for the cause, we judge other animals to be worthy of their debasement and deaths at our hands.

Farmed animals born with disabilities or who get sick or don't grow fast enough are seen not as vulnerable individuals, but as *Ballastexistenzen* to be disposed of, like the "worthless" humans the Nazis termed *unnütze Esser,* "useless eaters."[61] In 2020, when the COVID-19 pandemic shut down slaughterhouses and disrupted supply chains for meat, eggs, and dairy, the animal industry disposed of its sudden "surplus" of unproductive animals using ventilator shutdowns. Tens of millions of chickens and pigs were locked inside airless warehouses, heat was pumped in, and the animals were effectively baked alive, dying in agony of heat stroke and dehydration over the course of hours or days. The procedure was deemed "humane" by the American Veterinary Medical Association—an organization which, though popularly associated with one's friendly local vet, is in fact a ruthless appendage of animal agribusiness, a leading institutional culprit in collapsing the distinction between caring for animals and killing them.[62]

* * *

In his story "The Letter Writer," published in the *New Yorker* in 1968, the Nobel Prize-winning Yiddish author, Isaac Bashevis Singer, explicitly compared our treatment of animals to the Nazis' treatment of their victims. The story's protagonist is a New Yorker named Henry Gombiner, a vegetarian whose "parents, grandparents, sisters, brothers, aunts, uncles, and cousins" all died in the Holocaust. Like his story's protagonist, Isaac Bashevis Singer was himself a New Yorker, an ethical vegetarian, and a Holocaust survivor whose family was killed by the Nazis. Gombiner, who lives alone in an apartment building, befriends a mouse who lives there too. One day, watching the mouse sip from a saucer of water he has set out for her, he assures her: "Holy creature. No harm will come to you." Reflecting on the injustice of a world that would treat "even" a mouse as unworthy of life, Gombiner reflects:

> What do they know—all these scholars, all these philosophers, all the leaders of the world—about such as you? They have convinced themselves that man, the worst transgressor of all the species, is the crown of creation. All other creatures were created merely to provide him with food, pelts, to be tormented, exterminated. In relation to them, all people are Nazis; for the animals it is an eternal Treblinka.[63]

Charles Patterson, a former researcher at Yad Vashem, borrowed this last phrase of Singer's for the title of his book, *Eternal Treblinka: Our Treatment of Animals and the Holocaust*.[64] The French philosopher Jacques Derrida, one of the most influential philosophers of the late twentieth century, also saw parallels between Nazism and our treatment of other species. A Sephardic Jew raised in colonial Algeria—as a student he was expelled from a *lycée* under the antisemitic ordinances of the Vichy regime—Derrida maintained that there "are also animal genocides," and he went so far as to observe (with scandalous irony) that whereas the Nazis sought to slaughter the Jews once and for all, humans instead reproduce animals *ad infinitum* so that they might be "exterminated by means of their . . . overpopulation":

> As if . . . instead of throwing people into ovens or gas chambers (let's say Nazi) doctors and geneticists had decided to organize the overproduction and overgeneration of Jews, gypsies, and homosexuals by means of artificial insemination, so that, being more numerous and better fed, they could be destined in always increasing numbers for the same hell, that of the imposition of genetic experimentation or extermination by gas or fire.[65]

Do such comparisons offend us because they "reduce" human victims to "mere animals"? Or because they equate human civilization with the Third Reich?

Part of the unique horror of the Shoah was the victims' knowledge that they were being targeted not merely as individuals or families, but as an entire people or race. Like other genocides, the Shoah therefore inflicted a type of psychological and spiritual suffering that may be unique to human beings, owing to our capacity for complex language and historical understanding. In all other ways, however, the animals we kill suffer as we do. Furthermore, the empathic and social capacities of other species, coupled with their superior senses, enable them to experience the collective suffering of others. Elephant survivors of human violence exhibit signs of PTSD: rescued baby elephants who witnessed their mothers being killed by poachers wake up in the night screaming, and young adult elephants from decimated herds have been observed enacting sexual violence against hippopotamuses—a symptom of breakdown in the norms governing elephant culture.[66] During the annual massacre of dolphins in Taiji, when Japanese fishers kettle and then stab to death hundreds of dolphins at once, the dolphins cry out to one another using their unique names, while parents try frantically but in vain to protect their young. There can be no doubt that in their final moments during such pogroms, the dolphins suffer in the awareness of the collective murder of their clans.

In my introduction, I suggested that our treatment of animals is not merely wrong, but a form of radical evil. There is indeed no other term adequate to the scale of the extreme violence we inflict on the other beings, or the suffering that results from it. Nor is there another word that more aptly captures the horror of our own existential condition, which rests upon a universal crime in which we are all implicated, yet to which we are all indifferent. Sartre observed that while many antisemites "would not do [the Jews] the least harm" themselves, they also "would not raise their little fingers to protect them from violence."[67] Likewise, though many people would declare themselves against "factory farms," few would bother to "raise their little fingers" on behalf of the animals trapped within them. Most are instead content to coast along, without questioning how the chicken or pork on their plates got there.

The antisemite, Sartre writes, chooses "to find his being entirely outside himself," disappearing into the hateful mob in order not "to look within." What he "flees even more than Reason is his intimate awareness of himself."[68] Speciesism likewise shifts our gaze outward, away from moral reflection and self-knowledge. In our unchecked supremacy over other beings, we thereby apprehend ourselves as what we are *not*—the world's "only" intelligent life form, and the only being whose existence has worth—while pretending that we are *not* what we are—animals ourselves. In short, we use both our differences from other animals, and our similarities to them, as justification for our violence against them. As Mephistopheles observes to God in Goethe's *Faust*:

> The little god of earth, remains the same queer sprite
> As on the first day, or in primal light.
> His life would be less difficult, poor thing,
> Without your gift of heavenly glimmering;
> He calls it Reason, using light celestial
> Just to outdo the beasts in being bestial.[69]

If, as Sartre claimed, antisemitism is fear of the human condition, the same can be said of speciesism. We refuse responsibility for our freedom, telling ourselves that we have "no choice" but to go on hurting and killing the other beings, when instead we could choose compassion over violence. We choose speciesism, so to say, and in so doing we choose ourselves, but for the worse.

PART IV

BEYOND MEAT

10

ANIMAL, NOT VEGETABLE

In response to the endless cruelties I have outlined in this book, the obstinate meat-eater has one last recourse, and that is to maintain that other animals simply *are* unworthy of life. There is just something about the *nature* of other animals, that is, that renders them forever undeserving of our respect. It is this which permits us to go on killing them in the countless billions, not merely today or tomorrow, but for all eternity. Can the vegan offer a convincing reply to such a view?

So far in this work, I have been edging around the elephant in the room, which is the question of what an elephant *is*. When we talk about "animals," what do we actually mean? To ask what animals *are* is to inquire into *ontology*, the branch of philosophy that inquires into the "whatness" of things, or what makes something the sort of thing that it *is*. What makes dandelions, say, different from lions, or my friend Gerald different from my geranium? The answers we give to such questions have important ethical implications. It's fine for me to throw away an old rug, say, but not an elderly parent; and that's because a rug, unlike an aging relative, is not the *kind* of entity that can take an interest in not being put in a dumpster. If we are to arrive at a plausible account of our moral duties towards our fellow beings, then, we first need to know how they differ from other kinds of entities.

One reason why arguments over animal rights and the animal economy often seem to get nowhere is because vegans and meat-eaters set out from different starting points concerning the ontology of animals, and so end up talking past one another. Michael Pollan sums up these opposite starting points when he poses the question, "The pig or Pig?"[1] That is, are pigs and other animals unique individuals, deserving of our respect? Or are they mere instances of an eternal, faceless "type" (*Pig*), hence interchangeable? If animals are individual "someones," then we might hold killing them to be wrong. However, if we determine them to be "all alike," then killing them is no different than knocking down metal ducks in a shooting gallery—knock down one target, and an identical one pops up to take its place. No harm can be said to be done, that is, because there is no *one* being harmed. Hence Derrick Jensen's remark that while humans hunted the sea birds known as Great Auks for numerous generations, they did so without "causing appreciable *harm* to the birds."[2] Though millions of the animals died violently at human hands, none were "harmed" because the species was not exterminated outright.

This distinction between the uppercase and lowercase animal—Pig vs. "the pig," Auk vs. "the auk"—surfaces often in the discourses of hunters and critics defending the meat economy. "Before I began to hunt," writes journalist-turned-hunter Lily McCaulou, "I thought of animals as individuals, with families and emotions and a whole slew of anthropomorphic traits. This strikes me as the environmentalist, vegetarian animal lover's approach. Any death of any individual being is painful and bad."[3] Today, though, McCaulou sees her old views as childish. She views other animals now not as individuals, but as replenishable stock, and kills them with pleasure. Which is it, then? Pig or *the* pig?

WHY ANIMALS ARE NOT PLANTS

Sorting out what animals *are* from our stories and representations *about* animals can be difficult. The figure of the animal is probably the oldest, most complex symbol in human culture. Early cave drawings of horses, owls, bears, panthers, and others speak to the outsized role that other animals have played in the collective imaginary of our species from the start, as powerful spiritual emissaries and peers, on one side, and as prey, on the other. As we've grown more distant from nature, however, animals have lost much of their former mystery and power. Held captive on squalid industrial farms, or reduced to objects of public display in zoos, animals today have an abject status. The animals we are most likely to encounter in daily life are either the ones on our dinner plates or the ersatz animals of consumer culture—dancing penguins and singing lion kings. In this hall of mirrors, we seem to encounter only reflections of ourselves, never the animals themselves. So diverse and contradictory are our representations of animals that we may indeed come to doubt that animals *are* anything determinate at all, seeing them as blank screens upon which to project our own meanings.[4] Neither persons nor things, animals both exist and don't exist at the same time, like Schrödinger's cat. Like subatomic particles, said to assume a definite position only at the moment of observation, animals come to resemble a cloud of probabilities, with the figure of the animal occupying every possible cultural position at once, until the moment we fix some definite purpose upon it. We treat *this* kind of animal as meat, therefore it must *be* meat; we treat *this* kind of animal as a family companion, therefore it must *be worth* treating as a family companion.

Beneath this seeming indeterminacy, however, lies a rather more definite, and prejudicial, view of other beings. On this view, every animal is like every other, a timeless copy of an original forged by nature long ago. Animals come into the world with their repertoire of "behaviors" intact. Programmed by DNA and driven blindly by instinct and desire, animals are flotsam tossed on the sea of existence. Hobbled by primitive brains, they approach the threshold of intelligence without ever crossing over it. Though animals exhibit emotions, these are but crudely developed. Unable to recollect a past or to anticipate a future, they remain prisoners of time, trapped in an eternal Now. Life for animals in the "state of nature" is as Thomas Hobbes described it— "solitary, poor, nasty, brutish, and short." Lacking awareness of death, they cannot fear it. Animals are born, they struggle for survival, they die—that's all. And since every pig or chicken is like every other, their lives can be swapped out or exchanged without any loss, whether to nature or to our own moral sensibilities.

The trouble with this view, the sediment of centuries of archaic belief, is that it happens not to be true. Our fellow beings aren't instinctual machines, mindlessly enacting the scripts of their DNA. They aren't all the same, and they don't live in a perpetual Now. Nor are they insensible to death—they fear it and do everything they can to avoid it. We nevertheless persist in viewing other animals as so far beneath us as to be virtually indistinguishable from insentient organisms like plants. "What about plants?" is indeed one of the first things the skeptical meat-eater asks the vegan. Since all life requires death, the reasoning goes, it makes no difference whether we get our sustenance from animals or from plants, since both involve the taking of life. Vegans are therefore revealed to be hypocrites and sentimentalists. Writer Barbara Kingsolver takes this position in *Animal, Vegetable, Miracle*, asking rhetorically, "Who among us has never killed living creatures on purpose?" Kingsolver mocks vegetarians, as we saw, for objecting when farmers cut off the heads of "crops that blink their beady eyes," but not when they cut the heads off lettuces, comparing the killing of animals to "picking apples off trees"—or even killing bacteria. "When a child is sick with an infection we rush for the medicine spoon," she writes, "committing an eager and purposeful streptococcus massacre." In other words, killing plants, killing animals, killing germs—it's all the same thing.

But, of course, it's not the same thing. Cutting the head off a mammal or bird can no more be said to resemble "picking apples" or cutting lettuces than strangling an infant can be said to resemble wringing out the laundry or squeezing lemons to make lemonade. And to suggest that it *is* the same thing is to deliberately engage in a fallacious type of reasoning called a "category mistake." Category errors occur when we mistake one type of entity for another. Nonsense statements like, "the sofa is sad," or "my zinnias have been thinking about umbrellas again," are category errors because neither furniture nor plants are the *kinds* of entities capable of having thoughts or feelings. When Kingsolver compares decapitating birds to harvesting lettuces, or describes goats as "four-legged tools," or when poultry industry scientists call chickens "egg-laying machines," they too are committing category errors. Even very young children understand that animals and plants, sentient and insentient entities, are different *kinds* of beings. Other species, too, grasp the distinction. If a cat should appear in my yard, the squirrels and birds become suddenly watchful of him, while paying no heed to the swaying tree branches, the falling leaves, or the parked cars nearby. Octopuses disguise themselves most often as insentient nature—as kelp, coral, or rocks—to avoid being perceived as conscious prey.

Just how we and other animals are able to recognize one another is something of a mystery. Aristotle, however, believed that it had something to do with the fact that we and other sentient beings share an animal soul—what the philosopher Joel Sachs describes as "that inward depth of life that opens in perception." Sachs writes:

> If a bird lands on a branch near us and cocks its head in our direction, chances are we will smile and say "hello." This is sometimes described, dismissively, as anthropomorphism. . . . But is it not possible that this unguarded encounter might be of a more original significance? Might not the bird be one of many mirrors in and through which I begin to encounter myself? This is not an occasion of certainty or clarity, of deduction or hypothesis, but of an obscure inner accord. . . . I see the bird see me. I believe the bird perceives me, not because I have a theory to explain it, but because it makes immediate sense. I have a soul because I recognize a fellow soul; it takes one to know one.[5]

Encountering another embodied mind, I find myself bound up in a relation with an "other" whose interiority I only ever glimpse—like a sea creature whose mysterious form flashes up suddenly from the obscure depths, only to disappear again. In such moments, we experience a direct kinship with other animals that is absent in our encounters with plants.

To say this is not to demean plants or to deny their extraordinary natures. The more that scientists study plants—and fungi too—the more astonished they are by the complexity of their engagement with the world around them. Trees not only adapt and respond to environmental conditions but communicate information to the other trees around them, "warning" them of danger.[6] Nonetheless, plants lack a central nervous system or indeed any kind of neuronal structure—the minimal threshold necessary for consciousness, as far as we can tell. Though a small handful of scientists have speculated that plants possess a neurobiology, citing supposed evidence of "synapse-like" elements in their systems, their arguments have been refuted. In 2021, researchers at the University of Heidelberg conducted a thoroughgoing review of the relevant literature and concluded that "there is no evidence whatsoever that these [supposed] 'synapse-like domains' exert any of the functions of neuronal synapses." Plants simply "do not have any structures resembling animal synapses (neither chemical nor electrical)." The researchers added that researchers who speculate about plant "cognition" are misleading the public by "ignoring the distinct evolutionary history and ecological adaptation of plants and animals."[7] Simply, there is no evidence that plants are capable of the mental and emotional states we associate with first-person experiences. This point isn't merely important, it is all. For it is subjective experience, in a word, *consciousness*, that renders animals, including human ones, vulnerable to the kinds and qualities of harm that matter most, including trauma, suffering, loss of liberty, and death of a self.

WHAT IS IT LIKE TO BE A BAT?

Assuming that other animals, like us, do have subjective experiences of some kind, the question arises of how or whether we could ever know anything concerning them, given our different physiologies. This was the very question posed by the philosopher Thomas Nagel in his celebrated 1974 essay, "What Is It Like To Be a Bat?" Presumably, Nagel proposed, it must be "like" something to be a bat. But what? Bats are so radically *unlike* us that we would seem unable to model their internal lives. It would do no good, for example, for Nagel to imagine himself with wings, soaring about, echolocating and eating insects, because he'd still be himself, Tom Nagel, the human philosopher, doing these things. The problem isn't just that other animals can't tell us about their experiences; it's that those experiences must be so unlike ours as to defy understanding. Our form seems to leave us gazing at other beings across an abyss of mutual incomprehension. As Ludwig Wittgenstein famously observed, even if a lion could talk, we wouldn't be able to understand what he said.

Philosophers love to quote this line from Wittgenstein, I suspect because it confirms their own skepticism regarding animal minds. However, as Wittgenstein had no training in animal ethology (and didn't even get along well with other humans), we're under no obligation to give him the last word on this subject. If Wittgenstein's and Nagel's claim is that we can never *fully* know what it is like to be a bat or a lion, to say nothing of a more evolutionarily distant cousin like an orb spider, then they are undeniably right. Few of us can claim even to know our own spouse fully, either—to say nothing of someone from a different culture or historical epoch. But we need to distinguish between the claim that we can know *everything* about the subjective experiences of other beings, and the claim that we can know *nothing* about them. And in reality, there is a great deal we *can* know, or reasonably intuit, about what it's like to be a bat or an elephant, even though there is also a great deal we can't.

Broadly, there are two ways we can know something about the experiences of other animals: the first is through formal scientific inquiry, the second is by relying on our own senses and emotions in observing and forming personal relationships with them. While the first method has been with us for only a few centuries, our mammalian cognition and affect have been providing us with reliable ways of knowing the world and others in it for hundreds of thousands of years. Drawing on both approaches, the scientific and the personal-affective, we can grasp key aspects of the "being" of other animals (though, again, not all).[8]

Naturalistic study of other species dates back at least to Aristotle's *History of Animals*, written in the fourth century BCE. Like other ancient Greeks, Aristotle viewed other species within the context of a natural hierarchy, and he held the human mind to be superior to all others. However, in contrast to the Stoics who emphasized human separateness from other species, Aristotle acknowledged that where humans and other animals were concerned, "certain psychical qualities are identical with one another, whilst others resemble, and others are analogous to, each other." While humans may possess more of some qualities than other animals, other animals may likewise exhibit "more or less of some other." Just as "we find knowledge, wisdom, and sagacity" in us, "so in certain animals there exists some other natural potentiality akin to these." Animals, too, exhibit such temperaments as "gentleness or fierceness, mildness or cross temper, courage or timidity, fear or confidence, high spirit or low cunning." We are even similar developmentally: "psychologically a child hardly differs for the time being from an animal."[9]

The status of animals was greatly reduced in Judaism, which held that humans alone were made in the image of God. In *Genesis*, God instructs Adam and Eve to "replenish the earth, and subdue it, and have dominion" over all other animals, an injunction God repeats to Moses after the Flood, telling him that "the fear of you and the dread of you shall be upon every beast of the earth, and upon every fowl of the air, upon all that moveth upon the earth."[10] Christianity later adopted this view; it also accepted the Greek conception of natural hierarchy, while jettisoning Aristotle's view of continuity between humans and other species.[11] In the seventeenth century, animals lost even more ground, with philosopher René Descartes's depiction of animals as "machines"—soulless matter set in motion by God in obedience to natural laws. "I am not worried that people say that men have an absolute empire over all the other animals," Descartes wrote in a letter, because they lack reason. Even the supposed intelligence or "cunning" animals was an illusion—akin to "a clock which tells time better than our judgment does" due to the mechanical disposition of its parts.[12]

Charles Darwin challenged both of these ways of seeing animals—the monotheistic view that humans were uniquely made in the image of God, and Descartes's conception of animals as machines. Instead, he maintained that we and other animals share fundamental behavioral, emotional, and cognitive traits. Though Darwinism shook the pillars of human exceptionalism, however, it failed to topple them. In the twentieth century, behavioral psychologists, sociobiologists, and geneticists repackaged evolutionary theory within the traditional framework of human supremacy. The Cartesian view of animals as instinctual automata morphed into the view of animals blindly enacting behavioral scripts dictated by their DNA, in tandem with environmental and adaptive pressures. Hence the contention of Richard Dawkins, author of *The Selfish Gene*, that we ought to picture "the animal as a robot survival machine with a pre-programmed computer controlling its muscles."[13] Evolutionary biologists like Stephen Jay Gould and Richard Lewontin, and sharp-eyed philosophers like Mary Midgley, pushed back against this gross reductionism. Unfortunately, however, they failed to purge science of its residual Cartesianism.[14] To this day, many scientists still treat animals in the lab not as "someones"—embodied consciousnesses—but as animate matter to be manipulated and destroyed at the whim of the researcher.

Scientists have long sought to identify some special feature of our brains that might account for the unique complexity of our minds, and thus to distinguish us absolutely from other beings. However, every neurophysiological feature once believed to be unique to our species, including domain general intelligence, lateralization, encephalization quotient, and even number of cortical neurons, has now been observed in other species. Nor are our brains organized differently than other brains. In 2020, when researchers in Tel Aviv studied brain connectivity across 130 different mammalian species, including human beings, they discovered that "the brains of all mammals, from tiny mice through humans to large bulls and dolphins, exhibit equal connectivity, and information travels with the same efficiency within them."[15]

Since the brains of other animals are highly similar to our own, it is reasonable to suppose that some fundamental aspects of their subjective experiences are similar to our own, as well. Comparative psychology, pharmaceutical science, and veterinary medicine are among the fields that indeed assume we can reliably intuit the internal mental and emotional states of other animals. In hundreds of experiments—all of them, in my view, morally indefensible—researchers have tested antidepressants and anti-anxiety medications on other species, inducing and then "curing" despair, depression, and anxiety in mice, rats, apes, and even fruit flies, to assess their efficacy for humans. It is now routine for veterinarians to prescribe Prozac and other SSRIs to treat mood disorders in cats, dogs, birds, and many other species. We may never know what it is exactly like to be a bat. But evidently we know something about what it is like to be a *depressed* bat.

SETI PHONE HOME

"*Homo sapiens* has been walking the planet for 300,000 years. It's therefore all the more noteworthy that in the next 50 years we could learn that we are not the only intelligent species in the cosmos."[16] So observes astronomer Seth Shostake, a leading researcher with the Search for Extraterrestrial Intelligence project or SETI, an international team of researchers scanning the heavens in the hopes of detecting the radio waves that might indicate the existence of life on other worlds. If only SETI's scientists were to turn their powerful telescopes towards Earth, however, they might be amazed to discover a planet teeming with myriad other forms of intelligent life, other ways of feeling, perceiving, and thinking which, though alien to our own, are no less wondrous.

No one disputes that the perceptual abilities of other animals far outstrip our own. Bats and dolphins echolocate, birds "see" the magnetic field of the Earth, fishes and dolphins can sense electrical fields in other animals. The human eye contains three kinds of cone receptors;

bony fishes have four, enabling them to see colors we can't.[17] Dogs have two olfactory systems, including one we lack entirely, Jacobson's organ.[18] "If you make the analogy [of a dog's sense of smell] to vision," scientist James Walker explains, "what you and I can see at a third of a mile, a dog could see more than 3,000 miles away and still see as well."[19] Taking our dog on a brisk walk, we may mistake our companion's desire to linger and sniff everything for sheer obstinacy. But the dog takes a different view. Plunged into a world of sensorial riches, she turns her analytical interest to the complex relationships she perceives unfolding through time. Hurrying a dog on a stroll is like asking an art connoisseur to take in the Louvre's six miles of galleries on the back of a speeding motorcycle.

Nonhuman animals far outclass us not only in senses but in speed, agility, reflexes, strength, and endurance. Human runners collapse from exhaustion after completing the 26-mile Boston Marathon; the bar-tailed godwit, a small New Zealand seabird, flies 7,500 miles during its biannual migration, without stopping. Peregrine falcons achieve airspeeds of up to 240 miles per hour, executing turns so extreme that the G forces would render the crew of a fighter jet unconscious, if not kill them outright. Because we identify intelligence and consciousness with the mind, not the body (a prejudice dating back to the ancient Greeks), we tend to undervalue such feats, viewing them as "mindless." But the ability to discriminate objects in one's environment and to coordinate the movement of one's body in space takes intelligence and judgment. From the perspective of an outfielder, a baseball leaping off the end of a bat at eighty miles an hour appears as a mere speck rocketing upwards. How then is the fielder able to position him- or herself in space at just the right moment to catch it? The equation for calculating a ballistics trajectory is $y = h + x\tan(\alpha) - gx^2/2v_0^2\cos^2(\alpha)$. (I had to look that up.) However, I have yet to see an outfielder whip out a pocket calculator. Instead, the fielder works the problem through in an intelligent but "embodied" way, "feeling" his or her way into the ball's descending arc. Professional ball players catch about 80% of the balls that come their way; dogs probably do as well or better chasing frisbees and rubber balls.

Bodily-kinesthetic intelligence is one of seven forms of intelligence in humans identified by the psychologist Howard Gardner, the others being logical-mathematical, spatial, musical, linguistic, interpersonal, and intrapersonal. All seven forms have been observed in other species.[20] As it is beyond my scope to review the enormous research literature on the scientific study of animal minds, I will only touch on some highlights here. Let me say at the outset, however, that I do not condone the unethical methods used to obtain much of this data. All such research founders on a contradiction: we have "no choice" but to experiment on animals, scientists say, owing to the close similarities between their physiology, neurology, and psychology and our own. Yet we are morally permitted to exploit and kill them, they also say, because they are so *unlike* us as to be unworthy of our fundamental respect. But we can't have it both ways, weaponizing both their similarities to us, and differences from us, against them.

Most of us recall the "tree" of evolution from middle school science class, with protozoa at the roots, multicellular organisms higher up, then fishes and birds, then mammals, then apes, and, finally, *Homo sapiens* perched on the highest branch. All evolutionary roads are shown to lead to us, the pinnacle of creation. But this picture turns out to be wrong. There is no scientific evidence of a fixed hierarchy in cognition between different phyla and classes of animals. As the primatologist Frans de Waal observed, the notion that there is a "linear cognitive scale," in which intelligence proceeds from a "low" end to a "high" end, is simply a myth.[21]

In 1960, Jane Goodall, a young primatologist conducting field research in Gombe National Park in Tanzania, discovered that chimpanzees used twigs as tools to capture termites, upending centuries of prejudice about the capabilities of other species. Since her discovery, chimpanzees have been observed using many other tools in culturally variable ways. In Boussou and Gombe, for example, chimps use rocks as hammers and anvils, while in Fongoli chimps chew on leaves to rid themselves of hiccups.[22] Other chimps fashion "sandals" out of leaves and twigs to protect their sensitive feet. Tool use is also common among other apes. Gorillas have been observed breaking off tree branches to use while wading into water, to test the depth of the water in front of them, while female macaques have been seen using stones to masturbate.[23] Scientists long framed intelligent behavior in apes as "proto-human." Since apes are evolutionarily close to us, it was to be expected that they should be capable of doing some of the same things we can, if only in an inferior way. By studying apes, the thinking went, we can peer back into our own evolutionary past, seeing in the mirror of nature a cruder reflection of ourselves. We now know, though, that complex cognition and feeling are found not just in apes but in many other species. Snakes and other reptiles, for example, are able to "learn mazes and make visual discriminations as rapidly as most birds and mammals," while the cognitive abilities of some marine fishes "compare to or surpass those of apes."[24]

Tool use, too, has now been observed in many non-ape species. Orange-dotted tuskfish use rocks to break open shells. Octopuses have been observed carrying the half-shells of coconuts, then looking for other half-shells with which to create make-shift shelters. New Caledonian crows fashion twigs into tools for different purposes—and bring their tools with them when they move.[25] Green herons fish using bread as bait, exhibiting a subtle understanding of fish behavior and psychology.[26] Dolphins impale sea sponges on their beaks to shield themselves from the prickly spines of the urchins they forage, and teach one another how to use them.[27] A particularly innovative use of tools was observed in a captive dolphin named Kelly at the Institute for Marine Mammal Studies in Mississippi. After researchers rewarded the dolphins with fish for turning in scraps of paper littering their pool, Kelly began stashing pieces of paper under a rock at the bottom of the pool—then tearing off small pieces one at a time, to turn in for multiple rewards. As journalist Lisa Langley recounts, Kelly then upped the ante:

> One day, when a gull flew into her pool, she grabbed it, waited for the trainers and then gave it to them. It was a large bird and so the trainers gave her lots of fish. This seemed to give Kelly a new idea. The next time she was fed, instead of eating the last fish, she took it to the bottom of the pool and hid it under the rock where she had been hiding the paper. When no trainers were present, she brought the fish to the surface and used it to lure the gulls, which she would catch to get even more fish. After mastering this lucrative strategy, she taught her calf, who taught other calves, and so gull-baiting has become a hot game among the dolphins.[28]

Despite the fact that dolphins have been shown to be self-aware, have complex emotions, and transmit knowledge from one generation to the next—the definition of culture—scientists nonetheless continue to abduct them from the wild, to hold them captive against their will in tanks and pools, and to force them to participate in experiments.[29]

Animals also exhibit a practical awareness of causality and of the basic physical principles they need to survive. While only humans have quantum physics, other species needn't entertain formal scientific theories in order to understand the way natural objects behave, or to use that knowledge in an improvisatory and intelligent way. Apes confronted with a desirable object floating in a pool cast stones behind it, using the ripples to bring the object within reach.[30] At a zoo in Sweden, a chimp responding to a youngster being strangled by a rope carefully lifted him first to relieve pressure on his neck, before attempting to remove the rope. Seabirds drop shells onto rocks or other hard surfaces to break them open, showing an intuitive grasp of the relation between height, gravity, and force of impact on a falling body. (Good experimentalists, they try different heights and surfaces to achieve their desired results.) Corvids presented with a worm floating inside a narrow glass, beyond their reach, will toss pebbles into the glass to raise the desired object, showing an understanding of Archimedes's principle of volume displacement. The birds also appreciate the difference between objects with buoyant properties and ones that sink and displace water. Chimps too know to raise objects in a glass by pouring water into it, and will urinate into the glass if no other means are available. Human toddlers, meanwhile, fail the water displacement test entirely.

Many people now accept that chimps, elephants, gorillas, crows, parrots, dolphins, and whales are intelligent. Thanks to the documentary *My Octopus Teacher*, about a diver's friendship with a mollusk off the coast of South Africa, cephalopods too have been admitted into the exclusive pantheon of animals said to exhibit "human-like" intelligence. (Horrifically, a number of companies are developing octopus "farms" to raise and kill millions of octopuses in industrialized conditions.) The trouble with our obsession with so-called "smart" animals, however, is that it only reinforces the supposed general rule of animal stupidity. In reality, the evidence shows sophisticated cognition to be common throughout the animal realm.

One of our most prejudicial beliefs about other species is that they're trapped in an eternal present, like Clive Wearing, the famous British amnesiac who lost his ability to recall anything that happened more than thirty seconds before. Since temporality is the basis of the biographical self, an inability to navigate in time might suggest that other animals lack such a self. But we now know that other species, too, orient themselves by looking backwards and forwards in time. Only humans appear able to conceive of events in the extremely distant past or future, such as the extinction of the dinosaurs or the projected explosion of our sun billions of years from now. However, these are cultural experiences made possible by language. At an individual level, ethologist Lesley Rogers suggests, "the memory abilities of animals do not differ" qualitatively, in many cases, from those of humans.[31] Furthermore, our working memory isn't even the most advanced on

Earth.[32] At the Primate Research Institute at Kyoto University, a chimpanzee named Ayumu is able to recall the order and spatial location of the numbers one through nine when flashed for 210 milliseconds on a computer screen. Ayumu is able to get the right numbers, in the right order, nearly every time, with 80% accuracy—"something no human has managed so far."[33] Even when college students are given numerous practice sessions, Ayuma radically outperforms them.[34]

Many other animals also exhibit excellent episodic memory—the ability to recall things that happened to them. Mice recognize the faces, and even the perfume, of the laboratory researchers who experiment on them; chickens remember their mother and siblings their entire lives.[35] Clark's Nutcracker can stash and remember the location of up to 20,000 food caches, scattered over many square miles of the Rockies.[36] Male hooded warblers are able to recognize "the songs of birds that had been their neighbors the previous season."[37] Sheep, shown dozens of photographs of other sheep, can accurately identify their individual faces two years later—a level of facial recall rivaling that of primates.[38] Darwin noted that animals "often call to each other when separated and evidently feel much joy at meeting; as we see with a horse, on the return of his companion, for whom he has been neighing."[39] Captive dolphins respond to the unique signature whistles (names) of former tank mates, even if their shared confinement lasted only briefly. One dolphin recognized the call of a friend she hadn't seen in twenty years.[40] Two elephants who'd crossed paths in a circus twenty-three years earlier likewise recognized and excitedly greeted one another.[41]

Memory would be a useless adaptation, though, if animals couldn't use it to anticipate future events. Whales keep track of peak periods of phytoplankton density in distant feeding grounds; other species, too, may travel hundreds or thousands of miles to find mates or food, suggesting an ability to form a mental image of the future and to plan accordingly, in order to arrive at the right place at the right time.[42] Hammerheads know when and where to expect wrasses, the small fishes who swim into the mouths of larger fish to feed on parasites there, to be at their cleaning stations. Gobies stranded in a drying tidal pool know where the neighboring pools lie for them to leap into— suggesting that the fish commit the ocean floor's topography to memory during high tide (a feat unlikely to be achieved by any human).[43] Chimps make temporal maps of hundreds of fruit-bearing trees, traveling long distances to arrive when the fruit has ripened.[44] Primates have been observed gathering straw to be used as bedding later in the day, and assembling tools for later use in foraging. At a zoo in Sweden, one chimpanzee was observed in the early morning hours collecting and piling up rocks "to throw at zoo visitors later in the day." After zoo-keepers caught on and took away his rock stashes, the chimp was seen "breaking off pieces of brittle concrete from the walls in his enclosure" to store and throw instead.[45]

Animals also form detailed mental maps of their surroundings. Grey whales migrate thousands of miles between their nurseries off Mexico and their feeding grounds in the Arctic; elephants find their way to watering holes across hundreds of miles of savannah. Ocean-going fishes navigate in part using subtle changes in underwater sounds "caused by distant land formations and different water depths"—akin to finding your way from Manhattan to Boston listening for echoes off the Empire State Building and Fenway Park.[46] Birds too have an exceptional grasp of space. When I lived in Chicago, I saw pigeons riding the subway to get around, hopping off calmly at particular stations; pigeons in London have been seen doing the same thing using the Underground. Memorizing a subway route, though, is child's play compared to mapping a continent, something birds do routinely during their migrations. Birds are believed to take their bearings using not only the position of the sun and constellations, but also scent, acoustical cues, cloud movements, the Earth's magnetic field, and visual landmarks. They also make continuous in-flight decisions about which navigational cues to prioritize, adjusting their course to take into account weather and wind drift.[47]

For centuries, it was assumed that mammals were smarter than birds, whose evolutionary path diverged from our own some 280 million years ago. We now know, however, that avian brains are just made differently.[48] Though birds don't have a cerebral cortex, they have a homologous organ, the pallium, which exhibits a similar layered architecture.[49] Ounce for ounce, the avian brain is more powerful than the mammalian brain, exhibiting such elegance and efficiency in organization that scientists have compared it to a supercomputer.[50] Furthermore, the same capacities found in our brains, such as long-term memory and domain general intelligence, have been observed in avian brains too.[51] Avian minds show such astonishing depth of perceptual awareness and cognitive sophistication that they are now recognized as rivaling or exceeding those of primates. Pigeons outperform humans in some forms of statistical inference—like the Monty Hall problem—and can be taught to distinguish between different French Impressionists. They also understand the concepts of time and space.[52] Chickens learn from one another, have at least two dozen different "words" or vocalizations for warning one another of predators, and take account of their "own prior experience and knowledge" when working out problems.[53]

Our species appears to be peerless in its ability to dissociate from immediate context by manipulating abstract signs. Thanks to our capacity for language, we have evolved the protean ability to transform nature and ourselves in nearly limitless ways—for good and ill. But other animals, too, use signs to communicate thoughts and feelings to one another. The philosopher Montaigne observed in the sixteenth century that other animals "are able . . . to communicate with one another, that they understand one another, and not only those of the same species, but also those of different species":

Even in those creatures that have no voice we may easily infer, from the mutual services we see them rendering each other, that they have some other means of communication; their movements speak and negotiate. . . . Just as well our deaf-mutes dispute, argue and tell stories by means of signs. . . . Lovers use their eyes to express anger, reconciliation, entreaty, thanks, to make appointments, in short for every purpose. . . . With the head we invite, we dismiss, admit, disclaim, give the lie, welcome, honour, reverence, disdain, demand, show the door, we cheer, lament, caress, chide, submit, defy, exhort, threaten, assure, and inquire.[54]

Researchers have shown that dogs understand denotative as well as connotative speech—not only what is said to them, but how meaning changes according to context and emotional register.[55] (As Montaigne observed, a horse "knows that a dog is angry when it barks a certain way but is not afraid when it gives voice in another way.") Birds make urgent appeals to other birds for help in mobbing a predator like a hawk, with individuals of different species often joining the attack. Scientists have found that many animals pay close attention to the alarm calls of other species. Spying a hawk, say, a tufted titmouse or chickadee may broadcast that information to a wider public, in an alarm propagating through a forest at speeds of a hundred miles per hour or more. They often do this, moreover, at a frequency above the hearing of many predators, in what researcher Erick Greene terms a "private channel."[56]

While many scientists remain skeptical that other animals possess "true" language, others are open to the idea. Dolphins have been shown to understand syntax and compound sentences, and Kanzi, the bonobo, can understand hundreds of sentences spoken in English.[57] Alex, the captive African Grey parrot, could verbally describe, in English, objects he'd never seen before, identifying them by color, shape, and material.[58] Vervets have different warning cries for snakes, leopards, and eagles.[59] Prairie dogs likewise learn the "names" of different predators and can even vary the acoustical elements of their cries to communicate their "size, color, and shape." They also create new phonemes to refer to novel objects. One group of prairie dogs assigned the label "danger" to a man whom they'd seen fire a shotgun more than a month earlier.[60]

WHAT ABOUT INSECTS?

Until recently, scientists assumed that insects, spiders, mollusks, and other invertebrates—the vast majority of all animal species—lack sophisticated cognition. According to Roger D. Hanlon, however, an authority on cognition in cephalopods at the Woods Hole Oceanographic Institution, it is "nonsense" to suppose that "vertebrates are the smartest things around."[61] Some mollusks have indeed now been shown to be as intelligent as primates, and the cognitive abilities of arthropods like insects and spiders are getting a closer look, as well. Though we assume that a small being must correspondingly have only a "small" degree of consciousness, if any, we may just be too hung up on size.

In fact, the largest insects and spiders are larger than the smallest mammals and birds—exposing the fallacy of conflating brain size with cognitive ability. But even in extremely small creatures, scientists have uncovered evidence of astonishingly sophisticated cognition. Insect researchers Chittka and Niven observe that while early computers weighed a ton or more and occupied a whole room, yet were capable only of limited arithmetic, calculators today outperform such machines by orders of magnitude and fit inside our pocket. "It is the technology within which matters, not the size," and the "same principle applies to brains." The smaller scale of insects allows their neurons to send information more quickly and efficiently than bulkier brains, whose "longer connections increase conduction delays and energetic costs." There may thus be an inverse relationship between brain size and brain efficiency. Chittka and Niven speculate that the ability to learn rules and to form concepts emerged as "adaptive strategies because of, rather than despite, the miniaturisation of the insect brain," which may explain why scientists have found levels of neuronal plasticity in insects comparable to that of vertebrates. Furthermore, the neuronal "'circuits' of insects behave in much the same way as they do in vertebrates, performing similar functions."[62] Dozens of different kinds of learning have been identified in insects, including learning sequenced steps to achieve a goal, contextual learning, and the ability to generalize experiential knowledge to new phenomena. As one researcher notes, the number of cues used by ants to navigate, including "sun position, polarized light patterns, visual panoramas, gradient of odors, wind direction, slope, ground texture, step-counting" and others, "is probably greater than for humans."[63]

In *The Structure of Behavior* (1942), the philosopher Maurice Merleau-Ponty refuted the behaviorist view of animals as merely "reacting" to "stimuli."[64] Rather, animals actively maintain an "equilibrium" rooted in their own "general attitude toward the world."[65] Animals don't merely "receive" sense impressions, passively, but make meaning of their worlds. When challenged with a novel problem, for example, animals go "off script," improvising a solution. Merleau-Ponty described one cruel experiment performed by behaviorists in which the scientists took a beetle and taped together two of its legs to see whether it would move in the same way as before. Instead, the insect used different muscles to improvise an entirely new form of locomotion. Even an insect, then, will "resolve a problem posed by its milieu" in a non-stereotyped, creative way.[66] Subsequent research has proven Merleau-Ponty right—other animals simply don't behave in the mechanistic way that neo-Cartesianists have maintained.

Some scientists are at last coming around to Merleau-Ponty's view. "Insects are not the hardwired reflex automats they were once believed to be," one team of researchers recently announced.[67] In 2017, researchers at Queen Mary University in London taught bumblebees to roll a tiny "soccer" ball into a goal. Though rolling an object into a hole was a task no bee had been called upon to do in the previous 130 million years, the bees quickly mastered the task and even improved on the method they'd been taught. "Some bees," *Smithsonian* later reported, "succeeded at getting their ball into the goal with no demonstration at all, or by first watching the ball move on its own." The most successful bees were those who'd watched other bees solve the problem. However, the bees didn't just copy what they saw—after observing their companions they "then figured out on their own how to accomplish the task even more efficiently using their own techniques." The lead scientist on the study, Clint Perry, noted that while "people view insects as unthinking machines," the experiment showed that bees can think for themselves. In an interview, Perry conceded that the bees probably showed more creativity in solving the problem than he himself might have in a similar scenario.[68]

Other researchers have demonstrated that bees can count, grasp concepts of same and different, and can apply knowledge from one sensory context, like hearing, to another, like sight. (The rate at which honeybees can learn new colors, meanwhile, "is not just superior to human infants, but to all vertebrates that have been studied."[69]) The cognitive architecture of invertebrates in fact seems to resemble that of vertebrates, at least in some ways. Like us, they have been shown to perceive in gestalts, focusing their perception on specific objects while "blurring out" the rest of their sensory and experiential field, suggesting that they too ascribe meaning to their experiences. Sleeping jumping spiders exhibit signs of REM sleep—just like cats, dogs, parrots, cuttlefish, and us. Wasps and moths can recognize individual faces. When insects and spiders are given mood-altering drugs, they behave in much the same way that humans do: spiders given LSD build cockamamie webs, while bees given cocaine act impulsively, exhibit altered judgment, show exaggerated enthusiasm for things they like, and later exhibit symptoms of withdrawal. Such results raise disturbing questions about the ethics of treating "even" insects as disposable fodder in invasive experiments. We know enough already to call for a moratorium on all such research, to say nothing of the farming of insects for food. An estimated trillion or more insects are already raised and killed each year for human consumption and to feed animals raised for slaughter; plans by the meat industry (already under way) to raise and kill quadrillions more insects for commercial food purposes are simply unconscionable.[70]

OTHER NATIONS

In 1925, the naturalist Henry Beston built a small cottage on a beach in Eastham, Massachusetts, on Cape Cod. With the Nauset Marshes at his back and the Atlantic Ocean as his doorstep, Beston spent the next two years closely observing the comings and goings of the gulls, terns, crabs, sand spiders, and other denizens of the intertidal zone. Reflecting later on his experiences in his book *The Outermost House*, Beston wrote:

> We need another and a wiser and perhaps a more mystical concept of animals. Remote from universal nature and living by complicated artifice, man in civilization surveys the creature through the glass of his knowledge and sees thereby a feather magnified and the whole image in distortion. We patronize them for their incompleteness, for their tragic fate for having taken form so far below ourselves. And therein do we err. For the animal shall not be measured by man. In a world older and more complete than ours, they move finished and complete, gifted with the extension of the senses we have lost or never attained, living by voices we shall never hear. They are not brethren, they are not underlings: they are other nations, caught with ourselves in the net of life and time, fellow prisoners of the splendour and travail of the earth.[71]

We are not alone, but are surrounded by other consciousnesses, other worlds. And each such world is a singularity worth valuing on its own terms.

11

PERSONS, NOT THINGS

In 2014, New York State Supreme Court judge Barbara Jaffe issued a writ of habeas corpus in response to a suit filed by the non-profit Nonhuman Rights Project (NhRP) on behalf of Hercules and Leo, two chimpanzees being held captive by Stony Brook University. A habeas writ, which requires authorities holding a person in custody to present him or her before the court, is one of the most fundamental principles of jurisprudence, the bedrock of the protection of persons. For decades, Hercules and Leo had been kept in a basement laboratory at the university, where they were implanted with electrodes and subjected to locomotion studies requiring repeated anesthesia. In an unprecedented order, the judge now ordered Stony Brook's president to appear in court to answer the NhRP's allegations that the chimps were "being unlawfully detained." It was the first time a nonhuman had been granted habeas standing in a modern court of law.

After the judge's order was reported in the press, Judge Jaffe backtracked, removing the habeas writ. Yet as the case proceeded, Jaffe seemed skeptical of the university's arguments. Christopher Coulston, the Assistant Attorney General defending Stony Brook, maintained that since the chimps had the status of property, they had no standing to file a grievance through human representatives. "They have no ability to partake in human society, the society that has developed these rights," he told the court.[1] Coulston warned that "granting the chimps personhood would create a slippery slope regarding the rights of other animals."[2] But Judge Jaffe seemed unconvinced. "The law evolves according to new discoveries and social mores," she observed. "Isn't it incumbent on judiciaries to at least consider whether a class of beings may be granted a right?"[3]

In the end, the court decided against the plaintiffs. But the embarrassing publicity around the case led Stony Brook to quietly retire Hercules and Leo to an animal sanctuary a few years later, sparing them further suffering. Meanwhile, the profound metaphysical and ethical questions raised by Nonhuman Rights Project concerning the nature of "personhood" have remained unanswered by the courts.

Can a "mere animal" be considered a person? The dictionary suggests otherwise. "Emphatically, as distinguished from a thing, or from the lower animals," reads one definition of "person" in the *Oxford English Dictionary*. Historically, philosophers have tended to associate personhood with a capacity for reason and the qualities associated with it, such as freedom and autonomy. On this view, only "thinking" beings are free, as only they are capable of making choices about their lives and values. It was Aristotle's view, thus, that neither children nor animals could be considered good or bad, moral or immoral, since they lacked the rationality needed to exercise virtue. Later philosophers would expound some version of his view—most notably Immanuel Kant, who argued that only rational, self-determining beings—ones capable of evaluating and affirming objective moral principles—could rightly be considered persons. While humans exhibited such qualities, Kant held, other animals "are not rational [and] . . . they are therefore called things." Other animals can therefore only have value relative to the uses that we make of them.[4] To put the matter differently, the question of who gets to count as a "person" traces the bounds of permissible violence: only beings who are human are deemed worthy of life.

As critics have pointed out, however, if only "rational and autonomous" beings are persons, then it's not clear that many *humans* qualify, either. As the scholars Sue Donaldson and Will Kymlicka note, "the capacity to engage in rational argumentation and to conform to consciously understood principles" is "at best, a fragile achievement" even for humans, "a fluctuating characteristic that varies not only across human beings, but also across time within a life." By Kant's definition, dolphins and apes can't be considered persons, since they appear not to engage in formal moral reasoning; but "it is equally clear that many humans," including young children, the mentally disabled, and the severely mentally ill, wouldn't qualify as persons in Kant's sense, either. To ground human rights in Kant's narrow conception of personhood is therefore to "render human rights insecure for everyone."[5]

Constitutional law scholar Laurence Tribe made this very point in an amicus brief before the New York Supreme Court in 2020, on behalf of a different suit brought by the Nonhuman Rights Project—this one involving an elephant with the unfortunate name of Happy. Captured as an infant in Thailand in 1971, then sold to an abusive animal entertainment group in California, Happy was eventually bought by the Bronx Zoo, where she lived for decades in a desolate environment with other captive elephants, made to perform tricks for the zoo's visitors. By the 2000s, Happy was living in solitary confinement and exhibiting such severe symptoms of depression that the *New York Times* branded her "the world's loneliest elephant."[6] In his brief, Tribe chastised the Court for its earlier ruling in the Hercules and Leo case that "chimpanzees and all other nonhuman animals are not fit candidates for personhood on the mere ground that they are not human."[7] The Court had denied personhood to chimps on grounds that they lacked human language, and thus couldn't be bearers of "social responsibilities and duties"; Tribe, however, faulted the Court for affirming a "fundamentally flawed definition of legal personhood," one with the unintended consequence of placing human rights at risk, too.[8]

THE NARCISSIST IN THE MIRROR

The Nonhuman Rights Project has itself been criticized by some scholars sympathetic to animal rights for focusing its briefs on so-called "smart" animals, ones whose cognitive and behavioral repertoires can most closely be said to resemble our own. The NhRP's hope is that once *some* animals have been granted legal recognition as persons, it will eventually become possible to achieve legal personhood for members of other species, as well. However, even if the NhRP won legal recognition of orcas, elephants, chimps, and dolphins—the species that have so far been the focus of the NhRP's efforts—99.99% of all animal species would still retain the status of property or "things" under the law.

One of the ways the Nonhuman Rights Project has sought to challenge the exclusion of nonhumans from the legal category of persons is to introduce scientific evidence from the mirror test, which purports to demonstrate self-awareness. As its name suggests, the test was invented in the 1970s by Gordon Gallup, Jr., to assess the ability of chimpanzees to recognize themselves in a mirror. After showing the chimps a mirror and observing their behavior, Gallop anesthetized them and painted a mark on their foreheads. Once they had come to, Gallop gave them the mirror again. What he found is that chimps used the mirror to investigate the strange new spot on their foreheads, suggesting that they knew that the ape in the mirror was themselves. In subsequent experiments, chimps used mirrors to peer inside their mouths and investigate other parts of their bodies normally hidden from view. Scientists have since discovered that several other species, too, are able to recognize themselves in mirrors, including bottlenose dolphins, whales, gorillas, elephants, magpies, and cleaner wrasses. The NhRP argues that any species able to recognize themselves in a mirror must possess the quality of self-awareness, a key property of persons.

As with other cognitive litmus tests designed to separate persons from non-persons, however, the mirror test is flawed. First, it is unclear what passing the mirror test really means. Some have speculated that the ability to conceive of oneself as a distinct "self" may be limited to species with complex social orders in which the ability to see oneself as others do might be a useful adaptation. However, if so, it is unclear why wrasses, who don't have complex social networks, pass the mirror recognition test, while macaques and parrots, who do, fail it. Furthermore, it is unclear whether the ability to understand a *representation* of one-self, as in a mirror or photograph, is a necessary or sufficient condition for having or being a "self."[9] Cats fail the mirror test. But if I were to put a dab of paint on my cat's paw or some other part of her body within her sight while she is awake, she would immediately investigate it and try to lick it off. She would also wonder what I am up to, and look at me with bewilderment or suspicion. If animals lacked the ability to distinguish between themselves and others, they would not be such shrewd judges of the intentions of others, which, however, they are. Dogs and cats can tell the difference between someone who steps on them by accident, and someone who does so deliberately. When I tug on my cat's tail in a playful way, she knows I'm teasing; but if I were to pull her tail sharply, or suddenly shout at her, she would react with alarm; were I to repeat my aggressive behavior, our relationship would suffer, and she would stop trusting me altogether. My cat understands that *I* am not *her*, and that *she* is not *me*; and she interprets "tail-pulling" in the context of our relationship. If a stranger should visit my house and try to pull my cat's tail, she would likely react with some combination of fear, anger, and confusion—the way you or I would react if a stranger on an elevator were suddenly to grab at our face or leg.[10]

The ability to recognize oneself in a mirror, in short, ought not to be conflated with *having* a self. Nor is it clear why recognizing oneself in a mirror should be taken as the threshold for ascribing moral worth to a life. Children with autism can have difficulty recognizing themselves in a mirror. The age threshold for passing the mirror test, meanwhile, is culturally variable: in the US and other wealthy countries of the global North, most children pass the mirror test after the age of about twenty-four months, while some Kenyan children between the ages of two and six years fail it.[11] Does that mean that Kenyan children aren't "self-aware"? Should we cease treating them as persons, or grant them fewer rights?

My friend's adult daughter, Esther, has an undiagnosed neurologi-cal disability that makes it impossible for her to do most basic math, to grasp the difference between utilitarianism and Kantianism, or to live without constant assistance from others. Despite her disability, however, Esther is one of the most compassionate and emotionally perceptive people I know. She is also quite intelligent, even though her mind travels down quirkier paths than the ones traveled by the neurotypical person. Is she not a person? During my father's battle with Alzheimer's, there came a time in the progression of his disease when he was no longer able to recognize himself in the full-length mirror in the hallway outside his bedroom. Seeing his own reflection, he would mistake it for a stranger, and speak to it. By this time, too, my father had forgotten not only who I and my sisters were, but also who he was. So profound was his loss of self that, when he sneezed, he would say, "Bless you!," as if someone else had sneezed. My father's illness obliterated so much of his identity that it eventually made it impossible for him to care for himself. In the last year of his life, he came to exhibit less of a capacity for memory, self-and-other relations, practical autonomy, and situational awareness than Zorro and Sundance, the two Corgi dogs whom he and his partner Donna lived with. Yet until a stroke ended his life, my father remained an affable and loving presence who took pleasure and interest in life. Even in his diminished state, he hadn't ceased to be a "someone," despite his inability to recognize himself *as* a someone.

THINKING DIFFERENTLY ABOUT PERSONHOOD

It is clear that the traditional ways philosophers have gone about defining "persons" have been flawed. While moral deliberation, language, abstract reasoning, and the ability to conceive of oneself in the third person are worthwhile capacities to have, they in no way exhaust the qualities of *being-a-person*, whether in our species or any other. Nor is it self-evident why those capacities should be taken to be the most important, or sole, defining attributes of personhood—rather than, say, the ability to love and be loved, to experience loss, to possess *joie de vivre*, etc.

The philosopher Tom Regan proposed the term "subject of a life" as a work-around to Kant's overly strict conception of persons, suggesting that we see every animal as "the experiencing subject of a life, a conscious creature having an individual welfare that has importance" to that subject. We and other animals "want and prefer things, believe and feel things, recall and expect things," and "all these dimensions of our life, including our pleasure and pain, our enjoyment and suffering, our satisfaction and frustration, our continued existence or our untimely death—all make a difference to the quality of our life as lived, as experienced, by us as individuals."[12] It's because animals are "subjects of a life" that they have an integrity that we ought to respect. It follows, Regan maintained, that we ought to end our exploitation and killing of animals for food, medical experiments, and other uses.

I agree with Regan's approach, though "subject of a life" seems to me an unnecessarily baroque term to describe something as plain as *consciousness*. All of the following terms, therefore, seem to me equally good: consciousness, self, person, individual, singularity, subject of a life, embodied mind, being-in-the-world, "someone." Since *person* is a common term denoting the dignity and inviolability of an individual, I prefer that one.[13] However, any of the other terms will do nearly as well, since all are attempts to describe the same phenomenon—*a "singular" or unique existent with a subjective experience of the world.* Minimally, we may hold the following qualities to be constitutive of consciousness, hence of persons or "someones": subjective experience, emotions, intelligence, intentionality, practical autonomy, temporality, vulnerability, mortality, and "personality" (individuality). So defined, all vertebrates and most if not all complex invertebrates can be seen to exhibit the qualities of persons, while plants, bacteria, viruses, fungi, machines, and simple animal organisms without a nervous system—like amoeba, sponges, and Trichoplax—do not. Thus, you, your cousin, your cat, and the mice living under your sink can reasonably be characterized as persons, but not your rhododendron, your mountain bike, ChatGPT, or the bacteria living in your gut.

What makes animals persons is not that they have "human-like" characteristics but that they exhibit qualities of a *self*, i.e., of a being who possesses thoughts, perceptions, and feelings. To be a self or consciousness is not merely to *have* a perspective, it is to *be* a perspective—a "someone" who experiences the world from a point of view, an "I" who knows, who feels, suffers, desires, etc. And as every animal species has its own ontology or distinctive "style" of existence, there are as many different ways of being a "someone" as there are unique species. Being-an-otter, being-a-carpenter-ant, being-a-long-tailed-hawk, being-a-cuttlefish, and so on, are all ways of *being-a-person*, even if they differ in fundamental ways from *being-a-human*.

To be a person or "someone" is to be pleased or frightened, bored or curious, certain or doubtful. It is to seek freedom, and to flourish within one's capacities. Persons take sensuous joy in their embodiment, in the power and virtuosity of free movement—running, leaping, soaring, diving, bounding. Persons often seek out the company and comfort of others; many form enduring bonds of affection or love with others, particularly with their young. They enjoy sex and a languid nap in the sun. Persons go through similar stages of life, from the playful curiosity and impetuosity of youth to the world-weariness and infirmity of old age, approaching the end of the life cycle *sans* eyes, *sans* teeth, *sans* everything. (Some animals live only hours or days; others live longer than we do: crocodiles and orcas can live into their 90s, tortoises to 150 years, Koi fish to 200 years, and Greenland sharks and quahogs to 500 years—or more.) Persons fear death, and they experience anxiety or distress witnessing the death of others of their kind. (Scientists found that fruit flies who merely saw other dead fruit flies aged more quickly, and died 30% sooner, than flies spared the awful sight.[14]) To be a person is to be susceptible to cold and hunger, disease and disability, violence from others, etc.—in a word, to suffer the "heart-ache and the thousand natural shocks / That flesh is heir to." Persons feel the ache of hunger, the pain of toothaches, broken wings and injured fins, and the misery of viral infections, diarrhea, flu, and insomnia. To be a person is to be vulnerable, too, to loneliness and despair, trauma and grief.

INTENTIONALITY AND AUTONOMY

Though many philosophers have denied autonomy to other animals, the evidence shows that other species exhibit what the late animal law scholar Steve Wise, founder of the Nonhuman Rights Project, called "practical autonomy."[15] As Montaigne observed, other animals don't operate merely from "instinct," but with "reason and foresight":

> Do the swallows that we see at the return of spring, ferreting out all the corners of the houses, conduct their search without judgement? Do they choose without discrimination, out of a thousand places, that which is most commodious for their lodging? Are the birds, when they weave those beautiful and wonderful habitations of theirs, able to use a square figure rather than a round, an obtuse rather than a right angle, without knowing their properties and effects? Do they fetch, now water, now clay, without having concluded that hardness is softened by moisture? Do they line the floors of their palaces with moss or down unless they have foreseen that the tender limbs of their young will lie more softly and comfortably? Do they shelter themselves from rainy wind and build their cabins to the east, without knowing the different properties of the winds, and without considering which one is more healthy for them than the other? Why does the spider thicken her web in one place and slacken it another? Why does she use now one kind of knot, now another, unless she possesses thought, deliberation and the power of inference?[16]

The intelligent autonomy we see in other species—their ability to solve problems and make choices—is a manifestation of the "intentional" quality of consciousness.[17] Every consciousness, that is, is at every moment directed "towards" something of significance to that consciousness, some phenomenon, whether it be an unexpected sound in the forest, an aching tooth, or a tennis match. To have consciousness is not merely to be "in" the world, it is to "have" a world. That is, consciousness is always ascribing *meaning* to the world. The mouse who narrowly escapes an attack by an owl at night, fleeing to the safety of her burrow, experiences something of *significance* to her. Her emotional responses—her terror at being attacked, her relief at being safely home again, her uncertainty about when it will be safe to venture out again, etc.—arise from a personal existential situation. Having narrowly escaped an attack from the air, the mouse will subsequently experience the sky differently than before, as a newly vivid horizon of danger. Her heightened awareness of vulnerability—borne of an intelligence in no way separable from her feelings, memories, and the meaning with which she encounters and constitutes her world—will alter the structure of her subjective "lifeworld."

The significance that animals give to their worlds is evident in everything they do, from seeking new living quarters to forming emotional relationships with others. As Carol Gigliotti shows in her wonderful book *The Creative Lives of Animals*, animals confront the challenges of their lives in spontaneous, creative ways, with flair, innovation, and joy.[18] Play, a feature of this creativity, offers a clear example of "intentionality" in other animals. Bears blow air bubbles in streams, then pop them with their claws. Bored captive octopuses use their funnels to blow jets of water at plastic bottles, repeatedly sending them floating under the water purifier of their tank to be returned to them again.[19] Crows fashion sleds out of the lids of cans or other objects, then use them to ski down icy slopes or roofs. Beluga whales put stones or seaweed on their heads, daring others to knock them off.[20] Alaskan buffalo have been observed running down to a frozen lake and skating across the surface, keeping their limbs stiff to do pirouettes on the ice. Animals will create games even with members of other species—like sea otters striking up games of chase with dogs on California piers.[21]

Coyotes, armadillos, sheep, cows, and others have been seen rolling, pushing, or tossing a ball around, just for fun. By animating the ball as if it were alive, they imbue it with a *significance* that it did not have before. The animal knows that the ball isn't sentient or alive, yet pretends otherwise by attacking, nuzzling, or cuddling it. Once the animal turns his or her intentional gaze elsewhere, the object again resumes its place as merely a "thing" among other things.

SOMEONE HOME: CONSCIOUSNESS AS SINGULARITY

Every consciousness unfolds within the bounded conditions set for it by evolution—exhibiting the psychological, perceptual, cognitive, and emotional repertoire particular to its species. At the same time, every consciousness remains always itself alone, a *singularity*. Just as no two bodies can coincide in space and time, no two consciousnesses ever coincide—each remains its own horizon of possibilities. No "I" coincides even wholly with itself: every consciousness reaches beyond itself—beyond the horizon of what it is given. It remains always a free, spontaneous agent of its own existence.

Scientists were once skeptical of individuation in other species. When Japanese primate researcher Junichiro Itani toured the United States in the late 1950s, claiming to be able to recognize each of the more than one hundred monkeys he studied as a distinct individual, American scientists simply didn't believe him. "Monkeys look so much alike," Frans de Waal recounts, "that Itani obviously was making things up."[22] But he wasn't: each monkey was indeed unique, as his research showed. Even today, as ethologist Lesley J. Rogers observes, we tend to view other animals "as unitary entities," all possessing the same characteristics, "ignoring individual differences" (as in Pollan's eternal "Pig").[23] It has now been shown conclusively, however, that genetic and environmental variance ensures that no two members of any species are the same. Scientists studying captive octopuses have found each to be unique—some are curious and outgoing and crave human connection, while others are moody and hold grudges against individuals they dislike. Individual fish too have unique temperaments, preferences, and eccentricities. Even insects within the same species exhibit personality variance: some are bold while others are timid or easily discouraged, some are gregarious while others are antisocial.[24] We can only guess at what subtle aspects of temperament we are missing in studying beings whose evolutionary paths diverged from our own eons ago.

Personality variance has been demonstrated in dozens of species, from birds to spotted hyenas, sometimes using tests originally devised to measure personality traits in humans.[25] Researchers at the Weizmann Institute and the Max Planck Institute have developed an algorithm based on the Five-Factor Model (derived from the famous Myers-Briggs test) to sort mice into the same five types of personality as humans—"extroversion, agreeableness, conscientiousness, neuroticism and openness to experience." The scientists concluded that "each mouse could be seen to have a unique, individual personality that consistently informed its behavior."[26] The original Five-Factor Model was based on the assumption "that the fundamental traits of human personality have, over time, become encoded in language."[27] The fact that this same model has now been successfully adapted to identify personality types in other species confirms that personality is pre-linguistic in nature.[28]

Personality tests, though, offer only a crude measure of individuation. Anyone who has lived with cats or dogs knows that each exhibits unique likes and dislikes, aptitudes, temperaments, relationships, eccentricities, and so on—just as we do. When psychologist and ethologist Barbara Smuts first began conducting field research on a troupe of more than a hundred baboons, she initially tried to pass herself off to the baboons as "nothing more than a detached observer, a neutral object." But the baboons "knew better," treating Smuts herself as "a social subject vulnerable to the demands and rewards of relationship." Smuts realized that if she was to get the data she needed, she would have to relate to the baboons on their terms, as an equal. Eventually, after weeks living alongside the baboons, Smuts was accepted within the baboons' community. She in turn came to recognize each baboon as a unique individual. "Every baboon had a characteristic voice and unique things to say with it; each had a face like no other, favorite foods, favorite friends, favorite bad habits." A baboon Smuts called Lysistrata, for example, "liked to sneak up on an infant riding on its mother's back, knock it off (gently), and then pretend to be deeply preoccupied with eating some grass when mom turned to see the cause of the infant's distress." The experience changed the way Smuts saw other beings. Today, when she gazes into the eyes of an animal, Smuts sees "someone home," a "someone so like ourselves in their essence that we can co-create a shared reality as equals."[29]

My friend Karen Davis, the founder of United Poultry Concerns, a nonprofit advocating on behalf of chickens and turkeys exploited for food, once drove from Virginia to Maryland to rescue severely traumatized and injured hens raised in crowded battery cages so small that they had been unable to extend a single wing. After retrieving the birds, who were exhibiting shock, Karen didn't have the heart to put them in crates for the return journey, so she let them sit together on the back seat instead. As she drove, she spoke calmly and soothingly to the birds, and eventually they quieted down and began looking around them in curiosity. "Then, an astonishing thing happened," Karen recounted. "The most naked and pitiful looking hen began making her way slowly from the back seat, across the passenger seat separator, toward me. She crawled onto my knee and settled herself in my lap for the remainder of the trip."[30] No one, not even Karen, who worked closely with chickens for decades, could have predicted that this particular hen, who had previously known only violence and degradation in her short life, never a single kindness, would have sought out Karen's embrace as she did.

Consciousness, in sum, is an open rather than closed phenomenon; it is always its own "type." Neither energy nor matter, it cannot be reduced to the physical processes that somehow give rise to it. It is not a "thing." However much we attempt to contain "the animal" within an abstract scientific schema of "behaviors," it forever eludes categorization and prediction. The map is never the territory.

A WORD ON ANIMAL ETHICS

I have suggested that *consciousness* ought to be seen as the necessary and sufficient condition of personhood, as the ontological property that gives sentient beings their transcendent value. Any animal who exhibits the quality of singularity of consciousness ought therefore to be held worthy of our respect. My ethical position coincides with that of Donaldson and Kymlicka, who maintain that "whenever we encounter 'someone home,'" a "vulnerable self," we ought to respect that being's bodily and psychic integrity.

A "someone"-centered ethics of this kind, grounded in empathy and in practices of care and compassion, seems to me far superior to utilitarianism, which tends to view persons only as fungible "vessels" of pain and pleasure. Because utilitarians cannot muster an unqualified respect for vulnerable selves, they hold that the rights of the individual can or even should be waived when doing so is likely to maximize the greater happiness of all those potentially affected by our actions. This makes it hard for utilitarians to say just why killing persons is wrong— hence Peter Singer's callous views on euthanizing disabled human infants, and his qualified support of "humane" animal agriculture— provided, he says, that "we rear animals in ways that give them good lives" and don't cause them to "suffer when they are killed."[31] (Singer says he gives a "pass" to "conscientious omnivores."[32]) As we have seen, Singer's view that causing suffering to animals is worse than violently ending their lives is now also the "go to" argument for Michael Pollan, Temple Grandin, and other leading apologists for the animal system, all of whom maintain that animals can be killed without causing harm to their interests. It is clear, however, that any system that treats the lives of sensitive and emotionally complex beings as "disposable" will inevitably also cause them great suffering in the end: once the decision to kill has been made, everything else will be permitted. The utilitarian position is therefore self-defeating.

I have a great deal of respect for Peter Singer and for his past work in animal advocacy. It was reading *Animal Liberation* in college, in fact, that convinced me to become a vegetarian, setting me on the path that has led to the book you now hold in your hands. However, I am not alone among animal advocates today in thinking that Singer's theoretical approach has become an impediment to animal justice.

In her book *Justice for Animals*, philosopher Martha Nussbaum offers an alternative theory of animal rights, arguing that sentient beings have a right to flourish within the range of their natural capacities, as individuals and collectivities. It is therefore wrong, she holds, not only to cause animals to suffer, but to thwart the development of their potentialities. While Nussbaum's position is more ethologically informed than Singer's, and hence more attuned to animals' psychological and social needs, she nevertheless agrees with Singer that some animals "are not harmed by a painless death in the midst of a thriving life."[33] Into this latter category Nussbaum has placed all fish. Though she acknowledges that fish feel pain, are intelligent, have emotions, experience "a rich social life," and even may live "complicated and fascinating lives," Nussbaum denies that killing them harms them, supposedly because they lack "temporally extended projects."

Even if fish could be shown to lack a temporal self, however, Nussbaum has not satisfactorily explained why the lack of a "temporally extended project" should render a being's life worthless or disposable. Many humans, too, including those suffering from dementia or afflicted with a terminal illness, lack "complex temporally extended projects," yet we don't slaughter or test pharmaceuticals on them. Furthermore, there is no good reason to suppose that fish in fact do live in a "perpetual present."[34] Since some fish have been shown to have very good memories and to possess the ability to anticipate future events, wouldn't it be wiser to grant all fish the benefit of the doubt? Nussbaum instead errs in the opposite direction. Like other "enlightened omnivores" she clings to the baseless hope that fish can be killed in the billions "humanely" and "painlessly."[35] With similar unwarranted credulity, Nussbaum supports "well-designed" zoos and marine parks and the "humane" commercial exploitation of sheep for wool—notwithstanding, say, well-publicized undercover videos documenting workers viciously brutalizing sheep in the wool industries of Australia and the UK.[36] Surely a theory of "animal justice" that makes such ample room for indiscriminate killing of trillions of marine animals, and for the forced confinement, exploitation, and degradation of animals for human entertainment, remains woefully incomplete.

What is strikingly absent in both Singer's and Nussbaum's accounts of our relations with animals is any meaningful conception either of freedom or dignity. Freedom, however, is one of the constitutive elements of consciousness, a preference exhibited by all sentient organisms. To deprive an orca, penguin, lion, or shark of their freedom is therefore to show lack of respect for their autonomy. To treat such beings as spectacles of entertainment, as objects for the human gaze, is meanwhile to violate their integrity and dignity as persons or "someones."

Implicitly, Singer and Nussbaum assert a version of what I have elsewhere termed human "species right," or the right of every human to make violent use of every nonhuman.[37] Rather than mount an explicit defense of such a "right," however, the authors merely presume it. This fatally weakens the integrity of their respective projects, since rights are meaningless unless they serve as an inviolable protective cordon around "vulnerable selves."[38] It is because animals lack such a protective cordon that, while many US states have statutes against the abuse or torture of animals, they exempt commercially exploited animals—- i.e., the vast majority of all animals. In the absence of federal laws prohibiting exploitation of all other species for food, entertainment, hunting, science, and other purposes, animals will continue to suffer and die in unfathomably cruel ways. Alas, the courts will resist granting personhood or "someonehood" to other beings so long as we continue to take an interest in exploiting them as commodities—and as long as we presume the natural "right" to do whatever we like to them.

Skeptics of animal rights warn that if we grant personhood or the principle of inviolability to members of other species, we'll end up on a slippery slope. Where do we draw the line? Is killing a mosquito to be held equivalent to murder? It is necessary, first, to distinguish between moral injunctions and legal rights. It may be impractical to grant insects the same legal protections as humans; but we could certainly grant them serious moral consideration, following the least harm principle whenever we encounter even such a small "vulnerable self." We may be justified to kill a mosquito on our child's arm; but it would be better to apply DEET (which discourages mosquitos rather than killing them) and to avoid swampy areas with high mosquito counts. Meanwhile, we can, and should, seek the prohibition of all insecticides, which are killing trillions of endangered arthropods and poisoning all life on Earth.

There will occasionally be hard cases where human and nonhuman interests genuinely clash—as when locusts descend on a poor farmer's crops, or when bed bugs invade our bedchamber. In such instances, a principle of self-defense may reasonably apply—assuming, however, that all nonviolent means to remedy (or prevent) the situation have genuinely been exhausted. But the right to self-defense cannot plausibly be extended to justify animal agriculture, fishing, zoos, animal experimentation, or other exploitative practices. Nor can legitimate concern for endangered ecosystems trump respect for the sentient inhabitants who dwell within them. Environmentalists are quick to consign members of "invasive" species to their deaths, but slow to challenge the economic forces that lead to the introduction of those species in the first place. No "invasive" species is as harmful as our own, but I have yet to hear Sierra Club or Greenpeace advocating the mass slaughter of real estate developers or the CEOs of oil companies.[39] Wildlife officials must stop resorting to violence against animals as the first, rather than last, resort when coping with ecological disruptions created by our own failed institutions and bad choices.

So which moral theory is best for navigating our relations with our fellow beings? I have taken a pluralistic approach to ethics in this work, drawing insights from a variety of methods and traditions, including feminist care ethics, the phenomenology of empathy, post-Kantian deontology, Buddhist principles of *ahimsa*, Jewish existentialist ethics, and the philosophy of love. Yet after teaching moral philosophy to college students for twenty-five years, I have come to suspect that simply "doing unto others as we would have them do unto us" may be nearly as sound a moral principle as any. The Golden Rule may lack the sophistication of Kant's categorical imperative, or the solidity of Bentham's hedonic calculus. But by inviting us to imagine our way into the shoes—or wings, fins, or hooves—of other embodied beings, it has the advantage of shattering our habitual egoism. I may never know exactly what it is like to be a cow, a fish, or a lobster, but I *can* imagine what it would be like to be branded with a red-hot iron, or to suffocate slowly on the deck of a trawler, or to be plunged alive into boiling water. And since I would find all of these things to be terrible if they happened to me, I can intuit why they would also be terrible to happen to my neighbor, to a stranger in a foreign land, or to a "someone" from another species.[40] Exercising our empathetic imaginations, we can learn to recognize and respond to the interests and needs of other beings, other "someones." The vulnerability of the Other cries out to us for creaturely solidarity and redress. We have only to listen.

12

TWO WAYS OF LOOKING AT A BLACKBIRD

In the winter of 1878, a child was born to a Jewish family named Buber in the city of Vienna. At the age of three, following his parents' divorce, the child, named Martin, was sent to live on his paternal grandfather's country estate in Lemberg (what is today Lviv in Ukraine). With its orderly tree-lined streets and stately buildings, the old city might have been mistaken for a city in Austria—a number of Austrians had indeed migrated there in recent decades, lending the city a Viennese air. Yet Lemberg was also a thriving center of Polish and Jewish culture, and the boy's grandfather, a bank auditor, was a distinguished Talmudic scholar. As the boy grew, his grandfather tutored him in the Torah and Jewish lore, just as his own father had done before him. The child's greatest spiritual lesson, however, would be learned not in his grandfather's study, but in his stables. From a chance encounter with a horse on his grandfather's estate, the child, grown into a man, would later develop one of the most profound spiritual insights of the twentieth century.

Of all the animals on the estate, the one who most held the young boy's fancy was a majestic dappled-grey horse, and the boy would sometimes quietly slip into the horse's stall to brush him. One day, as he stood gently stroking the horse's great flanks, the boy looked up and saw to his amazement that the horse was looking at him, too. For a moment, the two gazed into each other's eyes, and a connection welled up suddenly between them. The horse, Buber later wrote, had "let me approach, confided itself to me." Boy and horse became bound up with one another in a communion of being more direct and honest than words. A moment later, however, as the boy became aware of his own hand brushing the horse's body, the horse turned away, sensing the boy's shift in attention. The moment of connection between them vanished. Brief though it had been, however, the encounter left a tremendous impression on the young boy. In that moment, he had realized that the world was more than a mere collection of "things." Existence had revealed itself to him instead as a community of singular beings, each with its own mysterious integrity.

It was this insight that Martin Buber, the child in the story, would eventually make the basis of his 1923 book, *I and Thou* (in the original German, *Ich und Du*). *I and Thou* remains one of the most important works in religious philosophy, a moving treatment of the human condition and of the nature of love. Though chiefly concerned with the relationship between humans and other humans—as an expression of our relation with God—the book also examines our spiritual relations with other animals. The two opposite modes I have outlined in this book vis-á-vis our treatment of animals—as subjects of our love, one moment, and as objects to be exploited or destroyed, the next—can broadly be seen to correspond to Buber's own distinction between two existential states—the *I-Thou* and *I-It*. The two modes of "address" represent not merely different ways of approaching other animals, but two different ways of being human. With apologies to poet Wallace Stevens, there are but two ways of looking at a blackbird. And the one we choose defines us as surely as it defines the blackbird. Which is the better way to live a human life?

I AND THOU

Drawing on the mystical Jewish tradition of Hasidism, whose adherents seek a direct, ecstatic experience of the divine, Buber held God to be a living presence in the world, one we might encounter in addressing others as "Thous." The English word "Thou" (the cognate of *Du* in German or *tu* in French) is an archaic form of "you," signifying an intimate, familiar form of address. To approach another being as a *Thou* is to relate to them with our whole being, without preconceptions or any desire to control them. When in this mode of address, we allow the other to rise up before us not merely as "a thing among other things," but as a being unlike all others whose exclusiveness resists our every attempt at categorization or reduction.[1] While Buber believed that we can address even trees and other plants as "Thous," only with other humans and nonhuman animals did he believe we could enter into a "two-sided" or reciprocal relation. While other animals may not have words, they nonetheless "speak" to us with their being. "An animal's eyes have the power to speak a great language," Buber writes. In a passage about his cat, Buber reflects:

> Sometimes I look into a cat's eyes. The beginning of this cat's glance, lighting up under the touch of my glance, indisputably questioned me: "It is possible that you think of me? Do I really not just want me to have fun? Do I concern you? Do I exist in your sight? Do I really exist? What is it that comes from you? What is it that surrounds me? What is it that comes to me? What is it?"[2]

While this moment between Buber and his cat lasts, the rest of the world—the banal realm of facts and practical matters—slips away. "The world of *It* surrounded the animal and myself," Buber writes, while "for the space of a glance the world of [*Thou*] had shone out from the depths."[3] Just as in his childhood encounter with his grandfather's horse, however, the connection is lost, and the world rushes in again. Human and cat are thrust once more back into the realm of ordinary experience. But something meaningful has occurred—they have encountered one other.

It is not possible to dwell forever in the pure moment of the *I-Thou*, because we also live in the realm of practical necessity. Much of the time, going about our daily affairs, we must treat the world and others in it as our objects—the mode of relation Buber terms the *I-It*. Strictly speaking, the *I-It* mode isn't really a way of "relating" at all. When I address the other as a "Thou," I do so with my whole being;

but when I address the other as a mere "it," I do so only with a narrow part of myself—the grasping, desiring, controlling part of my ego. *I* open a door, *I* order lunch, *I* investigate a plant cell with a microscope, etc. My *I* is always doing, assessing, measuring, judging, controlling. Though relating to the world as an *It* is inevitable, it is not the only mode available to us. And of the two modes of address, only the *I-Thou* relation affords spiritual and ethical truth.

While Buber saw the *I-Thou* relation as an experience of God, we needn't subscribe to his theology to appreciate the profound implications of these two modes of human existence. In approaching the other as a *Thou*, we *see* the other as they are, rather than as we merely imagine them to be. Meanwhile, in opening ourselves to the fullness of the "being" of the other, we achieve a deeper connection to ourselves, too. In its most complete sense, the *I-Thou* is a form of love. The one who "takes his stand in love," Buber writes, ceases to see others remotely, as mere "its" (or "dots," to borrow my language from a previous chapter). Love is bound up always with the *exclusiveness* of the other whom we love—with the particular person. In loving this other, we seek only what is best for them, rather than for ourselves. "Love," Buber writes, "is responsibility of an *I* for a *Thou*."[4] Love gives meaning to our existence, providing the ground for all true knowing and being. Every living being has limitless value, participating in the infinite, yet it is only in the relation of love that we can perceive that value.[5]

Ordinarily, we think of human consciousness alone as having absolute value. But there is irreducible value, too, in the "singularity" of every consciousness or "vulnerable self." A skeptic might ask whether this value is real or simply imagined. There is in fact an old debate in philosophy about whether we hold something to be worth loving because we love it, or whether we love it because it is worth loving, in itself. Aristotle's view, which I find persuasive, is that one "can't love just anything" but only "what's lovable."[6] Genuine love of another, that is, isn't merely a conceit on our part, something we "project" onto the object of our love, but a way of valuing something *worth* valuing.

"I love thee and thou art so lovely and so wonderful and so beautiful and it does such things to be with thee," murmurs Robert Jordan, the American protagonist of Ernest Hemingway's novel *For Whom the Bell Tolls*, to a Spanish woman named Maria after they first make love. Hemingway uses the archaic "thou" and "thee" to evoke the purity and exclusivity of his lovers' spiritual and sexual union. When we gaze into the eyes of our lover, the rest of the world slips away into an infinite distance. We find ourselves in a kind of bubble universe in which only we and our beloved exist: not you *and* me, but *I-and-Thou* uttered as one. I do not "lose" myself in the other person; yet here there is also no separation, as I and the other become bound up in a moment of communion. When we approach the "other" in openness and empathy, we open ourselves to the singularity of the other. "Only in feeling and in love," wrote the philosopher Ludwig Feuerbach, "does 'this'—as in 'this person' or 'this object,' that is, the particular—have absolute value."[7]

Like empathy, love is not merely a feeling but a way of "knowing." Love "gives" us our transcendent object, so to say, enabling us to see qualities in our beloved that would otherwise remain hidden from us. Only a loving parent *sees* the child as he or she *is*. The child remains a mystery, retaining a depth of being that always remains elusive and partially obscure. Yet through their love, the parent alone apprehends the child's singularity. And in that greatest of tragedies, the death of a child, the parent alone knows what has been lost—a value beyond all measure. As the scholar Arne Vetlesen observes, "what I find lovable in my beloved is his or her uniqueness"—the qualities, revealed in my love, that render my beloved "irreplaceable and unexchangeable."[8] This insight illuminates the love that we are capable of experiencing in our relations with members of other species, too. Only in relating to the animal other as a unique *Thou*, in a relation of mutual trust and vulnerability, is *this* particular being's "irreplaceable and unexchangeable" nature revealed to us. And through that relation, we discover a richer sense of our own existential and spiritual possibilities.[9]

THERE IS NO OTHER PROOF OF BEING BUT LOVE

To illustrate these concepts, and following in the vein of Martin Buber's description of his cat, I want to offer some brief reflections on my own experiences with companion animals.

My sisters and I grew up alongside a succession of adopted strays and shelter rescues, whom we and our parents treated as members of our family. This is not to say that we mistook our companions for humans: while their lifeworlds overlapped with ours, it was clear that they also inhabited different realms of experience. They saw and heard things we couldn't see or hear, smelled things we couldn't smell. When they slept, they moved their limbs and uttered suppressed cries; but what phantoms they chased in their dreams, we could not fathom. Despite our different evolutionary histories, we were nonetheless able to share a pleasant life together. Our companions sought out our affection and company as often as we sought out theirs. When they were unwell, we brought them to a doctor to be treated. And when we ourselves were laid up in bed, our companions would come lie with us. Our cats and dogs were able to interpret many of our moods and intentions, just as we were able to interpret many of theirs. If one of the cats wanted to go outside, she or he would stand by the door and give us a significant look. Each animal was unique, with quirks, preferences, and habits of their own. Tiki, our Siamese cat, had the habit of leaping up onto my father's shoulders as he sat at the kitchen table; the two would sit together like that for some time—my father eating or reading the newspaper, Tiki with his body draped around my father's neck, his legs dangling down—each silently enjoying the company of the other.

There were times when our behavior must have seemed baffling or irrational to our companions—as when we let them outdoors at some times but not others, or suddenly shooed them off the living room sofa, or boarded them in the dreaded kennel when we went on vacation (a trauma to them). By the same token, their behavior could be perplexing and exasperating to us, as well. Our cat Tiki had one vexing habit that deprived me of many a good night's sleep. Before we would all head to bed each night, we would go to the door and call Tiki, and most times he would dutifully come rushing in. Sometimes, though, if he was engrossed in his carousings, he would pretend not to hear us, even though we could plainly see him stalking through the underbrush of the backyard, not ten yards away. Eventually, we would give up and go to bed. Later, in the middle of the night, Tiki would scale a tall fence and leap up onto the roof, showing up outside my second floor bedroom window to be let in again, crying and noisily dragging his claws across the screen until I opened the window and let him in— along with mosquitos in summer and cold air in winter. Much as I tried to discourage Tiki from this practice, even spraying him with a water bottle, he persisted, evidently having concluded that his late-night liberties were worth the indignities he suffered getting back inside again. I hadn't trained Tiki to climb up onto the roof and awaken me; he had trained me to let him in.

Later, when I lived with cats as an adult, I began to peer more deeply into the lives and experiences of my companions.[10] After completing graduate school, my partner M. and I moved to Oak Park, Illinois, where we decided to adopt two cats from the local shelter—a long-haired, orange-and-white tabby with an elfin face, whom we named Alfie, and a long-haired black cat with bright eyes, whom we named Sasha. (A video of our cats can be found on my author's website.) Once installed in their new home, they proved inseparable. There was no nook or cranny of our apartment they didn't explore, and within weeks of their arrival they had together discovered a hidden crawl space in the ceiling above our bathtub, one we had not known about, which they accessed by leaping onto the top shelf of the bathroom linen closet and scaling an interior retaining wall.

It is the quotidian rather than the extraordinary that makes up the substance of our lives, and this was true of the four of us, a family of interspecies intimates whose shared habits formed the ground of a domestic existence. When we brushed our teeth before bed, the cats would come into the bathroom to watch. Alfie made a nightly game of leaping up and pulling the string of the bathroom light, turning it on and off, each time crashing down into the wicker wastebasket. At bedtime, the cats would join us in bed, Alfie settling on my chest and Sasha on M.'s. If Sasha made it onto the bed first, Alfie would become jealous, walking by the bed with feigned disinterest and ignoring our invitations to join us. Eventually, he would leap up and settle on my chest, pressing his face against mine. However, if I became so absorbed in reading a book that I began to pet Alfie in a distracted way, he would at once register my loss of attention and leap testily off the bed—digging me just enough with his claws, which he normally kept carefully retracted, to signal his displeasure.

Though we had planned to keep the cats indoors, a furnace malfunction one hot summer night forced us to evacuate the building and release the cats into the cool evening air. At once, powerful, febrile senses honed over the course of millions of years suddenly went online for the first time. Alfie and Sasha drank in the natural world in huge sensorial gulps, attentive to every scent and sound in the expanse of yards and gardens and streets. The world suddenly revealed itself to them in its full intoxicating splendor. From then on, they became indoor-outdoor cats, coming and going into the late evening, each new day offering fresh opportunities for adventure and exploration. With the exuberance and curiosity of all youth, they plunged through lush hedges, explored the secret tunnels of groundhogs, and frolicked for hours in the violent thunderstorms and blizzards of the Midwest. Turning up together at the front door soaked to the skin and covered in mud, they would saunter in with bright eyes, then head with nonchalance to their water and food bowls. Then they would make up their toilet for half an hour before throwing down somewhere to dry off.

Despite their great affinity for one another, there was a period when friction appeared in their relationship. Sometimes, Alfie would hide in our bedroom closet behind the floor-length curtain strung across the opening as a door, positioning himself just out of sight. There he would patiently lie in wait, sometimes for half an hour or more, hoping to catch Sasha unawares on his way to the bedroom window sill, where he liked to sit and gaze out onto the street. If Sasha didn't show, Alfie would eventually leave his hunter's blind and go looking for something else to do. Often enough, though, Sasha would fall into Alfie's ambush. If Sasha wasn't sure where Alfie was, he would walk past the closet slowly and cautiously, with his ears back and his head turned in the direction of a potential attack. Alfie would explode through the curtain just the same, hurling himself upon Sasha with sudden violence. Though it was mischievous fun for Alfie, it was plain from the desperate panic in Sasha's eyes that he hated it. Around this time, too, Alfie took to chasing and tackling his friend even after Sasha had lost interest in their game.

Alfie's attacks and rough play soon became a dark spot in what had previously been the cloudless sky of Sasha's existence. Once a place of safety, our apartment had become a place of anxiety and fear. I cannot prove, but have little doubt, that some version of these dark episodes haunted Sasha's dreams as he slept. Finally, after weeks of enduring this abuse, Sasha had had enough. A morning came when he simply refused to have anything to do with Alfie at all. When Alfie approached him to play, Sasha would hiss at him and stalk away with an ugly look, ears folded back. Baffled by his friend's new behavior, Alfie would sit on his haunches with a comically quizzical expression, tilting his head from side to side as if trying to make sense of Sasha's behavior. Ethologists have shown that other animals have a sense of fair play just as we do, negotiating their personal boundaries and rules of interactions with others. So it proved now. Sasha's refusal to engage with Alfie went on for days, and it was painful to watch.

Eventually, after days of getting the silent treatment from his companion, Alfie finally got the message. He became mindful of his claws and teeth during the cats' rough-housing, and he put an end to his ambush game (mostly). When Sasha grew tired of being chased, Alfie would now tactfully step away. The two cats again became inseparable comrades, and harmony was restored to our household.

This is but one story of many I might relate concerning our shared lives together. No account I might offer of Sasha and Alfie's experiences, however, could fully capture the complexity of their personalities, nor exhaust the meaning of their lives. Our cats remained emissaries from a world alien to our own. Yet notwithstanding the differences between our species—perhaps, indeed, because of them—we shared a rich and meaningful existence together, and we developed deep emotional bonds. And when those bonds were finally, ineluctably, sundered, we were left bereft.

Not long after the events I have described, M. and I moved with our infant son to Boston. A few weeks afterwards, Alfie disappeared, and our frantic efforts to recover him proved fruitless. One morning not long after Alfie went missing, I arrived at my office after my hour-long commute to find an anguished phone message from my partner, telling me that Sasha had been killed by a car. I cancelled my classes and got back on the road, crying most of the way. When I arrived home again, I found my partner with our two-year-old son huddled on the living room floor over Sasha's still-warm body. We later learned that a woman had struck Sasha down with an SUV in front of our house, then pulled over to see if he had survived. Finding him dead, the woman had wrapped his ruined body in a baby blanket from her car, then placed him on the sidewalk. It was there that my partner had found him, his eyes open but unseeing.

Alfie's disappearance and Sasha's death threw us into a grief as profound as any I had known before or have known since. The twin losses undid the invisible rituals woven into our existence, and our world seemed to tilt off its axis, making the familiar suddenly unfamiliar. The cats had filled our lives with relationality and wonder. Now a desolation filled our home. Turning a corner in our apartment, we would expect to encounter one of the cats, only to find our senses grasping at emptiness. Alfie and Sasha's absence had become a palpable presence.[11]

The mystical kabbalistic tradition tells us that every intentional action we take in a loving way can be the fulfillment of a *mitzvah*, or command from God. In this connection, even our everyday relations with our beloved animals, though ostensibly unfolding mostly in the realm of the *I-It*, had been suffused with love. As Lindgren Johnson notes, it is indeed the "repeated awakenings and openings" of attention and mutuality that constitute the ground of love, raising the otherwise banal realm of *I-It* into the transcendent realm of *I-Thou*.[12] Though some philosophers argue that other animals lack a "narrative life" through time, the lives of our animal companions unquestionably had a narrative and biographical structure. And had our cats been living in freedom, as "feral" cats outside a human domicile, their experiences would have been no less existentially significant, though their lives had gone unwitnessed by human eyes, and unregistered by any human heart.

Due to our species narcissism, we have come to think of our cats and dogs as somehow "special," as having qualities that set them apart from other species. But the same qualities that make our companion animals worthy of our love are to be found in other sentient beings. We know this partly because humans have also forged deep, enduring bonds of affection with members of dozens if not hundreds of other species, including horses, sheep, turkeys, pigs, mongooses, magpies, rhinos, elephants, otters, mynas, parrots, wolves, orcas, bears, dolphins, fish, and even—in the remarkable case of Costa Rican fisherman Gilberto Shedden's twenty-year friendship with "Pocho"—with a one-thousand-pound wild crocodile. Such friendships confirm the value to be found in every consciousness approached as a *Thou*.

In *Animal Liberation*, Peter Singer makes a show of the fact that he does not himself "love" animals. His sole concern as a utilitarian, he says, is to maximize the overall happiness of sentient beings, while reducing their overall unhappiness. However, we must ask what it can mean to seek the *happiness* of others without also finding *them* to be worth valuing in themselves, as being deserving of our loving concern. If I do not care about *you*, why should I care about what happens *to* you? The utilitarian way of formulating ethics, it seems to me, seriously misconstrues the meaning, purposes, and possibilities of human life. Surely a tradition that so openly scorns empathy and love cannot hope to summon within itself, or in us, the powerful resources needed to confront the evils of our time.[13] Nor can such a tradition, which admits no pride of place for empathy or love in our theories of moral life, offer a plausible account of the spiritual dimensions of our condition that make life worth living—by which I mean a sense of ethical and existential purpose grounded in loving connection with others. Because utilitarians fail to recognize love as a paramount value, they are helpless before the existential problem of death, which they tend to view in quantitative terms—i.e., purely as the realization or frustration of aggregate pains or pleasures over a lifetime. No one, though, who has cradled a dying animal or infant can fail to grasp the profundity of death, nor be insensible to the irrevocable harm it confers. It is in our very finitude that our own lives are rendered precious; and it is the vulnerability of those we love, their susceptibility to death, which renders us vulnerable to grief. And in that grief alone do we find confirmation of the limitless value of what we have lost.

THE BELL TOLLS FOR THEE

A life lived only in the mode of the *I-It*, Buber held, is so impoverished as to be a life not worth living. The individual unable to enter into authentic relations with others is "to be pitied," he wrote. Even worse, though, is the one who mouths the words "I-Thou" cynically, out of a desire to manipulate, control, or destroy others. Buber described such persons as "contemptible."[14] Those today who, though claiming to love and respect animals, seek out opportunities to exploit and inflict violence upon them, must be placed in this latter category. What the hunter or locavore mistakes for "respect" or even "love" of the animal he victimizes is malignant narcissism. When we reduce other animals to mere objects of our use, we encounter them only in their "thing-like" dimensions, obstructing our view of their true natures. We thereby lose the opportunity for the deeper communion with others—both human and nonhuman—that constitutes our highest good.

Buber conceived of the *I-Thou* relation as an opening out onto a wider world of universal compassion. The one who honors the *Thou* "can be effective, helping, healing, educating, raising up, saving." In the responsibility that I take for the other "lies the likeness . . . of all who love, from the smallest to the greatest."[15] It was essentially this injunction, Buber noted, that Christ made the centerpiece of his teaching—love of all humanity.

We do not need to enter into a personal *I-Thou* relation with every "other" in order to grasp the singular value of each. As feminist peace activist Barbara Demming observed, though it isn't possible for us to love every person individually, what "*is* possible is to act toward another human being on the assumption that all [human] lives are of value, that there is something about any [individual] to be loved, whether one can feel love for [that specific person] or not."[16] This same insight can be applied to our relations with other natural beings. I do not need to personally encounter every individual chicken, whale, or minnow to recognize their finitude and vulnerability, and hence to regard each as worthy of my respect as a *Thou*. Love indeed fails to obtain its universal, transcendent character so long as it remains parochial or private. Only in responding in solidarity and mutual aid to the needs of others even distant from ourselves is an authentic moral life possible. As John Donne wrote:

> No man is an island entire of itself; every man
> is a piece of the continent, a part of the main. . . .
> any man's death diminishes me,
> because I am involved in mankind.
> And therefore never send to know for whom
> the bell tolls; it tolls for thee.

Today, love for our fellow human beings can seem in such vanishingly short supply that it may seem counterintuitive, or simply quixotic, to urge that we extend our solidarity to other species as well. With each passing day, however, our own survival more and more depends on our learning to address all creatures of the Earth, too, from the smallest to the greatest, as "Thou." The freed Roman slave Terence famously remarked that nothing human could be alien to him; in affirming our common existential condition with other beings we might at last come to recognize that nothing animal is wholly alien to us, either. Our species is not "an island entire of itself" but a part of the biotic main, a "piece of the continent." And should a deer perish in a forest fire, a shark die on the deck of a ship, or a bird die of the flu, that death diminishes me, too.

CONCLUSION

AFTER DOMINION

Nine miles from my home as the blackbird flies, on the site of what is now City Hall Plaza in Boston, once stood the offices of the abolitionist newspaper *The Liberator*. It was here, from its perch overlooking the bustling cobblestone street of Cornhill, that William Lloyd Garrison and the free Black journalists who wrote for the paper hurled thunderbolts of rage and invective against the evils of slavery—and against those who profited by, or merely excused, the slave system.[1] Funds for the newspaper had been raised by a committee of Black women led by Bathsheba Fowler and Elizabeth Riley, and the paper was sustained in its early years by Black Bostonians and other Black Americans in the Northeast.[2] As late as 1829, Garrison, a white journalist raised in Newburyport, Massachusetts, had sided with the reformist wing of the abolitionist cause, which called for a gradualist approach to eliminating slavery. Two years later, however, he had changed his mind. In his inaugural address in *The Liberator* in January 1831, Garrison now denounced the "pernicious doctrine of gradual abolition," asking "pardon of my God, of my country, and of my brethren the poor slaves, for having uttered a sentiment so full of timidity, injustice, and absurdity."

Boston had been home to anti-slavery sentiment at least since the Revolution, when Prince Hall, a Black Bostonian and former slave, had agitated for the equal treatment of Blacks within the Continental Army. Garrison now framed abolitionism as a continuation of the same struggle for liberty as the Revolution, invoking the pitched battle between rebellious colonists and the British Army at Bunker Hill, fifty years before. For the next thirty years, *The Liberator* would be the most widely circulated abolitionist newspaper in the nation. So radical was the paper in its denunciation of the slave system that the slave-owning state of Georgia put a $5,000 bounty on Garrison's head, the equivalent to $150,000 today.[3] Only with the signing of the Emancipation Proclamation did *The Liberator* shut down.

No one in 1831 could have imagined that Garrison's anti-gradualist stance, so uncompromising that even Frederick Douglass at times found it extreme, would one day become the common sense of the nation. Yet it did. Today, few would hold that slavery should have been reformed rather than abolished, or that its evils should have been tolerated a moment longer than they were. In hindsight, we agree that the problem with slavery wasn't its "excesses"—the abuses inflicted by the cruelest of slave owners—but the slave system itself.

Today, a new "abolitionist" movement has taken shape. Like the abolitionists of old, who broke with the anti-slavery moderates who sought only a gradual phasing out of slavery over time, the new abolitionists view as misguided the efforts of animal gradualists or "welfarists" to ameliorate only the "excesses" of the system. From this new abolitionist viewpoint, animal agriculture, fishing, whaling, fur ranching, genetic engineering of animals, bull fights, and so on, are but symptoms of the same corrupt structure, the same total system of exploitation and violence. Where the animal welfarist seeks only "better" modes of confinement for hens, more "humane" gas chambers for pigs or "more sustainable" forms of killing marine life, the abolitionist seeks an end to the violent relation of domination itself.[4]

Will future generations one day look upon our treatment of animals today with the same degree of moral revulsion that we now feel gazing back at the horrors of slavery? Will they wonder, too, at our own apathy and indifference in the face of so plain and pervasive an evil?

If we have learned nothing else from 12,000 years of animal agriculture, it is that we cannot exploit and kill other sensitive beings ethically or "kindly." The idea of a "humane" omnivorism is as old as the hills. The Jewish injunction against *tzar ba'alei chayim*, causing "suffering of living creatures," dates back nearly three thousand years; yet kosher guidelines for "ethical" slaughter were nowhere in evidence in 2004 at the Agriprocessors plant in Iowa, the nation's largest kosher slaughterhouse, when an undercover investigation revealed cows being shocked in their "sensitive faces . . . with electric prods," having "their tracheas and esophagi ripped from their throats with meat hooks or knives" while conscious, and "[writhing] in pools of their own blood, trying desperately to stand up for up to three minutes as blood poured from their throats."[5] More than a thousand years have passed, too, since the Islamic scholars of the Brethren of Purity condemned human brutality towards animals in *The Case of the Animals vs. Man*; yet animals are still subjected to unspeakable cruelties throughout the Middle East, and there are few laws in Muslim societies protecting animals from even extreme abuse.

Secular appeals to mitigate the cruel use of exploited animals have meanwhile fared no better. In 1641, when the authorities of the Massachusetts Bay Colony published *The Body of Liberties*, the first bill of rights published in the New World, they extended protections to domesticated animals, too. "No man," the bill proclaimed, "shall exercise any Tirranny or Crueltie towards any bruite Creature which are usuallie kept for man's use."[6] Four centuries later, however, "Tirranny and Crueltie" towards animals here in my native state are as pervasive as ever. It is no longer considered acceptable to beat a horse to death in the streets of Boston; but even worse acts of cruelty are inflicted every day in private, outside the public's gaze, in rural slaughterhouses and in government-funded laboratories at Harvard and MIT.

At the end of the day, the problem is that animals don't consent to being used and brutalized by us. So long, then, as we choose to exploit and impose our will on them, it will always be necessary for us to wield violent force against them. Critics who persist in clinging to the fantasy of "painless" animal agriculture, fishing, and other exploitative practices are therefore deceiving themselves as much as their publics. The spurious distinctions they draw between "ethical" and "unethical" forms of animal exploitation, between "necessary" and "unnecessary" violence and suffering, will forever remain distinctions without a difference.

* * *

In Henrik Ibsen's play *An Enemy of the People*, a physician named Dr. Stockmann discovers that the supposed healing waters of his town's new spas, about to open to the public, are in reality dangerous, having been poisoned by a tannery upstream. When Stockmann informs the town's leadership of his shocking discovery, he expects them to shut down the spas and to thank him for having narrowly averted both a public health disaster and the town's reputational ruin. Instead, the town's citizens reject Dr. Stockmann's findings and try to drive him and his family out of town. A mob attacks the Stockmann's home, shattering its windows with stones.

Whenever I hear vegans and animal advocates mocked as idealists or utopians, or even denounced as threats to civilization, I think of Ibsen's play. We see a similar story playing out in public debates over meat today, as the informed few try to warn the public of the ecological, health, and ethical calamities of the animal system, only to be shouted down by the meat-eating majority. Apologists for the animal economy have assumed the tragicomic role of Aslaksen—the cautious town printer who urges "moderation" throughout the play, yet who sides with the angry mob against the Stockmanns—in warning the public against the stridency and "immoderacy" of vegans. In response to such critics, no more apposite reply could be offered than William Lloyd Garrison's rebuttal to the gradualists of his own day, in the inaugural issue of *The Liberator*:

I am aware, that many object to the severity of my language; but is there not cause for severity? I will be as harsh as truth, and as uncompromising as justice. On this subject, I do not wish to think, or speak, or write, with moderation. No! no! Tell a man whose house is on fire to give a moderate alarm; tell him to moderately rescue his wife from the hands of the ravisher; tell the mother to gradually extricate her babe from the fire into which it has fallen;—but urge me not to use moderation in a cause like the present. I am in earnest—I will not equivocate—I will not excuse—I will not retreat a single inch—AND I WILL BE HEARD.

Though Garrison's critics did what they could to silence him, their efforts proved fruitless; it is likewise in vain that meat apologists hope for the "abolitionists" of today to moderate their demands, or to retreat from their convictions.

Slave apologists who denounced abolitionists as dangerous utopians warned that any effort to overthrow so ancient and venerable an institution would lead to social chaos and economic collapse. And they were not wholly wrong. Six hundred thousand Americans lost their lives in a brutal civil war, and the dissolution of the Atlantic slave trade brought wrenching upheavals to the economy and culture of the nation. Slave auctioneers no longer had enslaved people to auction. Printers of handbills advertising rewards for "runaway" slaves lost business. Sailors employed on slave ships had to seek work on other vessels. Blacksmiths no longer produced leg-irons for human "chattel" (though they continued to make irons for Black laborers impressed through the Thirteenth Amendment). Yet abolishing slavery was unquestionably the right thing to do. And the overthrow of the old world made possible the invention of a new, superior world. Black Americans seized upon their changed condition to create flourishing Black communities and new forms of culture and experience; their subsequent contributions to science, art, literature, music, and every other domain of human culture are incalculable. It would take another century of struggle for freed African Americans to secure true voting rights, and even today, the ugly legacy of slavery lingers on in continuing patterns of economic inequality, struggles over racist gerrymandering, disproportionate rates of incarceration for people of color, and mass shootings of Blacks by white supremacists. Abolition remains an ongoing project.[7] Nonetheless, the abolition of *de jure* slavery vastly extended the rights of Blacks and expanded our existential possibilities as a species.

Were we in our own epoch to end our enslavement of our fellow creatures, we would likewise put an end to one world while engendering a new, superior one. And we would not lament the passing of the old order as much as we think.

It was not long ago that whaling and horse-drawn carriages were viewed as being as vital to the nation's economy and cultural identity as ranching and lobstering are to the Texan and New Englander today. Yet no one misses these earlier brutal practices, or even notices their absence. Change is therefore possible. Today, plant-based milks are competing with cow's milk at the supermarket. Ringling Brothers has retired elephants from its circus acts. Greyhound racing has been all but eliminated in the US; similar efforts to end horse-racing are gaining momentum in the wake of the deaths of numerous horses at race tracks.[8] In 2019, the California state assembly passed a law banning fur products in the state; Macy's followed suit the next year, announcing that it was ending all fur sales in its department stores. In 2023, the Food and Drug Administration ended its longstanding requirement that drugs be tested first on nonhuman animals, admitting for the first time that "cell-based assays, microphysiological systems, or bioprinted or computer models" are just as effective. None of these developments—all achieved through the courageous, persistent efforts of animal advocates—have imperiled significant human interests.

After passage of the Fugitive Slave Act in 1850, compelling free states to return those who had escaped their bondage to their owners, organized resistance to federal enforcement of the act sprang up in Northern states. Here in Massachusetts, the Boston Vigilance Committee and a secret group called the Anti-Man-Hunting League worked to shelter fugitives. In 1851, an escaped slave named

Shadrach Minkins was liberated from a Boston courthouse and safely conveyed to Canada—one of many enslaved persons aided by Black and white abolitionist activists in Boston. Today we find organized resistance growing against the animal system, too.[9] Open rescues, in which activists liberate animals being held in miserable forced confinement, are forcing the courts to reckon with the illegality of interspecies compassion. In 2017, several activists videotaped themselves rescuing two maimed and dying piglets who had been discarded in a dead pile on a Utah farm supplying pigs to Smithfield Foods. Though Smithfield claimed the commercial value of the discarded piglets to be only $84.40, the FBI assigned multiple agents to investigate the case, pursuing burglary and theft charges against the activists. At the trial in 2022, the pro-industry judge prohibited the defendants from introducing any expert testimony concerning animal sentience and welfare or the suffering of the dying animals. He also prohibited introduction of the necessity defense, which excuses a criminal act committed to prevent an immediate, more serious harm from occurring. Nonetheless, the jury acquitted the activists of all charges against them—a turn of events that stunned all concerned. It was one of the most significant legal setbacks of the animal industry ever.[10]

Isolated legal victories and piecemeal reforms alone, however, won't end the animal economy. The broader structure of violence and ecological desolation described in this work will endure so long as we continue to view nonhuman animals as our slaves and commodities. In the meantime, companies like Smithfield will continue to kill billions of animals, and they will do so not only with the official sanction of the state, but with the tacit consent of a public for whom the pleasures of bacon outweigh any nominal concern for "animal welfare."

* * *

In the summer of 2023, torrential rains in Vermont led to calamitous flash floods that left the state's major cities under water, briefly cutting the state capital of Montpelier off from the outside world. The flooding, the worst in the state's history, was another ominous reminder, in a summer of frightening natural disasters across the globe, of the expanding threat of global warming. The floods also served as an ironic if unremarked counterpoint to the state's own thriving dairy and meat industries, whose climate-changing emissions had contributed in some small way to the disaster. Even as Vermont officials were providing emergency funding to help animal farmers recover from the flooding, however, a determined community of animal advocates in Windsor County was quietly charting a different course, beyond dominion and outside the commodity logics of the capitalist system.

The summer before the floods, I accompanied the animal ethicist Zipporah Weisberg on a research trip to Vermont to visit VINE animal sanctuary, located in the small town of Springfield. After leaving the highway, we drove through gentle hillsides, pine forests, and sprawling farmland before finally arriving at a large house shaded by a towering oak, where we were welcomed by VINE's director and co-founder, pattrice jones. An unassuming queer woman in her early sixties, with close-cropped gray hair and glasses, pattrice (she prefers the lowercase, like the poet e. e. cummings) would spend the next two days showing us around and explaining VINE's unique philosophy. A feminist and former tenant organizer, pattrice had originally run a small animal sanctuary in Maryland with activist Miriam Jones (then her partner). Later, the women relocated the animals to Vermont and expanded their operation. It was pattrice and Miriam who had opposed Green Mountain College's plan to kill Bill and Lou, the draft oxen, and who had offered to adopt the animals. Today, there are over 500 residents at the sanctuary, including chickens, alpacas, pheasants, ducks, pigs, and other "vulnerable selves," cared for by a paid staff and a small network of volunteers.

At first glance, VINE has the appearance of an ordinary working farm, with much of the traditional farm work of feeding and providing water for the animals, patching fences, and shoveling chicken waste.

Unlike on a working farm, however, none of the animals on VINE are there to "produce" or to be slaughtered for humans. Instead, VINE is a haven for animals rescued or escaped from the animal industrial complex—chickens saved from factory farms and misguided school egg-hatching projects, pigeons saved from canned hunts, cows rescued from the butcher. The sanctuary is consciously organized around LGBTQ, feminist, and ecological principles. Among other things, this means that the animals aren't condescended to, but treated as co-equals within the community. The sanctuary's governing principle of nonviolent ecological community is meanwhile extended as well to the adjacent woodlands and fields.[11] Unlike traditional farms and ranches, VINE doesn't treat neighboring animals as "pests" to be exterminated. Here there are no traps or poisons, not even for the rats who pilfer the seeds and corn set out for the chickens each morning.

After welcoming us, pattrice left us in the hands of Rachel, a Vermont native in her forties who cares for the chickens. Rachel told us that when she first started working at VINE, she had seen farmed animals the way others did, as food, having grown up eating meat and dairy like other Vermonters. Over time, though, she began to see them differently. "Everything changed in the first week or so," she said, "watching the birds, watching the mammals, watching everybody . . . just—the way they interacted with one another, the way they interacted with us—I was like, what am I doing?" Before, she had thought of chickens as all alike; now she began to see them as unique individuals. Rachel told us about a hen named C. who had been rescued from an egg-laying operation. Another hen from the same facility had arrived at VINE at the same time, and the two birds had remained close companions. "When C. passed away," Rachel recounted, "her friend mourned her. She kept on going to the corner where she would always snuggle up in the shavings or the straw, just sit there and make this noise that I'd never heard before—and I've heard many noises come out of these birds. It was like she was crying. It was so sad. You have some [birds] that grow a bond with each other and love one another, and then you have some that are just like. . . . It's like people." Today, Rachel no longer eats meat or other products from animals. "I was completely wrong," she told us. "I was misled."[12]

Like other staffers we went on to meet, Rachel refers to the nonhuman residents at VINE as "persons." The practice arose informally, out of simple recognition that each animal is an individual with complex needs that are both species-specific and highly personal. Animals whose trauma history or temperament make them wary of touch and connection are given a respectfully wide berth.[13] When other animals actively seek out hugs or caresses from the staff, however, the humans are happy to reciprocate their affections (chores permitting). The animals are generally not segregated by species, but allowed to associate freely with the other animals, and interspecies friendships are common.

On the day of our visit, we were on hand for the rare introduction of a new "someone" to the sanctuary, a cow named Pupil who'd lost her home after the woman who'd kept her as a "pet" died. Standing outside the barn at the top of the lower pasture, we heard the low rumble of the cattle transport truck straining up the steep dirt road leading to the main property. Even before the truck had come into sight, the other animals had streamed out of the barn to see who was arriving. Either because they knew that the transport only brought cows to the sanctuary, or simply keen to be in on whatever was happening, the cows rather impolitely shoved aside the smaller animals in their haste to greet the newcomer. After the driver had backed his rig up to the barn, he and Cheryl Wylie, VINE's director of animal care, gently coaxed Pupil down the truck's ramp, as the other animals looked on with avid interest. Once on her own, Pupil began exploring her new surroundings, first tentatively, then with quiet curiosity, accompanied (or perhaps pestered) by a young male cow who had taken an immediate shine to her. The two explored the pasture contentedly together.

While VINE is utopian in its aspirations, it is not a utopia, and doesn't claim to be. Like persons everywhere, the inhabitants of VINE bring plenty of drama to their relationships, and there are occasional squabbles and misunderstandings. The staff must also make compromises in order to ensure the safety and well-being of their residents. While the animals are given as much liberty and autonomy as possible, staff rely on physical barriers and chicken coops to protect the vulnerable from outside predators, and to keep the cows from straying onto their neighbors' private property. Vaccines and other veterinary procedures are also a necessity. Inevitably, VINE staff must also sometimes make the painful decision to euthanize someone in the last stages of a terminal disease, or following a catastrophic accident. In such cases, however, death is meted out not to "save resources," nor to reduce "aggregate suffering," but as a mercy to a beloved individual—and then only reluctantly and as a last resort. Every loss is personally grieved, as the loss of an individual.

Many people fear that a world without meat, dairy, eggs, and fish would be one without pleasure, perhaps even without purpose. Yet the visitor to VINE would be hard pressed to say what is missing from the rich, purposeful lives of the staff there. VINE is a struggling nonprofit, and its personnel are underpaid. Yet even staff who've been on site for many years remain excited about their work—we found them eager to share their experiences with us. And because everything the staff does is grounded in a genuine ethos of care, rather than in the illusion of care, the work at VINE has an existential and moral authenticity that one never encounters on a working animal farm. For here there is no violence, and hence no betrayal.

We have come to view our relations with other animals as a zero-sum game, fearing that to promote "their" interests is to threaten or diminish "ours." But VINE and similar experiments show us what we ourselves stand to gain in addressing other beings as "Thous" rather than as "Its," as persons rather than things. Standing outside the barn that afternoon at VINE, watching the goats lazing about in the shade to escape the summer heat, the guinea fowl chasing one another through the tall grass, the cows nudging the staff for neck rubs, we felt we had caught a glimpse of the Peaceable Kingdom—the lineaments not of some mythic Eden, still less of a fraudulent past "Golden Era" of animal agriculture, but of a more advanced civilization—a future society which, having chosen to bury its whips, prods, and chains, to dismantle its slaughterhouses and to recall its trawlers, had won for itself the higher spiritual goods of compassion, mercy, and love.

ACKNOWLEDGMENTS

No man is an island—I could not have completed this book without the support of a great many people. I want to begin by thanking my supportive friend Jessie Klein for introducing me to Ilene Kalish, my incomparable editor at New York University Press, whose faith in this project made this book possible, and whose insights made it better. I am also grateful to the terrific production and marketing staff at NYU Press, including Priyanka Ray, Valerie Zaborski, Jenny Rossberg, Sydney Garcia, James Michael Reilly (whose incisive copy edits improved the book enormously), and to my fabulous publicist, Javier Perez.

My thinking about animals has been shaped in innumerable ways by my conversations with friends and colleagues in the animal advocacy movement over the years. I especially want to thank Loredana Loy, Arianna Ferrari, Michael Addario, Saryta Rodriguez, Phil Murphy, Marina Bolotnikova, Bennett McIntosh, Émilie-Lune Sauve, Christiane Bailey, Valéry Giroux, Livia Boscardin, Emily Moran Barwick, Robert Grillo, Ashley Capps, Sue Coe, Carol Adams, Alice Crary, Carol Gigliotti, Vasile Stănescu, Dinesh Wadiwel, Kostas Alexiou, Kim Stallwood, Harold Brown, Brenda Sanders, Alastor Van Kleeck, David Nibert, Ralph Acampora, Dennis Soron, Stephen Eisenman, Ritik Rao, and Crystal Heath. All have inspired me with their courage and emotional resilience, as well as their insights into the animal system. I want to give a special thanks to pattrice jones, both for her inspiring work and for permitting me to visit VINE animal sanctuary. She and her staff generously took time away from their important labors to discuss their work with me.

There are several individuals to whom I owe an especially heavy debt. Zipporah Weisberg supported this project, and me, from its earliest stages, and our conversations about animal ethics have informed this book in countless ways. (It was Zipporah's coaching, too, that helped me through the hardest part of the writing.) Andrea Levy provided me with comradeship and summer writing retreats in the lovely townships of Quebec, and I have been nourished by our close friendship and by our shared vision of *un besere velt*. Robert C. Jones helped me sharpen my philosophical positions, and I am deeply grateful for his unflagging personal support and love in difficult times. My colleague Roger Gottlieb has been an extraordinary help professionally as well as personally, and I cannot adequately thank him for his years of advice, friendship, and mentorship. I am grateful to Matt Goodman—the best writer in New York City—for his love and his encouragement of my writing. My friend Jennifer McWeeny helped me think through the structure of my manuscript at a key stage, and her solidarity when we were faculty colleagues together helped keep me sane. Finally, I want to thank Susan Siroty, without whose compassion and support this book would assuredly never have seen light of day. (Susan, this is your book.)

Among the careful readers whose feedback proved indispensable to me in writing this book, I especially want to thank Lindgren Johnson, whose brilliant editorial guidance improved this book beyond measure, as well as Ike Balbus, Troy Vettese, Holger Droessler, and Joel Brattin, all of whom improved this work with their close readings and feedback. The remarkable Anna Gold, meanwhile, helped me to understand what my book was really about, and I am deeply grateful to her for her encouragement of the project, and me, at a late stage in my writing process. I am also thankful to the anonymous reviewers at NYU Press for their criticisms of an earlier version of the manuscript.

In addition to those named above, I want to thank my friends Barbara Epstein, Thomas Hartl, Chris Bobel, Zoe Habel, Leslie Lebowitz, Laurie Prendergast, Annie Chen, Dominique Valek, Victoria Johnson, Diane DeRoo, Jessie Webb, Eric Begleiter, Kathy Caswell, Robin Cohen, Peter Kwiek, Catherine Chandrick and John Plummer, Miriam and Esther Greenspan, Erin Delaney, Valerie Sperling, Sam Diener, Mary Holmquist, Dirk Zastrow, Ron Loeffler, Tess Oliver, Gail Dines, David Levy, Matias Letelier, Jennie Evans, Curt Newton, Bob Fernandes, Michael Klare, Mona Elokda, Pat Sand, Adam Beresford, Patricia Whythe, Esme Perkell, and Jenna Nguyen. Margaret Cerullo and Carol Bengelsdorf mentored me when I was a student at Hampshire College, and it was they who showed me a larger world, and I thank them both. Svitlana Poleva, finally, brought me hope from afar when I most needed it.

I want to thank Hope Bohanec, John Sorenson, Wes DeMarco, Lori Gruen, Russ Powell, and A. K. Thompson for providing me with professional opportunities that helped me clarify my thinking on this book's themes. I am also indebted to Amanda Turner for suggesting a better title for this book, and to scientist Meghan Barrett for educating me about cognition in invertebrates.

Among the many faculty and staff at Worcester Polytechnic Institute who have supported me over the years, I especially want to thank Margaret Brodmerkle, Mary Cotnoir, Pam Paskalis, Jim Cocola, Dan DiMassa, Tanja Dominko, Michelle Ephraim, Glenn Gaudette, Karen Hassett, Aarti and Ryan Madan, V. J. Manzo, Wes Mott, Mark Richman, Penny Rock, Eunmi Shim, Ruth Smith, David Samson, David Spanagel, Kris Boudreau, Rebecca Moody, Geoff Pfeifer, Adrien Stoloff, Kate Moncrief, Jean King, and John Zeugner. To my students, who have taught me so much over the years: thank you, too.

Finally, I wish to thank my mother, Marianne Sanbonmatsu, whose compassion for wasps (if not for spiders) instilled in me a love of animals, and my late father, Yoshiro Sanbonmatsu, who instilled in me a love of justice: the influence of both can be seen in this work. In everything I do I am sustained by my extraordinary sisters, Lisa Sanbonmatsu and Kira Sanbonmatsu, by my niece Karina and nephews Vanya and Rohan, by my stepmother Donna Petrangelo and stepbrother Chris Petrangelo, and by my cousins.

This book is dedicated to my beloved son, Emmanuel Sullivan, and to the memory of my late friend Karen Davis, the animal activist and former director of United Poultry Concerns, who died while I was finishing this book. Karen, your moral compass always pointed North. And it has shown me the way.

NOTES

INTRODUCTION

1 Michael Pollan, *The Omnivore's Dilemma: A Natural History in Four Foods* (New York: Penguin Press, 2006), 322.

2 Charlotte Higgins, "The Age of Patriarchy: How an Unfashionable Idea Became a Rallying Cry for Feminism Today," *The Guardian*, June 22, 2018.

3 Bernard Lewis, *Race and Slavery in the Middle East: An Historical Inquiry* (New York: Oxford University Press, 1992), 3. Quoted in Seymour Drescher, *Abolition: A History of Slavery and Antislavery* (Cambridge: Cambridge University Press, 2009), 3–4.

4 Peter Singer, *Animal Liberation* (New York: HarperCollins, 1975), 6. "Speciesism" was originally coined by psychologist Richard Ryder in the 1970s to describe our belief that humans are superior to all other animals.

5 Pablo Rosado, "More than 80 Billion Land Animals Are Slaughtered for Meat Every Year," Our World in Data, May 31, 2024, ourworldindata.org. Though fisheries measure their catch only in tons, the number of wild-caught fish killed each year is estimated to be as high as 2.7 trillion. "Number of Wild-Caught Fish Killed for Food, 2016," Our World in Data, no date, ourworldindata.org. Billions more fish suffer and die in commercial aquaculture. See Hannah Ritchie, "The World Gets More Seafood from Aquaculture than Wild Catch," Our World in Data, August 8, 2024, ourworldindata.org.

6 Hannah Ritchie, "Half of the World's Habitable Land Is Used for Agriculture," Our World in Data, Nov. 13, 2019, ourworldindata.org.

7 Yinon M. Bar-on, Rob Phillips, and Ron Milo, "The Biomass Distribution on Earth," *Proceedings of the National Academy of Sciences (PNAS)* 115, no. 25 (June 19, 2018): 6506–6511, doi.org/10.1073/pnas.1711842115.

8 Daniel Pauly, et al., "Global Trends in World Fisheries: Impacts on Marine Ecosystems and Food Security," *Philosophical Transactions of the Royal Society of London, Series B, Biological Sciences* 360, no. 1453 (2005): 5–12, doi.org/10.1098/rstb.2004.1574. Cited in Jonathan Safran Foer, *Eating Animals* (New York: Little, Brown, 2009), 33.

9 Environmental Justice Foundation, *Squandering the Seas: How Shrimp Trawling is Threatening Ecological Integrity and Food Security Around the World* (report) (London: Environmental Justice Foundation, 2003), 2.

10 Unlike biases against other groups, animus against vegans is viewed as socially acceptable. Cara C. MacInnis and Gordon Hodson, "It Ain't Easy Eating Greens: Evidence of Bias toward Vegetarians and Vegans from Both Source and Target," *Group Processes & Intergroup Relations* 20, no. 6 (November 2017): 721–44. Cited by Emily Moran Barwick, "The Science of Why People Hate Vegans," Bite Size Vegan, Aug. 30, 2023, https://bitesizevegan.org.

11 Chuck Palahniuk, *Lullaby* (New York: Doubleday/Random House, 2002), 161.

12 Barbara Kingsolver, *Animal, Vegetable, Miracle: A Year of Food Life* (New York: HarperCollins, 2017), 222.

13 MacInnis and Hodson.

14 Perpetrators of genocide invariably denigrate their human victims first by comparing them to nonhuman animals. The Nazis referred to Jews as "rats" and "vermin"; in the months leading up to the Rwandan genocide, Hutu perpetrators depicted Tutsis as cockroaches and snakes, etc.

15 Syl Ko, in Aph Ko and Syl Ko, *Aphro-Ism: Essays on Pop Culture, Feminism, and Black Veganism from Two Sisters* (New York: Lantern Books, 2017), 45. For centuries, Blacks and other people of color have been compared to "beasts" by whites, with racial difference represented in "zoological" terms—see Aph Ko, *Racism as Zoological Witchcraft: A Guide to Getting Out* (New York: Lantern Books, 2019).

16 "A Difficulty in the Path of Psycho-Analysis," in the Standard Edition of the *Complete Psychological Works of Sigmund Freud*, vol. XVII (1917–1919): *An Infantile Neurosis and Other Works* (n.p., 1955), 135–144. Cited in Charles Patterson, *Eternal Treblinka: Our Treatment of Animals and the Holocaust* (New York: Lantern Books/Booklight, 2002), 2.

17 Charles Darwin, *The Origin of Species* and *The Descent of Man* (New York: The Modern Library, 1936), 494–495.

18 What I am calling an "interspecies community" is similar to Eva Meijer's notion of "interspecies democracy." See Meijer, *When Animals Speak: Toward an Interspecies Democracy*, vol. 1 (New York: New York University Press, 2019).

1. APOCALYPSE NOW

1 C. D. Harvell et al., "Disease Epidemic and a Marine Heat Wave Are Associated with the Continental-scale Collapse of a Pivotal Predator (*Pycnopodia helianthoides*)," *Science Advances* 5, no. 1 (January 2019): 119–145, doi.org/10.1126/sciadv.aau7042.

2 "Mass Fish Die-Off in Southern Russia Sparks Probe," *The Moscow Times*, Oct. 19, 2020, www.themoscowtimes.com.

3 Dr. Michelle Wille, quoted in Tom Hartley, "'Unprecedented Trail of Destruction,'" Australian Broadcasting Company (ABC), May 20, 2024, https://www.abc.net.au.

4 Dinesh Wadiwel, *The War Against Animals* (Leiden: Brill, 2015).

5 Gerardo Ceballos, Paul R. Ehrlich, Peter H. Raven, "Vertebrates on the Brink as Indicators of Biological Annihilation and the Sixth Mass Extinction," *PNAS* 117, no. 24 (Jun 2020): 13596–602, doi.org/10.1073/pnas.1922686117.

6 Tom Perkins, "Flame Retardant Pollution Threatens Wildlife on All Continents," *Guardian*, Oct. 19, 2023.

7 John Alroy, "Current Extinction Rates of Reptiles and Amphibians," *PNAS* 112, no. 42 (Oct. 2015): 13003–08, doi.org/10.1073/pnas.1508681112.

8 Sandra Laville, "Dumped Fishing Gear Is the Biggest Polluter in Ocean, Report Says," *The Guardian*, Nov. 5, 2019.

9 "We've failed big time," admits Canadian scientist David Suzuki. "We as environmentalists focused on issues: drilling in the Arctic National Wildlife Refuge, threats to the caribou herd, stopping a dam in the Amazon. But even when we won, we failed as a movement to change the underlying assumptions of society, the behavior of government and business people." Norimitsu Onisha, "He Warned Canada about Climate Change But Says, 'We Failed Big Time,'" *New York Times*, Oct. 20, 2023.

10 Frédérik Saltré, Joel Chadoeuf, Katharina J. Peters, et al., "Climate-Human Interaction Associated with Southeast Australian Megafauna Extinction Patterns," *Nature Communications* 10 (2019): 5311, doi.org/10.1038/s41467-019-13277-0.

11 Ed Yong, "In a Few Centuries, Cows Could Be the Largest Land Animals Left," *The Atlantic*, April 19, 2018.

12 Penn State, Eberly College of Science, "Humans and Climate Contributed to Extinctions of Large Ice Age Mammals, New Study Finds," *ScienceDaily*, November 3, 2011.

13 Matthew Stewart, W. Christopher Carleton, and Huw S. Groucutt, "Climate Change, not Human Population Growth, Correlates with Late Quaternary Megafauna Declines in North America," *Nature Communications* 12, no. 965 (2021).

14 Quoted in Michael Balter, "Archaeologists Say the 'Anthropocene' Is Here—But It Began Long Ago," *Science* 340 (April 19, 2013): 261–2.

15 Eric Guiry, Fiona Beglane, et al., "Anthropogenic Changes to the Holocene Nitrogen Cycle in Ireland," *Science Advances* 4, no. 6 (June 2018), doi.org/10.1126/sciadv.aas9383.

16 In *The Sixth Extinction: An Unnatural History* (New York: Henry Holt, 2014), Elizabeth Kolbert incorrectly cites industrialization rather than capitalism as the cause of the extinction crisis. She also fails to identify animal agriculture and fishing as leading forces of ecological collapse.

17 Carolyn Merchant, *The Death of Nature: Women, Ecology, and the Scientific Revolution* (New York: HarperCollins, 1990).

18 Charlotte McDonald, "How Many Earths Do We Need?," *BBC*, June 15, 2015, https://www.bbc.com.

19 For example, see Intergovernmental Science-Policy Platform on Biodiversity and Ecosystem Services (IPBES), *Global Assessment Report on Biodiversity and Ecosystem Services* (Bonn, Germany: IPBES Secretariat, 2019), https://www.ipbes.net/global-assessment.

20 Unchecked human population growth is a major ecological problem, a crisis being exacerbated by neoliberal pro-natalists. See Nandita Bajaj, Eileen Crist, and Kirsten Stade, "Confronting the United Nations' Pro-growth Agenda: A Call to Reverse Ecological Overshoot," *Journal of Population and Sustainability* 8, no. 2 (2024). The nonprofit Population Balance offers excellent resources on this issue, www.populationbalance.org.

21 James Phillipps, "The World's Wealthiest 1% Generate Half of the World's Global Aviation Emissions," *Forbes*, Nov. 17, 2020; World Tourism Organization and International Transport Forum (2019), *Transport-related CO2 Emissions of the Tourism Sector—Modelling Results*, UNWTO, Madrid, doi.org/10.18111/9789284416660.

22 Quoted in Yong, "In a Few Centuries." Human-instigated fires, coupled with warming temperatures, may have led to a mass extinction 12,000 years ago. Robin O'Keefe et al., "Pre-Younger Dryas Megafaunal Extirpation at Rancho La Brea Linked to Fire-driven State Shift," *Science* 381 (2023), doi.org/10.1126/science.abo3594.

23 John Bellamy Foster, *Marx's Ecology: Materialism and Nature* (New York: Monthly Review Press, 2000).

24 Dinesh Wadiwel, *Animals and Capital* (Edinburgh: Edinburgh University Press, 2023); Marco Maurizi, *Beyond Nature: Animal Liberation, Marxism, and Critical Theory* (Leiden: Brill, 2021).

25 "Tour D'Horizon with Nestlé: Forget the Global Financial Crisis, the World Is Running Out of Fresh Water," Center for Investigative Reporting (https://www.revealnews.org). The cable was originally published by Wikileaks (https://wikileaks.org/plusd/cables/09BERN129_a.html).

26 R. E. A. Almond, M. Grooten, and T. Petersen, eds., *Living Planet Report* (Gland, Switzerland: WWF, 2016 and 2018).

27 Janet Ranganathan, et al., "Shifting Diets for a Sustainable Food Future" (working paper, World Resources Institute, April 2016); Damian Carrington, "Avoiding Meat and Dairy Is 'Single Biggest Way' To Reduce Your Impact on Earth," *Guardian*, May 31, 2018; J. Poore and T. Nemecek, "Reducing Food's Environmental Impacts Through Producers and Consumers," *Science* 360 (2018): 987–992, doi.org/10.1126/science.aaq0216. Per 1,000 kilocalories, raising cattle for beef produces 36 kg of greenhouse gas emissions, and raising lamb produces 12 kg; by comparison, growing potatoes or wheat produces .6 kg in emissions, peas produce .3, and nuts produce only .07. Hannah Ritchie, Pablo Rosado, and Max Roser, "Environmental Impacts of Food Production," Our World In Data, 2022, ourworldindata.org.

28 Arjen Hoekstra, "The Water Footprint of Food," Swedish Research Council for Environment, Agricultural Sciences and Spatial Planning (2008), in Water for Food, ed. J. Förare, 49–61; Stockholm: The Swedish Research Council for Environment, Agricultural Sciences and Spatial Planning (Formas), 2008, waterfootprint.org/Reports; and P. W. Gerbens-Leenes, M. M. Mekonnen, A. Y. Hoekstra, "The Water Footprint of Poultry, Pork and Beef: A Comparative Study in Different Countries and Production Systems," *Water Resources and Industry* 1–2 (2013): 25–36.

29 Christopher Flavelle, "How America's Diet Is Feeding the Groundwater Crisis," *New York Times*, Dec. 24, 2023; O. Tompa, et al., "Is the Sustainable Choice a Healthy Choice? Water Footprint Consequence of Changing Dietary Patterns," *Nutrients* 12, no. 9 (Aug 2020): 2578, doi.org/10.3390/nu12092578.

30 J. Poore and T. Nemecek, "Reducing Food's Environmental Impacts Through Producers and Consumers," *Science* 360, (2018): 987–992, doi.org/10.1126/science.aaq0216. See also Damian Carrington, "Vegan Diet Massively Cuts Environmental Damage," *The Guardian*, July 20, 2023; Hannah Ritchie, "If the World Adopted a Plant-Based Diet We Would Reduce Global Agricultural Land Use from 4 to 1 Billion Hectares," Our World in Data, March 4, 2021, ourworldindata.org.

31 Troy Vettese, "To Freeze the Thames," *New Left Review*, May–June 2018, 63–86; M. N. Hayek, H. Harwatt, W. J. Ripple, and N. D. Mueller, "The Carbon Opportunity Cost of Animal-Sources Food Production on Land," *Nature Sustainability* 4 (2021): 21–24, doi.org/10.1038/s41893-020-00603-4.

32 A meta-analysis of 109 studies concluded that *"excluding* commercial agricultural grazers increases the abundance of plant and faunal biodiversity in most ecosystems." Jan Dutkiewicz and Gabriel N. Rosenberg, "The Myth of Regenerative Ranching," *The New Republic*, Sept. 23, 2021, citing A. Filazzola, C. Brown, M. A. Dettlaff, et al., "The Effects of Livestock Grazing on Biodiversity Are Multi-trophic: A Meta-analysis," *Ecology Letters* 23, no. 8 (Aug 2020): 1298–1309, doi.org/10.1111/ele.13527.

33 Vasile Stǎnescu, "Selling Eden: Environmentalism, Local Meat, and the Postcommodity Fetish," *American Behavioral Scientist* 63, no. 8 (2019): 1120–36.

34 Carrington, "Vegan Diet." See also P. Scarborough, M. Clark, L. Cobiac, et al., "Vegans, Vegetarians, Fish-eaters and Meat-eaters in the UK Show Discrepant Environmental Impacts," *Nature Food* 4 (2023): 565–74, doi.org/10.1038/s43016-023-00795-w.

35 "Overview of Veganic Techniques," Veganic Agriculture Network, accessed May 5, 2024, https://goveganic.net.

36 Michael J. Orlich et al., "Vegetarian dietary patterns and mortality in Adventist Health Study 2," *JAMA Internal Medicine* 173, no. 13 (July 2013): 1230–38, doi.

org/10.1001/jamainternmed.2013.6473; J. Clem and B. Barthel, "A Look at Plant-Based Diets," *Missouri Medicine* 118, no. 3 (May–Jun 2021): 233–38.

37 Some worry that without animal products, there would be "nothing left to eat." However, we consume only a miniscule portion of the estimated 200,000 edible plant species available to us. Even if we stayed within our existing narrow range, the number of possible plant-based recipes is essentially infinite: the hundreds of different rices, grains, legumes, nuts, fruits, and vegetables we eat can be combined in limitless ways. (Consider that a fifty-two card deck of playing cards can be shuffled into 8×10^{67} possible orders, more than the number of atoms in the galaxy.)

38 The film *Cowspiracy: The Sustainability Secret*, directed by Kip Anderson and Keegan Kuhn, (Appian Way, 2004), documents the environmental movement's reluctance to address the role of animal agriculture in global warming. In *The End of Nature* (New York: Random House, 1989), Bill McKibben fails even to mention the subject.

39 Arthur Nelson, "Ex-Officials at UN Farming Body Say Work on Methane Emissions Was Censored," *Guardian*, Oct. 20, 2023. More recent reports by the FAO have been criticized by experts for downplaying the impacts of animal agriculture on climate. Cleo Verkuijl, Jan Dutkiewicz, et al., "FAO's 1.5°C Roadmap for Food Systems Falls Short," *Nature Food* 5 (April 2024): 264–266.

40 M. J. Martin, S. E. Thottathil, and T. B. Newman, "Antibiotics Overuse in Animal Agriculture: A Call to Action for Health Care Providers," *American Journal of Public Health* 105, no. 12 (Dec. 2015): 2409–10, doi.org/10.2105/AJPH.2015.302870.

41 D. Carroll, B. Watson, E. Togami, et al., "Building a Global Atlas of Zoonotic Viruses," *Bulletin of the World Health Organization* 96 (2018): 292–94. Destruction of habitat forces animals into closer contact with humans and one another, creating new disease vectors. Runoff of animal blood and waste from industrialized animal facilities meanwhile spreads pathogens to marine wildlife.

42 Joe Fassler, "The Revolution that Died on Its Way to Dinner," *New York Times*, Feb. 9, 2024. My objections to cultured meat technology can be found on my website, www.CleanMeat-Hoax.com.

43 "Protein Innovation," Cargill, August 23, 2017, https://www.cargill.com.

44 Private correspondence with Carsten Gerhardt, lead author, *How Will Cultured Meat and Meat Alternatives Disrupt the Agricultural and Food Industry?* (Chicago: AT Kearney, June 2019).

45 Henry David Thoreau, *Thoreau's Animals*, ed. Geoff Wisner (New Haven, CT: Yale University Press, 2017), 23.

46 Quoted in Wes Mott, "Henry David Thoreau (1817–1862): Capturing the *Anima* in Animals," in *Animal Theologians*, ed. A. Linzey and C. Linzey (Oxford: Oxford University Press, 2023), 142–43.

47 Raphael Lemkin, *Totally Unofficial: The Autobiography of Raphael Lemkin* (New Haven, CT: Yale University Press, 2013), 33.

2. DEFENDING YOUR DINNER

1 "Defending Your Dinner," *New York Times Magazine*, March 20, 2012. The online edition of the contest was entitled, "Calling All Carnivores: Tell Us Why It's Ethical To Eat Meat: A Contest."

2 Rush Limbaugh, "A Meaty Response to the New York Times," The Rush Limbaugh Show, March 21, 2012, https://www.rushlimbaugh.com.

3 Nick Fiddes, *Meat: A Natural Symbol* (New York: Routledge, 1991), 65.

4 Colin Barras, "Paleo Diet Was a Veggie Feast with a Side of Meat," *New Scientist* 232, no. 3103 (Dec. 2016): 10–16.

5 The total rises to 10% when insects are included. Rob Dunn, "How To Eat Like a Chimpanzee," blog, *Scientific American*, Aug. 2, 2012, https://blogs.scientific american.com.

6 "Seventy percent of U.S. Calories Consumed in 2010 Were from Plant-Based Foods," USDA Economic Research Service, 2011, updated Jan. 2017, ers.usda. gov.

7 Portions of this chapter appeared in John Sanbonmatsu, "Why 'Fake' Meat Isn't," *St. Louis Post-Dispatch*, Jan. 13, 2020.

8 In 2024, the highest administrative court in France, bowing to pressure from French agribusiness, voted to ban the use of twenty-one plant-based meat words in product marketing, including "steak," "grill," "ham," and "butcher." Koh Ewe, "France Becomes Latest Government to Regulate 'Meat' Labels for Plant-Based Foods," *Time*, Feb. 28, 2024.

9 Charles W. Mills, *The Racial Contract* (Ithaca, NY: Cornell, 1999).

10 Troy Vettese, "A Marxist Theory of Extinction," *Salvage Zone*, May 25, 2020, www.Salvage.Zone.

11 David Nibert, *Animal Rights/Human Rights* (New York: Rowman & Littlefield, 2002), 38.

12 David Nibert, *Animal Oppression and Human Violence: Domesecration, Capitalism, and Global Conflict* (New York: Columbia University Press, 2013); Virginia DeJohn Anderson, *Creatures of Empire: How Domestic Animals Transformed Early America* (Oxford: Oxford University Press, 2006).

13 Horses and dogs alike were crucial "not only for military campaigns but also for maintaining control of the conquered populations and forcing them to labor under brutally oppressive conditions." Mary Norton, *The Tame and the Wild: People and Animals after 1492* (Cambridge, MA: Harvard University Press, 2024), 78.

14 For its Philip Morris account in 1954, the Leo Burnett agency swapped out its "Mild as May" campaign for the more masculine "Marlboro Man." With its iconic image of a rugged cowboy with a craggy, care-lined, sun-tanned face, the campaign ran nearly half a century (1954–1999). Ranching is still associated in popular culture with masculine prowess and control over nature.

15 William Cronon, *Nature's Metropolis: Chicago and the Great West* (New York: W. W. Norton, 1992); Dominic Pacyga, *Chicago's Union Stock Yard and the World it Made* (Chicago: University of Chicago Press, 2015).

16 Upton Sinclair, *The Jungle* (New York: Doubleday, Page & Co., 1906), 40–42.

17 A. Smith, "Chicago: The Dark and Insanitary Premises Used for Slaughtering of Cattle and Hogs—the Government Inspection," *The Lancet* (Jan. 14, 1905): 120–22. Quoted in Upton Sinclair, *The Jungle*, Second Norton Critical Edition, ed. C. V. Eby (New York: W. W. Norton, 2022), 343.

18 Some reviewers of *The Jungle* ridiculed its sympathetic portrayal of the pigs. Upton Sinclair claimed that critics had mistaken his satire for moral earnestness.

19 "Upton Sinclair's *The Jungle*: Muckraking the Meat-Packing Industry," *Bill of Rights in Action* 24, no. 1 (Fall 2008), http://www.teachdemocracy.org.

20 Lauren Aratani, "'They Were Little': Photos Show Children Illegally Working in US Slaughterhouses," *The Guardian*, May 9, 2023.

21 Hannah Dreier, "The Kids on the Night Shift," *New York Times*, Sept. 18, 2023.

22 Gail A. Eisnitz, *Slaughterhouse: The Shocking Story of Greed, Neglect, and Inhumane Treatment Inside the U.S. Meat Industry* (New York: Prometheus Books, 2009); Rachel MacNair, *Perpetration-Induced Traumatic Stress: The Psychological Consequences of Killing* (London: Praeger, 2002).

23 Prabhu L. Pingali, "Green Revolution: Toward 2.0," *PNAS* 109, no. 31 (July 2012): 12302–08, doi.org/10.1073/pnas.0912953109.

24 "McDonald's History," McDonald's Corporation, https://www.mcdonalds.com. Accessed August 9, 2024; Joel Stice, "The Truth About How Many Burgers McDonald's Has Sold," *Mashed*, Feb. 2, 2023, Mashed.com, accessed August 9, 2024.

25 François Truffaut, *Hitchcock/Truffaut* (New York: Simon & Schuster, 1983), 288.

26 Frances Moore Lappé, Diet for a Small Planet (New York: Ballantine, 1971). In *Omnivore's Dilemma*, his own 400-page book about industrialized agriculture and America's changing diet, Pollan mentions Lappé's work only once—and without providing any details.

27 Singer, *Animal Liberation*, 25–94.

28 Eric M. Greene, "A Reassessment of the Early History of Chinese Buddhist Vegetarianism," *Asia Major*, Third Series 29, no. 1 (2016): 1–43. In the Laṅkāvatāra Sūtra, the Buddha tells his disciple, "I look on all beings as I would a child. And why would I approve eating the flesh of children?" *The Lankavatara Sutra*, trans. Red Pine (Berkeley, CA: Counterpoint Press, 2011), 418–19. See also Tristram Stuart, *Bloodless Revolution: Radical Vegetarians and the Discovery of India* (New York: W. W. Norton, 2006).

29 John Kieschnick, "Buddhist Vegetarianism in China," in *Of Tripod and Palate: Food, Politics, and Religion in Traditional China*, ed. Roel Sterckx (London: Palgrave Macmillan, 2005), 186–212.

30 Ovid, *Metamorphoses*, in Kerry S. Walters and Lisa Portness, eds., *Ethical Vegetarianism: From Pythagoras to Peter Singer* (New York: SUNY Press, 1999), 22.

31 Leonardo da Vinci, in *Notebooks* and *Codex Atlanticus*. Quoted by Jennie Richards, "Leonardo da Vinci, A 15th Century Animal Rights Activist and Vegetarian," Humane Decisions website, Feb. 11, 2016, www.humanedecisions.com.

32 "'85 Salmonella Outbreak Largest Ever, Study Says," *The Chicago Tribune*, December 11, 1987.

33 "Last Patient Is Released In Jack in the Box Case," *New York Times*, July 1, 1993.

34 S. L. Gottlieb, et al. (Listeriosis Outbreak Working Group), "Multistate Outbreak of Listeriosis Linked to Turkey Deli Meat and Subsequent Changes in US Regulatory Policy," *Clinical Infectious Diseases* 42, no. 1 (Jan. 1, 2006): 29–36, doi.org/10.1086/498113.

35 Roger I. Roots, "A Muckraker's Aftermath: The Jungle of Meat-packing Regulation after a Century," *William Mitchell Law Review* 27, no. 4 (2001).

36 Tony Weis, "The Meat of the Global Food Crisis," *Journal of Peasant Studies* 40, no. 1 (2013): 65–85, doi.org/10.1080/03066150.2012.752357; Bill Winders and Elizabeth Ransom, eds., *Global Meat: Social and Environmental Consequences of the Expanding Meat Industry* (Cambridge, MA: MIT Press, 2019).

37 C. R. Daniel et al., "Trends in Meat Consumption in the USA," *Public Health Nutrition* 4, no. 4 (April 2011): 575–83, doi.org/10.1017/S1368980010002077.

38 L. DeRose, E. Messer, and S. Millman, *Who's Hungry? And How Do We Know? Food Shortage, Poverty, and Deprivation* (New York: United Nations University Press, 1998); Jeremy Rifkin, *Beyond Beef: The Rise and Fall of Cattle Culture* (New York: Plume, 1993).

39 Mark Tatge, "Vegetarian Foods Plant Stronger Sales," NBC News, Sept. 17, 2004, www.nbcnews.com, accessed July 1, 2024.

3. THE OMNIVORE'S DECEPTION

1 James Derek Sapienza, "We Need To Talk about the Hummer H2," *Motor Biscuit*, Dec. 11, 2016, https://www.motorbiscuit.com; Dan Shope, "Fear Drives Sales of Hummer H2," *The Morning Show*, Dec. 8, 2002; Joseph B. White, "The Hummer Lives!," *Wall Street Journal*, Nov. 14, 2005.

2 In one of many moments of legerdemain in *Omnivore*, Pollan implied that the industrialization and "urbanization" (concentration) of farmed animals occurred after World War II, when the US government began subsidizing monocrop corn production, which was then used to raise animals on feedlots (Pollan, 67). To make this argument, however, Pollan ignored the earlier concentration and industrialization of animals at the Chicago Yards.

3 Lewis Mumford, *Technics and Civilization* (New York: Harcourt Brace & Co., 1934), 267.

4 Craig Upright, *The Radical History of Food Cooperatives in Minnesota* (Minneapolis: University of Minnesota Press, 2020).

5 Carolyn Dimitri and Catherine Greene, "Recent Growth Patterns in the U.S. Organic Foods Market," Agricultural Information Bulletin No. 777, US Department of Agriculture (2000).

6 C. L. Weber and H. S. Matthews, "Food-miles and the Relative Climate Impacts of Food Choices in the United States," *Environmental Science and Technology* 42, no. 10 (May 2008): 3508–13, doi.org/10.1021/es702969f; Hannah Ritchie, "Less Meat Is Nearly Always Better than Sustainable Meat," Our World in Data, Feb. 4, 2020, https://ourworldindata.org.

7 Pollan, *Omnivore*, 263.

8 Jim Weaver, *Locavore Adventures: One Chef's Slow Food Journey* (Newark, NJ: Rivergate/Rutgers, 2012), 77.

9 Julie Guthman, *Agrarian Dreams: The Paradox of Organic Farming in California* (Berkeley: University of California Press, 2014), 33.

10 Kingsolver, 223.

11 Kim Severson, "Celebrity Chef Announces Strict Animal Welfare Policy," *New York Times*, March 22, 2007.

12 Hampshire College, *Non Satis Scire*, Spring 2011, 10.

13 John Stauber, Sheldon Rampton, et al., *Toxic Sludge is Good for You: Lies, Damn Lies and the Public Relations Industry* (Monroe, Maine: Common Courage Press, 2002), 67.

14 James LaVeck, "Invasion of the Movement Snatchers," *Satya*, October 2006. Excerpted on Animal Rights Zone, http://arzone.ning.com. Recently, wealthy individuals associated with Effective Altruism, a philanthropic movement funded by tech billionaires and inspired by Peter Singer's utilitarianism, have flooded the "realists" with money while starving grassroots activist "idealists" of funding, damaging animal advocacy. See John Sanbonmatsu, "Effective Altruism and the Reified Mind," in *The Good It Promises, the Harm It Does*, ed. Carol J. Adams, Alice Crary, and Lori Gruen (Oxford: Oxford University Press, 2023), 204–24.

15 Andrew Martin, "Meat Labels Hope to Lure the Sensitive Carnivore," *The New York Times*, Oct. 24, 2006.

16 Initially appointed Director for Rural Development and Outreach at HSUS, Maxwell would later become political director of The Humane Society Legislative Fund, the HSUS's powerful lobbying arm.

17 Shapiro cast capitalist biotechnology as the "salvation" of animals and in 2018 created a startup, the Better Meat Company, promising to help meat companies achieve their "corporate sustainability goals," improve "the health profile" of their products, and improve their bottom lines by selling hybridized products that mix plant proteins with animal meats. Thanks to his efforts, Perdue's Chicken Plus™ combines vegetables with meat from factory-farmed chickens. "Perdue® Foods Launches Chicken Plus™ with Vegetable Nutrition: New

Chicken Nuggets, Tenders and Patties Meet Demand for Flexitarian Families," *PR Press Wire*, June 12, 2019.

18 Ariel Kaminer, "The Main Course Had an Unhappy Face," *New York Times*, March 19, 2010.

19 Jacqueline Turner, "Grass-fed Cows Won't Save the Climate, Study Says," *Science*, Oct. 2, 2017, www.science.org; Tara Garnett et al., *Grazed and Confused?* (Oxford: Food Climate Research Network, Oct. 2017). Though grazing cattle sequesters some carbon, cows produce more carbon gasses than they store.

20 James McWilliams, "The Myth of Truly Sustainable Meat," *Dallas News*, April 20, 2012.

21 "Amazon: Lame Duck in the Foie Gras Fight," Mercy for Animals, accessed Oct. 20, 2023, https://mercyforanimals.org.

22 Lauren Gazzola, "Don't Buy the Chipotle Hype: There's No Such Thing as 'Humane' Slaughter," *Salon*, March 2, 2014.

23 "Former Chipotle Employee Details Animal Abuse and Inhumane Practices," Yahoo News, Dec. 6, 2018, news.yahoo.com.

24 "Chipotle Claims 'No Animal Cruelty,' But a New Investigation Reveals Their Suppliers Are Factory Farms," World Animal News, Dec. 7, 2018, www.sentientmedia.org.

25 Chris Chase, "Americans Consumed a Record Amount of Seafood," *SeafoodSource*, June 7, 2022, https://www.seafoodsource.com.

26 Andrew Martin, "Meat Labels Hope to Lure the Sensitive Meat-Eater," *New York Times*, Oct. 24, 2006.

27 Grace Hussain, "Meat Consumption in the U.S.: Is It Increasing or Decreasing?," Sentient Media, Dec. 2023, sentientmedia.org.

28 Vis-á-vis animals, the capitalist state is by no means a neutral institution, but plays an integral role in defending corporate animal interests. C. Stache and C. Bernhold, "The Bourgeois Meat Hegemony," *Österreich Z Soziol* 46, no. 2 (2021):167–186, doi.org/10.1007/s11614-021-00454-z.

29 Michael Moss, "US Research Lab Lets Animals Suffer in Quest for Profit," *New York Times*, Jan. 19, 2015.

30 Erin McCormick, "Santa Monica 'Farm to Door' Purveyor Admits to Mislabeling Meats," *Guardian*, May 27, 2021.

31 In 2011, the TV show *Portlandia* satirized the predicament of "conscientious" consumers in a skit depicting a couple at an upscale organic restaurant going to absurd lengths to investigate the former living conditions of a chicken they want to eat.

32 Stijn Bruers, "Animal-welfare-labelled Meat Is Not a Stepping Stone to Animal-free Diets: Empirical Evidence from a Survey," *Journal of Environmental Economics and Policy*, March 20, 2024.

33 Once in office, the "compassionate" Bush proposed cuts to Medicare and other forms of aid for the poor, reserving his "cruelest health care cuts [to be] targeted at kids: programs to provide child care, prevent child abuse and train doctors at children's hospitals." Bill Press, "Bush Cuts Children's Health to Pay for Tax Cut," *Tribune Media Services*, April 6, 2001.

34 Roger Scruton, "A Carnivore's Credo," *Harper's* 312, no. 1872 (May 2006): 21–24, 26. "The consensus among the monotheistic religions has been that animals exist for our purposes and that we are entitled to use them, domesticate them and eat them, subject only to God's inscrutable dietary laws." Roger Scruton, *A Political Philosophy: Arguments for Conservatism* (New York: Bloomsbury, 2006), 47.

35 Vasile Stănescu, "Crocodile Tears: Compassionate Carnivores and the Marketing of 'Happy Meat,'" in *Critical Animal Studies*, ed. Jon Sorenson, 216–233 (Toronto: Canadian Scholars Press, 2014).

4. ROMANCING THE FARM

1 Karl Marx, *Contribution to a Critique of Hegel's Philosophy of Right*, in *Early Writings*, trans. Rodney Livingstone and Gregon Benton (New York: Penguin, 1992), 224. Marx depicted religion as a balm for the oppressed that failed to alter existing material conditions or relations of power; the same can be said of "enlightened" omnivorism.

2 Jenna Woginrich, *Made from Scratch: Discovering the Pleasures of the Handmade Life* (North Adams, MA: Storey, 2010), 115.

3 In his revisionist history, *Genghis Khan and the Quest for God* (New York: Penguin, 2017), Jack Weatherford argues that Khan instituted liberal reforms, including religious pluralism. However, Weatherford downplays the well-documented sadism and violence of Khan's rule.

4 Already by the colonial period, the nation's "cardinal image" was that of "a chaste, uncomplicated land of rural virtue," consisting of a "pasture" and "a twisting brook with cattle grazing nearby"—with elms and hills in the distance. Leo Marx, *The Machine in the Garden* (London: Oxford, 1978), 141.

5 Anonymous, *American husbandry. Containing an account of the soil, climate, production and agriculture, of the British colonies in North-America and the West Indies: With observations on the advantages and disadvantages of settling in them, compared with Great Britain and Ireland*, vol. 1 (London: J. Bew, 1775), 67.

6 White wryly suggested that Highstone had things backwards. "Pressure of city living? No pressure which I ever knew in town compares with the pressure of country living." E. B. White, "The Practical Farmer" (1940), reprinted in *One Man's Meat* (New York: Harper and Brothers, 1944), 172–73.

7 "[O]ur eating turns nature into culture, transforming the body of the world into our bodies and minds." Pollan, *Omnivore*, 10.

8 Ibid., 202.

9 Ibid., 219.

10 Only once in *Omnivore* does Pollan implicitly concede that converting sunlight into grass and then into animal protein to feed humans is less efficient than converting sunlight into plants to feed directly to humans. Pollan quotes rancher Allan Nation as writing that there are "only two ways" to convert sunlight into food: "One is for you is to walk out in your garden, pull a carrot and eat it. This is a direct transfer of solar energy to human energy. The second most efficient way is for you to send an animal out to gather this free solar food and then you eat the animal" (quoted in Pollan, 188). Readers of *Omnivore* were nonetheless given the false impression that the most efficient, direct, and ecologically benign way to grow food for human consumption is to raise ruminant animals on pasture. See Dutkiewicz and Rosenberg.

11 See Leo Marx, *Machine in the Garden.*

12 Pollan, *Omnivore,* 125.

13 Thomas Jefferson, *Notes on the State of Virginia,* ed. William Peden (Chapel Hill: University of North Carolina Press, 1955), 164–5.

14 Temple Grandin compares touching the walls of a Swift slaughterhouse to "touching a sacred altar" and describes restraining animals to be shot in the head with a captive bolt gun as "almost a religious experience." Temple Grandin, *Thinking in Pictures and Other Reports from My Life with Autism* (New York: Vintage Books, 2006), 25. Locavore farmer Jenna Woginrich buys an animal farm as a way, she writes, to be "a part of an infallible religion: Traditional Agriculture." Woginrich, *One-Woman Farm: My Life Shared with Sheep, Pigs, Chickens, Goats, and a Fine Fiddle* (North Adams, MA: Storey, 2013), 16. "If an agnostic has a herd of Brown Swiss, the twice-daily milking comes as ritualistically as Islamic calls to prayer. . . ." Ibid., 207.

15 Pollan, *Omnivore,* 233, 215.

16 Ibid., 260.

17 Ibid., 261.

18 Ibid., 241.

19 Ibid., 238. Pollan claims that "turning [a] pile of blood and guts into a savory salami . . . [thereby] symbolically redeems it, making good our karmic debts." Ibid., 405.

20 Jefferson, *Notes on the State of Virginia,* 165.

21 Pollan, *Omnivore,* 204.

22 Jefferson, 165.

23 Pollan, *Omnivore,* 243.

24 Ibid., 203, 130.

25 *Progressive Farmer* in 2015; cited by Tom Philpott, "Joel Salatin's Unsustainable Myth," *Mother Jones,* Nov. 19, 2020; "Joel Salatin, Cows, Carbon, and Climate" (video file, YouTube, 2016, https://www.youtube.com/

watch?time_continue=7&v=4Z75A_JMBx4), cited by Vasile Stănescu, "Selling Eden," 10. See also Pollan, *Omnivore*, 228.

26 Pollan, *Omnivore*, 192.

27 Ibid., 203–4.

28 Quoted in Ibid., 260.

29 Ibid., 254.

30 Pollan himself has written of the need to "liberate" small producers from federal regulations—specifically ones designed to protect consumers from poisoning by animal products. "Food-safety regulations must be made sensitive to scale and marketplace," he insisted. "Farmer in Chief," *New York Times*, Oct. 12, 2008.

31 "Joel Salatin, Responding to a Question on Gay Marriage and the Education Department," YouTube, 2012, accessed May 25, 2024, https://www.youtube.com/watch?v=Q4ayABZoizs.

32 Pollan, *Omnivore*, 236.

33 If someone wants to buy his products, Salatin tells Pollan, "that should be none of the government's business." Ibid., 233. Salatin's aversion to regulation of any kind may explain why Polyface is not an organic farm, since the "organic" label requires a certification process.

34 Ibid., 236.

35 Ibid., 132.

36 Between 1870 and 1920, agrarian resistance to capitalism only "enabled a stronger and more resilient capitalist state to emerge, while in the process co-opting and disarming opposition movements by integrating them into developing industrial capitalist social relations." Brad Bauerly, *The Agrarian Seeds of Empire* (Leiden: Brill, 2017), 105. Today's populist agrarianism has arguably done the same thing, reinforcing capitalist relations and compromising more radical movements.

37 Cited by Philpott, "Joel Salatin's Unsustainable Myth."

38 Monica Pronkzuk and Claire Moses, "Labeled Climate Culprits, European Farmers Rebel Over New Standards," *New York Times*, Aug. 26, 2023.

39 Roger Cohen, "For Farmers in France, a Fierce Battle to Survive," *New York Times*, April 1, 2024, A11.

40 In 2023, Senate Republicans introduced the Ending Agricultural Trade Suppression or "EATS" Act, hoping to end "the authority of states and localities to set animal welfare and food safety standards." The bill threatened over a thousand "state and local health and safety laws that set food-quality require-ments and stop the spread of invasive species and zoonotic diseases like avian flu." Marin Scotten, "From Cage-Free Chicks to Puppy Mills and Avian Flu: Republicans Are Trying to Roll Back Animal Protections," *The Guardian*, Sept. 22, 2023.

41 "Governor De Santis Signs Legislation to Keep Lab-Grown Meat Out of Florida," Office of the Governor of Florida (May 1, 2024).

42 Guthman, *Agrarian Dreams*, 263.

43 Weaver, 195.

44 Vasile Stănescu, "'Green' Eggs and Ham? The Myth of Sustainable Meat and the Danger of the Local," *Journal for Critical Animal Studies* VIII, no. 1/2 (2010): 8–32.

45 Leo Marx, 132.

46 Catherine Friend, *Sheepish: Two Women, 50 Sheep, and Enough Wool to Save the Planet* (Boston: Da Capo, 2011), 143, 144, 147.

47 Philpott, "Joel Salatin's Unsustainable Myth."

48 Historically, advocacy for animals has been closely intertwined with advocacy for human rights and progressive social reforms. In the seventeenth century, for example, the English reformer and early vegan Thomas Tryon "attacked not just cruelty to animals, but also negro slavery, war-games, the criminal code, the harsh treatment of the insane, and even the practice of making all persons behave as if they were naturally right-handed." Keith Thomas, *Man and the Natural World* (New York/London: Oxford, 1983), 291.

49 Dan Nosowitz, "Here Are Five Issues That Caused Farmers To Vote For Trump," *Modern Farmer*, Nov. 23, 2016.

50 Cited by Crystal Heath, "Avian Influenza's Threat to Chickens and Public Health," Humane Hoax Chicken Webinar, May 4, 2024, www.HumaneHoax.org. Joel Salatin expressed nearly identical sentiments in his interviews with Michael Pollan. "The USDA is being used by the global corporate complex to impede the clean-food movement. They aim to close down all but the biggest meat processors, and to do it in the name of biosecurity." Quoted in Pollan, *Omnivore*, 230.

51 Pollan, "Farmer in Chief."

52 Explaining why he and other high-end chefs seek out raw, unpasteurized milk, Daniel Patterson, a chef at Coi, an upscale restaurant in San Francisco, observed: "Raw milk is a primary touchstone of . . . [the] sort of agrarian, old-fashioned life." Dana Goodyear, "Raw Deal," *New Yorker*, April 30, 2012, 33. In 2024, right-wing pundits continued to encourage raw-milk consumption, despite urgent FDA and CDC warnings that raw cow's milk might be infected with avian flu.

53 Pollan, *Omnivore*, 314.

54 Judith Capper, "Meatless Mondays . . . Or More Veg Mondays?," blog, posted Oct. 9, 2012, accessed Oct. 28, 2023, bovidia.com.

55 Lierre Keith, *Vegetarian Myth* (Berkeley, CA: PM Press, 2009), 22, 249.

56 Pollan, *Omnivore*, 126.

57 Julie Bosman, "North Dakotans Reconsider a Corporate Farming Ban, and Their Values," *New York Times*, June 12, 2016.

58 Paul Kristiansen, Acram Taji, and John Reganold, *Organic Farming: A Global Perspective* (Ithaca, NY: Comstock/Cornell, 2006), 177.

59 Kim Severson, "With Goat, a Rancher Breaks Away from the Herd," *New York Times*, Oct. 15, 2008, D4.

60 Michael Pollan credits Bill Niman as one of his main sources of information about the cattle industry. Niman and his wife Nicolette have profited from their exploitation of thousands of animals in several operations spanning two continents—pigs in Iowa, cattle in the Midwest, and turkeys in Latin America. All this intercontinental traffic in the bodies of animals has made the Nimans millionaires. In 2012, the *New York Times* ran an opinion piece by Nicolette Niman entitled "The Carnivore's Dilemma," in which the rancher's wife and bestselling author of the memoir *The Righteous Porkchop* defended meat-eating. Killing and eating animals was *better* than sparing their lives, so long as one took pains to "avoid processed foods and those from industrialized farms." Nicolette Hahn Niman, "The Carnivore's Dilemma," *New York Times*, Oct. 31, 2012, A17.

61 Manuela Andreoni, "Brazil Sues Meatpacker for Millions in Damages," *New York Times*, Dec. 21, 2023, B3.

62 "JBS Profit at Four-Year High on Grass-Fed Beef: Corporate Brazil," *Bloomberg*, Oct. 1, 2012, Bloomberg.com.

63 Leaving aside hunting's unethical nature, organizing our food system around hunting would not even be feasible. Since there are thirty-six million deer and a million elk left in the US, and 330 million humans, every large mammal in North America would be extinct within a week.

64 Pollan, *Omnivore*, 84.

65 On the case for a transition to an ecologically informed, democratic socialism, see John Sanbonmatsu, *The Postmodern Prince: Critical Theory, Left Strategy, and the Making of a New Political Subject* (New York: Monthly Review Press, 2004). See also Andrea Levy, "Degrowth: A Snail's Eye View of Social Transformation and Ecological Preservation," *Science for Peace Bulletin* 35, no. 1 (May 2015): 24–28.

66 "They know what's up," the yeshiva student tells the reporter. "You can feel their feathers plump when you reach in. They all hide in the corner." Samantha M. Shapiro, "Kosher Wars," *New York Times*, Oct. 9, 2008.

67 Quoted by Alex Williams in "Slaughterhouse Live: You Be the Butcher," *New York Times*, Oct 23, 2009.

68 Ariel Kaminer, "The Main Course Had an Unhappy Face," *New York Times*, Nov. 19, 2010.

5. FREEDOM IS SLAVERY

1 Charles Darwin, Notebook B (1837–38), in *Charles Darwin's Notebooks 1836–1844*, ed. P. H. Barrett et al. (Cambridge: Cambridge University Press, 1987).

2 Emma Marris, "Modern Zoos Are Not Worth the Moral Cost," *New York Times*, June 11, 2021.

3 Pollan, *Omnivore*, 321.

4 Quoted in Pollan, 217.

5 Wes Jackson, "The Agrarian Mind," in *The Essential Agrarian Reader*, ed. Norman Wirzba (Lexington: University Press of Kentucky, 2003), 149–50. Farmers "have found a renewed logic in draft power," since "animals can be cheaper to board and feed than any tractor," Tess Taylor writes in "Brute Force: On Small Farms, Hoof Power Returns," *New York Times*, May 3, 2011.

6 Kingsolver, 223.

7 David Brion Davis, *The Rise and Fall of Slavery in the New World* (New York: Oxford University Press, 2006), 34.

8 Aristotle, *Politics*, trans. by Ernest Barker (Oxford: Oxford University Press, 1970), 4.

9 Davis, *The Rise and Fall*, 34.

10 Maryanne Cline Horowitz, "Aristotle and Woman," *Journal of the History of Biology* 9, no. 2 (Autumn 1976): 187.

11 George Fitzhugh, *Southern Thought* (1857), cited in Drew Gilpin Faust, ed., *The Ideology of Slavery: Proslavery Thought in the Antebellum South, 1830–1860* (Baton Rouge: LSU Press, 1981), 291.

12 Marjorie Spiegel, *The Dreaded Comparison* (Gabriola Island, BC: New Society Press, 1988), 39.

13 Aristotle, *Politics*, 21.

14 Pollan, *Omnivore*, 320.

15 Woginrich, *Made from Scratch*, 99, 105, 111.

16 William Harper, *Memoir on Slavery* (1852), in Faust, ed., 118.

17 On the natural status of (pre-racialized) slavery, see Aristotle, *Politics*, 21.

18 Harper, Faust, ed. Just as the "most ignorant farmer or laborer . . . knows the natures of [farm] animals . . . and governs them accordingly," wrote another apologist, so too does the slaver know and govern his slaves. J. H. Van Evrie, *Negroes and Negro "Slavery": The First an Inferior Race, the Latter Its Normal Condition* (1863), quoted in Spiegel, *Dreaded Comparison*, 36.

19 Pollan, *Omnivore*, 320.

20 Alyssa Jumars, "Beasts," in *Greenhorns: The Next Generation of American Farmers: 50 Dispatches from the New Farmers' Movement*, ed. Z. Bradbury, S. von Tscharner Fleming, and P. Manalo (North Adams, MA: Storey Press, 2012), 143.

21 Plato, *The Republic*, trans. and ed. by Raymond Larson (Arlington Heights, IL: Harlan Davidson, 1979), 221.

22 Aristotle, *Politics*, 17.

23 *Politics*, 3.

24 *Politics*, 11. Slaves "whose function is bodily service . . . produce their best when they supply such service"; for such "natural slaves . . . it is better for them . . . to be ruled by a master" (I.3, 13). Slavery for them is "beneficial and just" (Ibid., 14).

25 Thomas R. Dew, "Abolition of Negro Slavery," in Faust, ed., 65.

26 Ibid.

27 Harper, in Faust, 99.

28 Kathy Rudy, *Loving Animals: Toward a New Animal Advocacy* (Minneapolis: University of Minnesota Press, 2011), 8. Rudy defends scientific experimentation on animals so long as we remain "attuned . . . to their emotions, languages, needs, predilections, tendencies, desires, wishes, and hopes." She does not explain how such "attunement" to animals is to be shown while giving them electric shocks, infecting them with cancer, or inducing psychosis in them. "Such a *deep bond* in the realm of experimentation will push all to honor their gifts and sacrifices" (196; emphasis added).

29 Keith, *Vegetarian Myth*, 24.

30 Ibid.

31 Orwell spent most of his boyhood not on an animal farm but at a cruel boys preparatory school in East Sussex; yet he grasped that the animals we raise on farms in no way consent to the violent uses we make of them. "We are born," Major tells the animals, "we are given just so much food as will keep the breath in our bodies, and those of us who are capable of it are forced to work to the last atom of our strength; and the very instant that our usefulness has come to an end we are slaughtered with hideous cruelty." The enraged animals stage a successful rebellion, driving Jones and his men away. Then they rush around the farm to "wipe out the last traces of Jones's hated reign": "The harness-room at the end of the stables was broken open; the bits, the nose-rings, the dog-chains, the cruel knives with which Mr. Jones had been used to castrate the pigs and lambs, were all flung down the well. The reins, the halters, the blinkers, the degrading nosebags, were thrown on to the rubbish fire which was burning in the yard. So were the whips. All the animals capered with joy when they saw the whips going up in flames." George Orwell, *Animal Farm* (New York: Harcourt, Brace, Jovanovich, 1974), 18–30.

6. LOVE ME, BEAT ME, KILL ME, EAT ME

1 Michael Pollan writes that "domestication took place when a handful of especially opportunistic species discovered, through Darwinian trial and error, that they were more likely to survive and prosper in an alliance with humans than on their own." *Omnivore*, 320. One wonders how chickens, born of kings—the domesticated chicken is the closest living descendant of Tyrannosaurus Rex—managed to survive for millions of years before finally hitting through "trial and error" on the idea of forming an "alliance" with humans a mere 8,000 years ago.

2 Stephen Budiansky, "In from the Cold: Since the Ice Age, It Has Been in the Interests of Some Animals To Ignore the Call of the Wild," *New York Times Magazine*, Dec. 22, 1991, 17, 23. "The 'deal' that domesticated animals have made

over time with humans is that some of their freedoms would be curtailed in return for food, shelter, belonging, and love," writes Kathy Rudy (*Loving Animals*, 5).

3 Though quick to accuse animal advocates of anthropomorphism, Pollan has no hesitation imputing agency and foresight to the animals for having "chosen" to partner with us, saying that we "provided the animals with food and protection in exchange for which the animals provided the humans with their milk, eggs, and—yes—their flesh." *Omnivore*, 320.

4 Madeline Ostrander, "Joel Salatin: How To Respect Animals and Eat Them Too," *Yes!* magazine, March 28, 2011.

5 Jenna Woginrich, *Barnheart: The Incurable Longing for a Farm of One's Own* (North Adams, MA: Storey Publishing, 2011), 139. Emphasis added.

6 "Awareness of emotions involved *for both parties* is crucial." Rudy, *Loving Animals*, 194.

7 See Carol Adams, *The Sexual Politics of Meat* (Boston: Beacon, 1990).

8 Quoted in Jeffrey Moussaieff Masson and Susan McCarthy, *When Elephants Weep* (New York: Bantam Doubleday Dell, 1995), 39–40.

9 Rebecca Ryan, "The Sex Right: A Legal History of the Marital Rape Exemption," *Law & Social Inquiry* 20, no. 4 (1995): 954.

10 Weaver, 6. Emphasis added.

11 Friend, *Sheepish*, 236.

12 Ibid., 243.

13 Keith, *The Vegetarian Myth*, 26.

14 Rudy, *Loving Animals*, 100.

15 Benjamin Godwin, *Lectures on Slavery* (Boston: James B. Dow, 1836; reprinted Negro Universities Press/Greenwood, 1969), 49, 138.

16 Godwin, 136.

17 Anonymous, *American husbandry*, 80–81.

18 Locavores fetishize animals in ways that recall the fetishization of Blacks by slave owners. After selling a bull calf, Kristin Kimball boasts that "the black calf and his untouched testicles were sold at a tidy profit." *The Dirty Life: A Memoir of Farming, Food, and Love* (New York: Scribner/Simon and Schuster, 2010), 219. When two "Nigerian bucks" on Suzanne McMinn's farm prove "full of personality and spunk," she has them killed so that she won't have to deal with their "constant nuisance." *Chickens in the Road: An Adventure in Ordinary Splendor* (New York: Harper and Row, 2013).

19 Godwin, 136.

20 Ibid., 137.

21 Catherine Lee, "Foot-and-Mouth Disease Outbreak's Parallels with Covid Pandemic," *BBC*, Feb. 19, 2021.

22 Numbers Rabbah 20:15 (Midrash exposition of the Book of Numbers), quoted in *The Case of the Animals vs. Man before the King of the Jinn*, trans. Lenn E.

Goodman and Richard McGregor (London: Oxford, 2009), 5. The exposition explains a passage in Numbers in which a donkey is made to speak by God.

23 Plutarch (46–119 CE), "On the Use of Reason by 'Irrational' Animals," *Essays*, trans. Robin Waterfield (New York: Penguin, 1993), 387.

24 Richard McGregor, ed., *The Case of the Animals versus Man Before the King of the Jinn*, trans. Lenn Goodman (Oxford: Oxford University Press, 2012), 107, 100.

25 Ibid., 107, 118.

26 Ibid., 103. Emphasis added.

27 Ibid., 115.

28 Wajeeha Malik, "Inky's Daring Escape Shows How Intelligent Octopuses Are," *National Geographic*, April 14, 2016.

29 "Runaway Cow Escapes Slaughterhouse to Live on Polish Island," *BBC News*, Feb. 19, 2018. Plans to shoot the cow were called off when local villagers objected out of sympathy for the "hero cow" (as she became known).

30 Hal Whitehead, Tim D. Smith, and Luke Rendell, "Adaptation of Sperm Whales to Open-Boat Whalers: Rapid Social Learning on a Large Scale?," *Royal Society*, March 17, 2020. In 2023, it was reported that orcas had been attacking and sinking boats around the world, evidently sharing their tactics with other orcas. Sascha Pare, "Orcas Have Sunk 3 Boats in Europe and Appear To Be Teaching Others to do the Same," *LiveScience*, May 18, 2023.

31 *Earthlings*, dir. by Shaun Monson (Nation Earth, 2005).

32 Kingsolver, 222.

33 Quoted in Spiegel, *Dreaded Comparison*, 65.

34 Dew, "Abolition of Negro Slavery," 55.

35 Farmed animals are untroubled by their "loss of autonomy," Pollan claims. *Omnivore*, 320.

36 Hammond in Eric McKitrick, 123.

37 Ibid. Cf. Thomas Dew: "A merrier being does not exist on the face of the globe than the negro slave of the United States" (Dew, "Abolition of Negro Slavery," in Faust, 66).

38 Quoted in Ostrander.

39 Ewen Callaway, "When Chickens Go Wild," *Nature*, Jan. 20, 2016.

40 Woginrich, *Barnheart*, 144.

41 Kimball, *The Dirty Life*, 179.

42 Ibid., 217.

43 Ibid., 180.

44 Jefferson, *Notes on State of Virginia*, 265.

45 Renee King-Sodden, a Texas rancher's wife, became so heartbroken seeing cows chasing after the trucks taking their calves to slaughter that she convinced her husband to give up ranching altogether. The couple now run the Rowdy Girl animal sanctuary, Rowdygirlsanctuary.org.

46 Pattrice jones, *The Oxen at the Intersection: A Collision (or, Bill and Lou Must Die: A Real-Life Murder Mystery from the Green Mountains of Vermont)* (New York: Lantern Publishers, 2014).

47 Steven Fesmire, public comment on the VINE sanctuary website, Oct. 15, 2012, www.Blog.Bravebirds.org.

48 Harper, in Faust, 127.

49 Ibid., 115.

7. MURDER, SHE WROTE

 1 HeliBacon Company (www.HeliBacon.com). In an email (May 2024), the company confirmed to me "that this is a majority male experience," with women on hand typically as "partners of male guests."

 2 M. Kheel, "The Killing Game: An Ecofeminist Critique of Hunting," *Journal of the Philosophy of Sport* 23, no. 1 (1996): 40.

 3 Adams, *Sexual Politics of Meat*.

 4 Burger King, "Manthem—I Am Man," produced by the Crispin Porter + Bogusky agency (2006). The "Manthem" both reinforced and satirized the association of masculinity and meat: the "protest" movement in the ad featured men of all races, ethnicities, and classes—implying that only *meat-eating* can plausibly lend gender coherence to the newly embattled and fragmented category of "men."

 5 Vasile Stănescu, "The Whopper Virgins: Hamburgers, Gender, and Xenophobia in Burger King's Hamburger Advertising," in *Meat Culture*, ed. Annie Potts (Leiden: Brill, 2016), 90–108.

 6 Iselin Gambert and Tobias Linné, "From Rice Eaters to Soy Boys: Race, Gender, and Tropes of 'Plant Food Masculinity,'" *Animals Studies Journal* 7, no. 2 (2018): 128–79.

 7 Since much has already been written on the relationship between men, animals, and meat—see Brian Luke, *Brutal: Manhood and the Exploitation of Animals* (Champaign: University of Illinois Press, 2007)—I have decided to focus here instead on the changing role of women in the meat economy. An earlier version of this chapter appeared as "Murder, She Wrote: Legitimating the Meat Economy with 'Femivorism,'" in *The Humane Hoax*, ed. Hope Bohanec (New York: Lantern Books, 2023), 61–84.

 8 Lily McCaulou, *The Call of the Mild: Learning to Hunt My Own Dinner* (New York: Grand Central Publishing/Hachette, 2012), 238.

 9 Quoted in Adams, *Sexual Politics of Meat*, 123.

10 Peggy Orenstein, "The Femivore's Dilemma: Can Chickens Save the Desperate Housewife?," *New York Times*, March 14, 2010.

11 Betty Friedan, *The Feminine Mystique* (New York: W. W. Norton and Co., 1963), 15–21. Friedan mostly interviewed educated white, heterosexual, middle- or upper-class women, making her analysis all the more relevant for my discussion

here, since most "femivore" authors are drawn from much the same demographic.

12 Camas Davis, *Killing It: An Education* (New York: Penguin, 2019).

13 Woginrich, *Barnheart.*

14 Woginrich, *One-Woman Farm*, 45.

15 Ibid., 16.

16 Jessie Knadler, *Rurally Screwed: A Memoir of Losing Myself for Love* (New York: Berkley/Penguin, 2013).

17 McMinn, *Chickens in the Road*, 127, 165.

18 Kimball, *Dirty Life*, 4.

19 Woginrich, *One-Woman Farm*, 80.

20 Kimball, *Dirty Life*, 92.

21 McMinn, *Chickens in the Road.*

22 Woginrich, *One-Woman Farm*, 119.

23 Josh Kilmer-Purcell, *The Bucolic Plague: How Two Manhattanites Became Gentlemen Farmers* (New York: Harper Perennial, 2011).

24 Kingsolver, 93.

25 Other media outlets quickly took up Orenstein's neologism, and "femivore" found its way into the Urban Dictionary.

26 Catherine Friend, *Hit By a Farm: How I Learned to Stop Worrying and Love the Barn* (Boston: Da Capo Press, 2006), 27.

27 Woginrich, *One-Woman Farm*, 111.

28 Ellen Stimson, *Mud Season: How One Woman's Dream of Moving to Vermont Raising Children, Chickens, and Sheep & Running the Old Country Store Pretty Much Led to One Calamity After Another* (Woodstock, VT: Countryman/W. W. Norton, 2013), 163, 165.

29 Friend, *Hit By a Farm*, 113.

30 McMinn, *Chickens*, 116.

31 Friend, *Hit By a Farm*, 217; Friend, *Sheepish*, 72.

32 Friend, *Sheepish*, 76.

33 Woginrich, *One-Woman Farm*, 109.

34 Woginrich, *Barnheart*, 102.

35 McMinn, *Chickens in the Road*, 156.

36 Woginrich, *Made from Scratch*, 119.

37 Susan McCorkindale, *500 Acres and No Place to Hide: More Confessions of a Counterfeit Farm Girl* (New York: Berkley/Penguin, 2011), 300.

38 Friend, *Sheepish*, 90.

39 McMinn, *Chickens in the Road*, 156.

40 Kingsolver, 89.

41 Novella Carpenter, *Farm City: The Education of an Urban Farmer* (New York: Penguin, 2010), 92.

42 Friend, *Hit By a Farm*, 153.

43 Carpenter, *Farm City*, 194.

44 Ibid., 224.

45 James Baldwin, *Notes from a Native Son* (Boston: Beacon Press, 1951), 14.

46 Gabrielle Hamilton, *Blood, Bones & Butter: The Inadvertent Education of a Reluctant Chef* (New York: Random House, 2012), 19.

47 Kimball, *Dirty Life*, 128.

48 McMinn, *Chickens in the Road*, 223.

49 Friend, *Sheepish*, 8.

50 McMinn, *Chickens in the Road*, 87.

51 McCaulou, *The Call of the Mild*, 112, 114, 185.

52 Keith, *The Vegetarian Myth*, 5, 79.

53 Carpenter, *Farm City*, 94.

54 Ibid., 245–46.

55 Ibid., 76.

56 Ibid, 158.

57 Friend, *Sheepish*, 4.

58 Ibid., 68.

59 Woginrich, *One-Woman Farm*, 93.

60 Kimball, *Dirty Life*, 35; Carpenter, *Farm City*, 55. On the close association between hunting, sexual desire, and masculinity, see Kheel, 38–39.

61 McCaulou, *Call of the Mild*, 185.

62 McMinn, *Chickens in the Road*, 219.

63 Kimball, *The Dirty Life*, 10.

64 Ibid., 196.

65 Nancy Hartsock, *Money, Sex, and Power* (Boston: Northeastern University Press, 1983), 177, 176.

66 Herbert Marcuse, "Aggressiveness in Advanced Industrialized Society," in *Negations* (Boston: Beacon Press, 1970), 257.

67 Meredith Leigh, *The Ethical Meat Handbook* (Gabriola Island, BC: New Society Publishers, 2015), 84. Kristin Kimball similarly tells her fiancée that if she should die, she wants him to *compost her*. "And I hope something eats my heart and my liver. After I've eaten so many other creatures' hearts and livers, *it's the least I can do*." (Kimball, 197, emphasis added).

68 Christine Lennon, "Why Vegetarians Are Eating Meat," *Food & Wine*, June 26, 2017.

69 Adrienne Rich, "Toward a Woman-Centered University," in *On Lies, Secrets, and Silences* (New York: W. W. Norton, 1980), 130.

70 Susan Faludi, *Backlash: The Undeclared War Against American Women* (New York: Crown, 1991), 1.

71 Kimball, 22.

72 "All of these gals—these chicks with chicks—are stay-at-home moms, highly educated women who left the work force to care for kith and kin. I don't think

that's a coincidence: the omnivore's dilemma has provided an unexpected out from the feminist predicament, a way for women to embrace homemaking without becoming Betty Draper," the alienated housewife from the TV series *Mad Men*. Orenstein, "The Femivore's Dilemma."

73 Laura Ingalls Wilder's *Little House on the Prairie* is cited by several memoirists as a source of inspiration for their rural experiments.

74 Kim Severson, "Young Butchers with Cleavers Rule the Stage," *New York Times*, July 7, 2009.

75 Camas Davis has little to say about her relationship with her mother, but a great deal about her relationship with her father, "a lifelong hunter and fisherman, who handed me my first pocketknife" and who taught her to kill. *Killing It*, 14.

76 Friend, *Hit by a Barn*, 13, 171–72.

77 McCorkindale, *500 Acres*.

78 Kimball, *Dirty Life*, 28.

79 McCaulou, *Call of the Mild*, 41.

80 "Animal Well Being," Tyson Foods, accessed Jan. 30, 2020, http://34.202.97.133/sustainability/animal-well-being.

81 "Bovidiva" is short for "Bovine Diva." Judith Capper, "Do Moms Have Instant Beef Credibility?," Bovidiva, posted Nov. 14, 2013, accessed January 2020, https://bovidiva.com.

82 Curators at the Museum praised the aesthetics of Grandin's "serpentine ramp." Even Ingrid Newkirk, the director of PETA, contributed an essay on the MOMA website, praising Grandin's design. Discussion of *Design and Violence*, a MOMA book by Paula Antonelli, https://www.moma.org.

83 *She Was There for Me: The Story of Jenny Brown & Woodstock Farm Sanctuary*, directed by Andy Stepanian (FitzGibbon Media, 2015), https://vimeo.com/137158633.

84 Sixty percent of vegans in Britain, and nearly 80% of vegans in the US, are women. Alex Lockwood, "Why Aren't More Men Vegan?," *Plant-Based News*, Feb. 21, 2018.

85 Kate Millett, *The Loony-Bin Trip* (New York: Simon & Schuster, 1990), 114.

86 Ibid., 115.

87 Ibid., 122–23.

8. HARRY LIME DISEASE

1 Pollan, *Omnivore*, 68.

2 Psychopathy and sociopathy both denote an inability to empathize with others, a disregard for laws and rules, and an incapacity for remorse. However, sociopaths tend to be more emotionally volatile than psychopaths, and some are able to form emotional attachments with others. Some researchers believe that psychopathy has a strong genetic component, unlike sociopathy.

3 Heidi L. Maibom, in Thomas Schramme, ed., *Being Amoral: Psychopathy and Moral Incapacity* (Cambridge, MA: MIT Press, 2014), 91.

4 Maurice Hamington, *Embodied Care: Jane Addams, Merleau-Ponty, and the Caring Imagination* (Champaign: University of Illinois Press, 2004).

5 Jérôme Englebert, "A New Understanding of Psychopathy: The Contribution of Phenomenological Psychopathology," *Psychopathology* 48, no. 6 (2015): 368–75, doi.org/10.1159/000437441.

6 On the phenomenology of empathy in moral performance, see Arne Vetlesen, *Perception, Empathy, and Judgment: An Inquiry into the Nature of Moral Performance* (University Park: Penn State University Press, 2004).

7 "Ask a Psychopath—What Are Some of the Things You've Done?," PsychopathyIs channel on YouTube, posted 2021, accessed Nov. 2023, https://www.youtube.com/watch?v=fzfVtDPRzto.

8 Gwen Adshead, "The Words But Not the Music: Empathy, Language Deficits, and Psychopathy," in Schramme, 117. "For psychopaths," observes Heidi Maibom, "an action's harmfulness does not appear to count against, and sometimes counts in favor of, performing it." Maibom, 91.

9 Adshead, 117.

10 Ibid.

11 Pollan, *Omnivore*, 359.

12 J. H. Johns and H. C. Quay, "The Effect of Social Reward on Verbal Conditioning in Psychopathic Military Offenders," *Journal of Consulting Psychology* (1962), cited by Adshead, 116.

13 Pollan, *Omnivore*, 330.

14 Kerrin A. Jacobs, "Psychopathic Comportment and Moral Incapacity," in Schramme, 147.

15 "Interview with Psychiatrist Dr. Park Dietz," *The Iceman and the Psychiatrist*, directed by Arthur Ginsberg, HBO, 2003.

16 Kimball, *The Dirty Life*, 196.

17 Interview with Tommy Lynn Sells, "Cold-Blooded Killers," *Most Evil*, season 1, episode 2, Discovery Channel, 2006.

18 Scott Bonn, "How To Tell a Psychopath from a Sociopath," *Psychology Today*, Jan. 22, 2014.

19 Dawl Drzal, "'Eating Skillfully': An Englishwoman Falls in Love with China and Its Food," *New York Times Book Review*, July 20, 2008, 17.

20 Quoted by Julia Moskin, "Chef's New Goal: Looking Dinner in the Eye," *New York Times*, Jan. 1, 2008, Dining Section, 4.

21 Schwartz Media, "Food Fighters: AA Gill and Anthony Bourdain in Conversation," video, at 49:54, May 3, 2013, https://www.youtube.com/watch?v=F2tjvTmbEVw.

22 Robert C. Jones, "Modern Foodie Culture: A Celebration of Violence," in Bohanec, *Humane Hoax*, 275–90.

23 "Locavore Learns to Slaughter and Butcher His Own Pork," *Oregonian*, Feb. 1, 2010.

24 Judith Herman, *Trauma and Recovery: The Aftermath of Violence—from Domestic Abuse to Political Terror* (New York: Basic Books, 2022), 10.

25 Charles Darwin, *Expression of the Emotions in Man and Animals* (New York: Philosophical Library, 1955), 10, 85.

26 Frans de Waal, *Are We Smart Enough To Know How Smart Animals Are?* (New York: W. W. Norton, 2016), 67.

27 Ibid., 135.

28 Marc Beckoff, *Minding Animals* (Oxford: Oxford University Press, 2002), 102.

29 "Monkey Saves Dying Friend at Indian Train Station," *Guardian* (courtesy Reuters), Dec. 22, 2014.

30 Felicity Muth, "Can Pigs Empathize?," blog, *Scientific American*, Jan. 13, 2015, https://blogs.scientificamerican.com.

31 De Waal, 133. See also de Waal, *The Age of Empathy: Nature's Lessons for a Kinder Society* (New York: Crown, 2010).

32 Masson and McCarthy, 159.

33 Emily Underwood, "Rats Forsake Chocolate to Save a Drowning Companion," *Science*, May 12, 2015.

34 Konrad Lorenz, *Here I Am—Where Are You? A Lifetime's Study of the Uncannily Human Behavior of the Greylag Goose* (New York: HarperCollins, 1992).

35 Masson and McCarthy, 117.

36 "20 Years Ago Today: Brookfield Zoo Gorilla Helps Boy Who Fell into Habitat," *Chicago Tribune*, Aug. 16, 2016.

37 Masson and McCarthy, 155.

38 Pollan, *Omnivore*, 66.

39 Ibid., 66.

40 Ibid., 80. Pollan has repeatedly claimed, without scientific evidence, that farmed species are "stupid." "Meat birds are not like hens. Their brains have been bred right out of them, they're really nasty and stupid. . . . [B]y the time they were mature, I couldn't wait to kill them." In Ruth Reichl, "Michael Pollan and Ruth Reichl Hash Out the Food Revolution," *Smithsonian*, June 2013.

41 Harold Brown, "Farmkind," in *Turning Points in Compassion: Personal Journeys of Animal Advocates*, ed. Gypsy Wulff and Fran Chambers (n.p.: Spiritwings, 2014), 1–3.

42 Pema Chödrön, *Welcoming the Unwelcome: Wholehearted Living in a Brokenhearted World* (Boulder, CO: Shambhala, 2019), 17.

9. BLOOD AND SOIL

1 Portions of this chapter were originally published in "The Animal of Bad Faith," in *Critical Animal Studies: Thinking the Unthinkable*, ed. John Sorenson (Toronto: Canadian Scholars Press, 2014), 29–45.

2 Ian Austen, "Canadians Outraged After Report of Mass Killing of Sled Dogs," *New York Times*, Feb. 1, 2011.

3 Robert Matas and Sunny Dhillon, "Post-Olympic Slaughter of 70 Sled Dogs Prompts Rage, Embarrassment," *The Globe and Mail*, Jan. 31, 2011.

4 Ibid.

5 Saul Friedlander, *The Origins of Nazi Genocide* (Chapel Hill: University of North Carolina Press, 1997), 15.

6 Friedlander, 287.

7 Nestar Russell, *Willing Participants: Milgram's Obedience Experiments and the Holocaust*, vol. 2 (New York: Springer/Palgrave MacMillan, 2019), 245.

8 Ibid., 253.

9 *Shoah*, directed by Claude Lanzmann (New Yorker Films, 1985).

10 Quoted in Daniel Winters, "Tell Your Story But Keep It Real: Temple Grandin," *Canadian Cattlemen: The Beef Magazine*, June 1, 2012 (courtesy GFM Network News).www.canadiancattlemen.ca. A print version of this article originally appeared in *The Cooperator* (Oak Lake, Manitoba), May 31, 2012.

11 Ibid. Grandin seems unaware that the very neurological condition that she claims has given her special access to the experiences of animals would have landed her in the gas chambers of the Third Reich: Hans Asperger, the Nazi scientist who coined the term "autism" and was the first to describe the condition clinically, sent scores of autistic children to their deaths in the T4 program.

12 Karen Davis, "Black Eagle: An Organic Egg Farm Revisited," *Poultry Press* 21, no. 4 (Winter 2011–12), available at United Poultry Concerns website, www. upc-online.org.

13 "Thank You, Temple Grandin," blog, Dalla Terra Ranch, accessed June 2016, http://www.dallaterraranch.com. My emphasis.

14 Martin Gilbert, *Final Journey: The Fate of the Jews in Nazi Europe* (New York: Mayflower Books, 1979), 63.

15 Raul Hilberg, *Documents of Destruction* (Chicago: Quadrangle Books, 1971), 87.

16 C. R. Browning, *Ordinary Men: Reserve Police Battalion 101 and the Final Solution in Poland* (New York: Harper Perennial, 1998). Cited in Russell, *Willing Participants*, 253.

17 Russell, *Willing Participants*, 247, citing J. Toland, *Adolf Hitler* (New York: Doubleday, 1976).

18 Robert Payne, *The Life and Death of Adolf Hitler* (New York: Praeger, 1973).

19 Mathieu Ricard, *A Plea for the Animals: The Moral, Philosophical, and Evolutionary Imperative to Treat All Beings with Compassion* (Boulder, CO: Shambhala, 2016), 90.

20 Peter Singer and Helga Kuhse, *Should the Baby Live? The Problem of Handicapped Infants* (Oxford: Oxford University Press, 1985), 18, 30.

21 Ibid., 89, 93.

22 Ibid.

23 William P. Alford, "The Discordant Singer: How Peter Singer's Treatment of Global Poverty and Disability Is Inconsistent and Why It Matters," *American Journal of Law and Equality* 1 (2021): 194–220, doi.org/10.1162/ajle_a_00014.

24 Singer and Kuhse, 170.

25 Ibid., 192.

26 Martha Nussbaum, *Justice for Animals* (Chicago: University of Chicago Press, 2023), 156.

27 Adam Beresford, "Introduction," in Aristotle, *Nichomachean Ethics*, ed. and trans. Beresford (New York: Penguin Random House, 2020), xxxiv.

28 Killing and eating an animal "is a deep way to connect with an animal's spirit," Kathy Rudy avers in *Loving Animals*, 84.

29 Jason Mark, "The Moral Case for Meat," *Sierra*, Feb. 24, 2017.

30 Hence Kathy Rudy's assertion that, while "farm animals pay their dues in life with their products and flesh," it is a fair exchange, since "animals would rather have been alive for a while," having "lived and loved and played in the sun and the dirt and the rain, than not to be born at all." Even violent death is a small "sacrifice" for the animals to make in exchange for "the joy of living." Rudy, *Loving Animals*, 99. The same argument was also a staple in Antebellum apologia for slavery: slavery apologist William Harper, e.g., maintained that "man gives the boon of existence to myriads who would never otherwise have enjoyed it, and the enjoyment of their existence is better provided for while it lasts." *Memoir on Slavery* (1852), cited in Faust, *Ideology of Slavery*. The Nazis held similar views. "[M]an is the master; he has taken into his household the animals and plants which he keeps either for his use or for his pleasure. He gives them shelter, food, and care . . . and he holds their lives in his hands. Without him most of the organisms he keeps as domestic animals or indoor plants would perish." Paul Brohmer (Nazi biologist), *Biologieunterricht und völkische Erziehung* (Frankfurt: Verlag Moritz Diesterweg, 1933), translated and published as "The New Biology: Training in Racial Citizenship," in George L. Mosse, *Nazi Culture: Intellectual, Cultural, and Social Life in the Third Reich* (New York: Schocken Books, 1966), 86.

31 Keith, *The Vegetarian Myth*.

32 Quoted in Corrina Treitel, *Eating Nature in Modern Germany: Food, Agriculture, and Environment* (Cambridge: Cambridge University Press, 2017), 212. See also Ben Kiernan, *Blood and Soil: A World History of Genocide and Extermination from Sparta to Darfur* (New Haven, CT: Yale, 2007).

33 David Welch, *Propaganda and the German Cinema, 1933–1945* (London: I. B. Taurus, 2001), 90.

34 Kiernan, 429.

35 Filippo Tommaso Marinetti's aestheticization of masculine violence and war in *Manifesto of Futurism* (1909) influenced Mussolini's conception of fascism. On

Hitler's aestheticization of violence, see Frederic Spotts, *Hitler and the Power of Aesthetics* (Woodstock, NY: Overlook Press, 2003), especially his chapter "Purification by Death," 113–20. See also *Architecture of Doom*, dir. by Peter Cohen (Sandrew Film & Teater AB, Stockholm, 1989).

36 Tim Snyder, "Hitler's World," *New York Review of Books*, Sept. 24, 2015.

37 Dan Stone, "The Far Right and the Back to the Land Movement," in Julie V. Gottlieb and Thomas P. Linehan, eds., *The Culture of Fascism: Visions of the Far Right in Britain* (London: I. B. Taurus, 2004), 186–88. See also "John Sanbonmatsu Replies to Derrick Jensen," *Upping the Anti* (Sept. 9, 2011).

38 Rudolf Höss, *Kommandant in Auschwitz: Autobiographische Aufzeichnungen* (1958), quoted in Stangneth, *Eichmann Before Jerusalem: The Unexplained Life of a Mass Murderer* (New York: Knopf, 2014), 224.

39 Ibid, Stangneth.

40 Pollan, *Omnivore*, 232.

41 Ibid., 271, 237.

42 Karen Davis, "Do Chickens Mind Seeing Other Chickens Killed?," United Poultry Concerns podcast, March 10, 2023, https://upc-online.org/. Scientific studies have confirmed empathy in chickens. Lori Marino, (2017). "Thinking Chickens: A Review of Cognition, Emotion, and Behavior in the Domestic Chicken," *Animal Cognition* 20 (2), 2017: 127–147, doi.org/10.1007/s10071-016-1064-4.

43 Pollan, *Omnivore*, 233, 236, 271, 234.

44 Russell, *Willing Participants*, 257.

45 Quoted in Kiernan, 427. As a fugitive after the war, Adolph Eichmann made a furtive living in Germany and Argentina raising chickens and Angora rabbits for slaughter. Stangneth aptly describes Adolph Eichmann, the Nazi bureaucrat who arranged the logistics of the Holocaust, as "hostile to life."

46 Quoted in A. Arluke and B. Sax, "Understanding Nazi Animal Protection and the Holocaust," *Anthrozoös* 5, no. 1 (1992): 20.

47 Treitel, 206. Compare Michael Pollan's polemic against "processed" corporate foods with Himmler's desire to wrest control over agriculture out of "the hands of the food industries" because "the artificial is everywhere, everywhere food is adulterated, provided with ingredients which are said to make it last longer or look better or enrich it or anything else that the advertisers of the food industry care to say." "Artificial fertilizers," Fritz Wirz similarly warned, "interrupt the natural metabolism between man and his environment, between blood and soil." Both quoted in Treitel, *Eating Nature*, 204, 212.

48 Broadside issued in Nowy Sacz (Poland) announcing a meat rationing order. Anordnung / Zarzadzenie, Neu-Sandez, March 6, 1940. United States Holocaust Memorial Museum Collection.

49 Treitel, 8, 1–2.

50 Patterson, *Eternal Treblinka*, 125–129.

51 Ian Kershew, *Hitler: A Biography* (New York: W. W. Norton & Co., 2008), 952.

52 Jean-Paul Sartre, *Anti-Semite and Jew* (New York: Schocken, 1995), 17.

53 Ibid., 27.

54 Ibid., 38, 20.

55 Ibid., 150.

56 Allison Callahan, "Quiz: Test Your Protein," *New York Times*, Nov. 16, 2023. Thanks to years of propaganda by the US meat industry, many Americans worry that they may not be getting enough protein. In fact, most Americans already get more protein than they need. Kenny Torrella, "You're Probably Eating Way Too Much Protein," VOX, Jan. 30, 2024, vox. com. A further objection to veganism is that it is "too expensive." But food staples like pasta, legumes, flour, potatoes, etc., are cheaper than most animal products, notwithstanding government subsidies to the beef, pork, dairy, and egg industries that keep the prices of animal products artificially low.

57 The rhetorical plausibility of Orwell's allegory (a satire of Stalinism) rests on our ability to recognize the similarities between animal agriculture, on one side, and slavery and totalitarianism, on the other. Only beings capable of freedom are capable of being *unfree*, even in literary fiction: not even a writer of Orwell's talents could have drawn a convincing analogy between Stalinism and a brutal state run by, say, orange trees or cucumbers.

58 Primo Levi, *Survival in Auschwitz*, trans. Stuart Woolf (New York: Macmillan Publishing Co., 1986; originally published 1958), 121.

59 "Not every being with a human face is human," the Nazi jurist Carl Schmitt declared. Quoted in Claudia Koonz, *The Nazi Conscience* (Cambridge, MA: Harvard University Press, 2003), 2.

60 Concentration of a population by force is the prelude to killing them. In a notable lapse, Michael Pollan mistakenly (and repeatedly) misdefines CAFO in *Omnivore's Dilemma* as "Confined" Animal Feeding Operation, rather than Concentrated Animal Feeding Operation.

61 Friedlander, 81.

62 The nonprofit group Our Honor (www.OurHonor.org), founded by veterinarian Dr. Crystal Heath, is working to get the American Veterinary Medical Association to stop participating in animal exploitation.

63 Isaac Bashevis Singer, "The Letter Writer," *The New Yorker*, Jan. 13, 1968.

64 The Nazis not only applied principles of animal husbandry to their eugenics program, but borrowed techniques from the American system of mechanized animal slaughter to effect their genocide. Patterson, *Eternal Treblinka*.

65 Jacques Derrida, "The Animal That Therefore I Am," in *Animal Philosophy: Essential Readings in Continental Thought*, ed. Matthew Calarco and Peter Atterton (New York: Continuum, 2004), 120. Originally published in French (1999).

66 Charles Siebert, "An Elephant Crackup?," *New York Times Magazine*, Oct. 8, 2006.

67 Sartre, 49.

68 Ibid., 21.

69 Goethe, *Faust*, Part One, trans. Philip Wayne (Harmondsworth, UK: Penguin Books, Ltd., 1949), 40.

10. ANIMAL, NOT VEGETABLE

1 Pollan, *Omnivore*, 323.

2 Derrick Jensen, *A Language Older than Words* (New York: Chelsea Green, 2004), 104. Emphasis added.

3 McCaulou, 174.

4 "People will see very different things when they look into the eyes of a pig or chicken or a steer: a being without a soul, a 'subject of a life' entitled to rights, a receptable of pleasure and pain, an unambiguously tasty lunch" (Pollan, *Omnivore*, 332). Without argument, Pollan suggests that we cannot meaningfully decide between these different ontological and ethical claims.

5 Joel Sachs, in Aristotle, *On the Soul and On Memory and Recollection*, trans. Joel Sachs (Santa Fe, NM: Green Lion, 2004), 4, 6.

6 Rebecca Giggs, "A Better Way To Look at Trees," *Atlantic*, Aug./Sept. 2021.

7 David G. Robinson, and Andreas Draguhn, "Plants Have Neither Synapses Nor a Nervous System," *Journal of Plant Physiology* 263 (2021), doi.org/10.1016/j.jplph.2021.153467.

8 The phenomenological method is another means for knowing the experiences of other animals. See Corinne Painter and Christian Lotz, *Phenomenology and the Non-human Animal* (Dordrecht, Germany: Springer, 2007); Jennifer McWeeny, "Sounding Depth with the North Atlantic Right Whale and Merleau-Ponty," *Journal of Critical Animal Studies* 9, no. 1–2 (2011): 144–66.

9 Aristotle, *History of Animals*, Book VIII, http://classics.mit.edu.

10 Quoted in Peter Singer, *Animal Liberation*, 187.

11 Some authors have nevertheless found a basis for animal ethics in Christian teachings. See Andrew Linzey, *Animal Theology: Respecting the Worth and Rights of Animals* (Champaign: University of Illinois Press, 1995), and Matthew Scully, *Dominion: The Power of Man, the Suffering of Animals, and the Call to Mercy* (New York: St. Martin's Press, 2003).

12 René Descartes, Letter to the Marquess of Newcastle (1646), quoted in S. J. Armstrong, and R. G. Botzler, eds., *Environmental Ethics: Divergence and Convergence* (New York: McGraw Hill, 1993), 281–85.

13 Quoted in Masson and McCarthy, 165. B. F. Skinner chastised scientists who shrank from violence against animals in the lab, advocating "a language of control and domination" and "behavioral engineering and manipulation." De Waal, *Are We Smart Enough*, 37.

14 Mary Midgley, *The Solitary Self: Darwin and the Solitary Gene* (New York: Routledge, 2014).

15 Yaniv Assaf, Arieli Bouznach, Omri Zomet, Assaf Marom, and Yossi Yovel, "Conservation of Brain Connectivity and Wiring Across the Mammalian Class," *Nature Neuroscience* 23, no. 7 (2020): 805, doi.org/10.1038/s41593-020-0641-7.

16 "Are We Alone? PBS's NOVA Wonders," SETI Institute, May 9, 2018, https://www.seti.org.

17 Jonathan Balcombe, *What a Fish Knows: The Inner Lives of Our Underwater Cousins* (n.p.: Scientific American/Farrar, Straus, Giroux, 2017), 31.

18 David Tayman, "Howard Pets: Whose Nose Is Keener, Cat or Dog?," *Baltimore Sun*, April 1, 2011.

19 Peter Tyson, "Dogs' Dazzling Sense of Smell," *PBS Nova*, Oct. 4, 2012, https://www.pbs.org/wgbh.

20 Howard Gardner, *Frames of Mind* (New York: Basic Books, 1983).

21 De Waal, *Are We Smart Enough.* Beckoff, *Minding Animals,* 152.

22 "Jane Goodall," *National Geographic* 188, no. 6 (Dec. 1995): 107.

23 Gretchen Vogel, "Wild Gorillas Pick Up Tools," *Science,* Sept. 30, 2005.

24 R. G. Northcutt, "Variation in Reptilian Brains and Cognition," *Brain, Behavior, and Evolution* 82, no. 1 (2013): 45–54; A. L. Vail, A. Manica, and R. Bshary, "Fish Choose Appropriately When and with Whom to Collaborate," *Current Biology* 24, no. 17 (2014): R791–R793, Correspondence.

25 De Waal, *Are We Smart Enough,* 93.

26 See, for example, "Green Heron Catching Fish," YouTube, https://www.youtube.com/watch?v=Porp5v5lLKk, Accessed June 17, 2022.

27 Liza Langley, "Dolphins Learn How to Use Tools from Peers, Just Like Great Apes," *National Geographic,* June 25, 2020; Mark Peter Simmonds, "Into the Brains of Whales" in S. J. Armstrong and R. B. Botzler, *The Animal Ethics Reader* (New York: Routledge, 2008), 195.

28 Anuschka de Rohan, "Deep Thinkers: The More We Study Dolphins, the Brighter They Turn Out To Be," *The Guardian,* July 3, 2003.

29 David Grimm and Greg Miller, "Is a Dolphin a Person?," *Science,* February 21, 2010.

30 De Waal, *Are We Smart Enough,* 76.

31 Lesley J. Rogers, *Minds of Their Own: Thinking and Awareness in Animals* (New York: Routledge, 1998), 74.

32 Johan Lind, Magnus Enquist, Stefano Ghirlanda, "Animal Memory: A Review of Delayed Matching-to-sample Data," *Behavioural Processes* 117 (2015): 52–58.

33 De Waal, *Are We Smart Enough,* 119–20.

34 "Chimp vs. Human! Memory Test," *BBC Earth.* Posted on YouTube Dec. 25, 2013. https://www.youtube.com/watch?v=zsXP8qeFF6A. Accessed August 4, 2022.

35 Rogers, *Minds of Their Own,* 73.

36 Russell P. Baldo and Alan C. Kamil, "Long-term Spatial Memory in Clark's Nutcracker, *Nucifraga columbiana*," *Animal Behaviour* 44, no. 4 (Oct. 1992): 761–69.

37 Jane E. Brody, "Not Just Music, Bird Song Is a Means of Courtship and Defense," *New York Times*, April 9, 1991.

38 De Waal, *Are We Smart Enough*, 72.

39 Darwin, *Expression of the Emotions*, 165–66.

40 De Waal, 263.

41 James Ritchie, "Fact or Fiction? Elephants Never Forget," *Scientific American*, Jan. 12, 2009.

42 W. F. Fagan, "Migrating Whales Depend on Memory to Exploit Reliable Resources," *PNAS*, 116, no. 12 (2019): 5217–19.

43 Balcombe, *What a Fish Knows*, 106–7.

44 Rogers, *Minds of Their Own*, 72.

45 P. Carruthers, "Evolution of Working Memory," *PNAS* 18, no. 110 (suppl. 2) (June 2013): 10371–78, doi.org/10.1073/pnas.1301195110.

46 Balcombe, *What a Fish Knows*, 43.

47 Theodore Xenophon Barber, *The Human Nature of Birds* (New York: St. Martin's Press, 1993), 58–70.

48 Johan J. Bolhuis and Martin Everaert, *Birdsong, Speech, and Language: Exploring the Evolution of Mind and Brain* (Cambridge, MA: MIT Press, 2013).

49 Martin Stacho, Christina Herold, Noemi Rook, et al., "A Cortex-Like Canonical Circuit in the Avian Forebrain," *Science* 369, no. 6511 (Sept. 2020), doi. org/10.1126/science.abc5534.

50 The brains of birds are packed with "six times as many nerve cells as humans per cubic millimetre of brain." "Pigeons Better at Multitasking Than Humans," *ScienceDaily*, September 26. 2017. Note: the researchers at the Ruhr-Universitaet-Bochum who conducted this study later retracted their earlier findings: pigeons and humans in fact have comparable multitasking skills.

51 "Bird Brain? Birds and Humans Have Similar Brain Wiring," *Science Daily* (July 2013).

52 B. De Corte, V. M. Navarro, and E. A. Wasserman, "Non-cortical Magnitude Coding of Space and Time by Pigeons," *Current Biology* 27, no. 23 (2017): R1264–R1265. Pigeons taught to distinguish Bach from Stravinsky were later able to correctly identify "Buxtehude and Scarlatti as Bach-like and Eliot Carter and Walter Piston as Stravinsky-like." Jane E. Brody, "Not Just Music, Bird Song Is a Means of Courtship and Defense," *New York Times*, April 9, 1991, C1.

53 Carolynn L. Smith and Sarah Zielinski, "Brainy Bird," *Scientific American*, Feb. 2014, 62.

54 Montaigne, "Apologies for Raymond Sebond," in *The Essays of Montaigne*, trans. E. J. Trenchman (New York: Modern Library, 1946), 382–83.

55 Psychologist John W. Pilley taught Chaser, his border collie, to remember the names of over a thousand different plush toys. Chaser also demonstrated a capacity for inferential logic.

56 Christopher Solomon, "When Birds Squawk, Other Species Seem To Listen," *New York Times*, May 18, 2015.

57 Sue Savage-Rumbaugh, William M. Fields, and Jared Taglialatela, "Ape Consciousness—Human Consciousness: A Perspective Informed by Language and Culture," in *Animal Ethics Reader*, ed. Armstrong and Botzler, 161.

58 Ewen Callaway, "Parrot's Posthumous Paper Shows His Mathematical Genius," *Nature* (Feb. 2012), doi.org/10.1038/nature.2012.10071.

59 Rogers, *Minds of Their Own*, 38.

60 Con Slobodchikoff, "Animal Language and Prairie Dogs," Australia Animal Studies Association, posted March 2, 2021, cited in *Chasing Doctor Dolittle: Learning the Language of Animals* (New York: St. Martin's Press, 2012); Ferris Jabr, "Can Prairie Dogs Talk?," *New York Times*, May 12, 2017.

61 Quoted in *Chris Packham's Animal Einsteins*, series 1, episode 5, dir. by Dan Slee, BBC, 2021.

62 Lars Chittka and Jeremy Niven, "Are Bigger Brains Better?," *Current Biology* 19, no. 21 (2009): 995–1008. Note, however, the residual Cartesianism in Chittka and Niven's mechanistic descriptions of insect brains.

63 Antoine Wystrach, "We've Been Looking at Ant Intelligence the Wrong Way," published in *The Conversation*, reprinted in *Scientific American*, August 30, 2013.

64 Zipporah Weisberg, "Biotechnology as End Game: Ontological and Ethical Collapse in the 'Biotech Century,'" *NanoEthics* 9, no. 1 (2015), 39–54, doi.org/10.1007/s11569-014-0219-5.

65 Maurice Merleau-Ponty, *The Structure of Behavior* (Boston: Beacon Press, 1963; originally published in French in 1942), 148.

66 Ibid., 45.

67 Mario Pahl, Aung Si, and Shaowu Chang, "Numerical Cognition in Bees and Other Insects," *Frontiers of Psychology* 4 (2013), doi.org/10.3389/fpsyg.2013.00162.

68 Brian Handwerk, "Bees Can Learn to Play 'Soccer,'" *Smithsonian*, Feb. 24, 2017.

69 Chittka and Niven.

70 Meghan Barrett and Bob Fischer, "Challenges in Farmed Insect Welfare: Beyond the Question of Sentience," *Animal Welfare* 32 (2023): e4, doi.org/10.1017/awf.2022.5. Matt Reynolds, "Insect Farming Is Booming. But Is It Cruel?," *Wired*, March 16, 2023.

71 Henry Beston, *The Outermost House: A Year of Life on the Great Beach of Cape Cod* (New York: Viking Press, 1962; originally published 1928), 25.

11. PERSONS, NOT THINGS

1 Quoted in Jake Pearson, "Lawyer: Confinement of Chimps for Research Akin to Slavery," Phys.Org, May 27, 2015, https://phys.org.

2 Paraphrased by Pearson, Ibid.

3 Brandon Keim, "Chimpanzee Rights Get a Day in Court," *Wired*, May 27, 2015.

4 Immanuel Kant, *Grounding for the Metaphysics of Morals*, 3rd ed., trans. James W. Ellington (Indianapolis: Hackett Publishing, 1981), 35.

5 Sue Donaldson and Will Kymlicka, *Zoopolis: A Political Theory of Animal Rights* (Oxford: Oxford University Press, 2013), 27.

6 Tracy Tullis, "The World's Loneliest Elephant," *New York Times*, June 26, 2015.

7 "Brief of Amicus Curiae Laurence H. Tribe, The Nonhuman Rights Project, Inc., on Behalf of Happy, Appellate-Petitioner" (New York Supreme Court, Appellate Case No. 2020–02581, 2020).

8 Kant's conception of personhood relied on a hidden category of "sub-persons" that excluded non-European peoples from the category of "persons." Charles W. Mills, *Black Rights/White Wrongs: The Critique of Racial Liberalism* (New York: Oxford, 2017).

9 One problem with the mirror test is that it relies on a single sense modality—sight—even though many species rely more on other sensory modalities. Maggie Koerth-Baker, "Kids (and Animals) Who Fail Classic Mirror Tests May Still Have Sense of Self," *Scientific American*, Nov. 29, 2010.

10 Animals who see others being harmed may themselves exhibit symptoms of trauma, suggesting that their sense of self is connected to the well-being of others. (Psychologist Lori Marino speculates that orcas may have social emotions we lack entirely.) The sled dogs massacred at Whistler Adventures in Vancouver had come to trust their human overseers; yet when they saw Robert Fawcett, an employee they had long worked with, suddenly start shooting and stabbing dogs to death, they knew what was happening and fought valiantly for their lives.

11 V. Reddy, E. Williams, C. Constantini, and B. Lan, "Engaging with the Self: Mirror Behaviour in Autism, Down Syndrome and Typical Development," *Autism* 14, no. 5 (2010): 531–46, doi.org/10.1177/1362361310370397. See also Koerth-Baker, Ibid.

12 Tom Regan, "The Case for Animal Rights," in *In Defense of Animals*, ed. Peter Singer (New York: Harper Collins, 1986). Regan initially limited the term "subject of a life" to mammals, but later expanded it to include birds and other classes of animals.

13 Among others, Paola Cavalieri, *The Animal Question: Why Nonhuman Animals Deserve Human Rights*, trans. by Catherine Woollard (New York: Oxford University Press, 2001), and Gary Francione, *Animals as Persons* (New York: Columbia University Press, 2009), have made the case for personhood in other animals. In *Animals as Legal Beings: Contesting Anthropocentric Legal Orders*

(Toronto: University of Toronto, 2021), Maneesha Deckha argues instead that "person" is too loaded and anthropocentric a term to be used in reference to the legal status of nonhuman animals, and suggests the term "being" as an alternative. My argument here, however, concerns the ontology of animals, rather than their legal status.

14 Darren Incorvaia, "These Flies Age Faster After Witnessing Death," *New York Times*, June 13, 2023; and C. M. Gendron et al., "Ring Neurons in the Drosophila Central Complex Act as a Rheostat for Sensory Modulation of Aging," *PLoS Biology* (2023), doi.org/10.1371/journal.pbio.3002149. Other researchers have found that flies and spiders lapse into a state resembling despair or depression when thwarted in repeated efforts to achieve a goal.

15 The late Steve Wise defined "practical autonomy" as the ability to have desires and "to act intentionally and to have some sense of self." "'Practical Autonomy' Entitles Some Animals to Rights," *Nature* 416 (2002): 785.

16 Montaigne, "Apologies," 383–84.

17 The phenomenologist Edmund Husserl developed his theory of intentionality in *Logical Investigations* (London: Routledge, 2001; originally published 1900–1901).

18 Carol Gigliotti, *The Creative Lives of Animals* (New York: New York University Press, 2022).

19 Masson and McCarthy, *When Elephants*, 126–7; de Waal, *Are We Smart Enough*, 250.

20 Masson and McCarthy, Ibid.

21 Even insects enjoy manipulating objects for fun. See H. Samadi, G. Dona, C. Solvi, A. Kowalewska, et al., "Do Bumble Bees Play?," *Animal Behaviour* 194 (2022): 239–51. Sofia Quaglia, "Do Bees Play? A Groundbreaking Study Says Yes," *National Geographic*, October 27, 2022.

22 De Waal, 60.

23 Rogers, *Minds of Their Own*, 183.

24 S. Kralj-Fišer and W. Schuett, "Studying Personality Variation in Invertebrates: Why Bother?," *Animal Behaviour* 91 (2014): 41–52. Researcher Jason Watters has found that some water-striders get along well with others, while some are aggressive bullies and others are passive and "shy." As in us, individual temperament in insects appears to be a mix of heritable and environmental characteristics.

25 Charles Siebert, "The Animal Self," *New York Times*, Jan. 22, 2006.

26 "For the first time: A Method for Measuring Animal Personality," Weizmann Institute of Science, reported in *Science Daily*, Nov. 11, 2019.

27 James W. Grice, "Five-Factor Model of Personality," *Encyclopedia Britannica*, https://www.britannica.com.

28 Siebert, "Animal Self." To give one example, forty different traits, including scapegoating, calmness, aggressiveness, curiosity, warmth, deceitfulness, and

moodiness have been observed in hyenas. Samuel D. Gosling, "Personality Dimensions in Spotted Hyenas (*Crocuta crocuta*)," *Journal of Comparative Psychology* 112, no. 2 (1998): 107–18.

29 Barbara Smuts, "Reflections," in *Animal Ethics Reader*, ed. Armstrong and Botzler, 84–86.

30 Karen Davis, *For the Birds* (New York: Lantern, 2019), 112.

31 Madeleine Cuff, "We Can't Go on with Business as Usual and Think We Are Ethical," *New Scientist* 258, no. 3441 (June 3, 2023).

32 Zoë Corbyn, "Philosopher Peter Singer: 'There's No Reason to Say Humans Have More Worth or Moral Value than Animals,'" *Guardian*, May 21, 2023.

33 In an email exchange with me, Nussbaum pointed out that even humans can't always be considered "harmed by a painless death after a flourishing life," as in euthanasia. I replied that there is a world of difference between administering a "painless death" to a loved one out of compassion, at the end of a long life, and subjecting billions of sensitive, healthy beings to a needless violent death for our purposes. Martha Nussbaum, private correspondence (Jan. 8, 2023).

34 Nussbaum has said she is willing to revise her opinion about fish if more conclusive scientific evidence emerges concerning their temporal horizons.

35 Nussbaum, 168, 141. For a review of the scientific evidence for suffering in fish, see Jennifer Jacquet, Becca Franks, and Troy Vettese, "The Great Fish Pain Debate," *Issues in Science and Technology* 36, no. 4 (Summer 2020).

36 Undercover videos have revealed workers punching sheep in the face with fists and with sharp shears, stomping on them, and treating them with such extreme violence that they sometimes rupture their torsos, causing their intestines to spill out. Oliver Milman, "Sheep Cruelty Video Sparks RSPCA Investigation," *The Guardian*, July 10, 2014; Harriet Grant, "Secret Videos Reveal Workers Beating Sheep on English and Scottish Farms," *The Guardian*, Nov. 16, 2018. See author's website for these and other videos documenting the prevalence of extreme abuses in the animal agriculture system.

37 John Sanbonmatsu, ed., *Critical Theory and Animal Liberation* (New York: Rowman & Littlefield, 2011), 13.

38 Donaldson and Kymlicka (*Zoopolis*) make a persuasive case for ascribing differential rights to nonhumans on the basis of their status as citizens, denizens, and "liminal" animals.

39 Marina Bolotnikova, "It's Time to Stop Demonizing 'Invasive Species,'" *Vox*, Nov. 28, 2021.

40 Feminist ethicists have shown that we are always-already dependent upon the care of others, while phenomenologists have revealed empathy and sympathy to be the basis of care. See Josephine Donovan, "Sympathy and Interspecies Care," in *Critical Theory and Animal Liberation*, ed. Sanbonmatsu, 277–94. Perhaps a

better formulation of the Golden Rule might be, "Do unto others as you would have them do unto those you love."

12. TWO WAYS OF LOOKING AT A BLACKBIRD

1 Martin Buber, *I and Thou* (New York: Charles Scribner's Sons, 1958), 8.
2 Ibid., 97. Though Buber never fully broke with the anthropocentric prejudices of monotheism, his great sympathy for animals complicated his effort to affirm a humanism that might otherwise have excluded them. Ryan Brand, "Martin Buber (1878–1965): Encountering Animals, a Prelude to the Animal Question," in Linzey, *Animal Theologians*, 334–43.
3 Buber, 97.
4 Ibid., 15.
5 Only in love "is the finite in the infinite; in this alone, and only in this, is the infinite depth, divinity, and truth of love constituted." Ludwig Feuerbach, *Principles of the Philosophy of the Future*, trans. Manfred H. Vogel (New York: Bobbs-Merrill, 1966), 52.
6 Aristotle, *Nichomachean Ethics*, 191.
7 "Only sensuous beings affect one another. I am an 'I' for myself and simultaneously a 'thou' for others." Feuerbach, 52.
8 Vetlesen, *Perception, Empathy, Judgment*, 204.
9 See Roger Gottlieb, *A Spirituality of Resistance: Finding a Peaceful Heart and Protecting the Planet* (Lanham, MD: Rowman & Littlefield, 2003).
10 While living with animal companions can open our eyes to the depth of nonhuman experience, there are also compelling ethical and environmental objections against keeping such companions. Cats are among the most lethal of predators, possessing such extraordinary speed, strength, agility, and heightened senses that, loosed outdoors, they can empty a neighborhood of its songbirds, small mammals, and other creatures. However, keeping cats indoors brings its own problems. Like Aubrey Hepburn's cosseted princess in *Roman Holiday*, the indoor cat is forced to endure a tedious existence within a confined, artificial, unchanging environment. A further consideration in the ethics of keeping companion species is the meat economy: if cats and dogs were a country, they'd be the fifth biggest consumers of meat on Earth. Dogs, as omnivores, can thrive on a vegan diet as easily as we can, but few people think to feed their dogs a vegan diet (which may in fact be healthier for them). Unlike dogs, cats are obligate carnivores. There is some evidence that even cats can thrive on a balanced vegan diet, provided it is supplemented with essential amino acids like taurine, but research on the topic is thin.
11 Note to philosophers: in Heideggerian terms, our *care* for the lifeworld we shared with our cats made possible their absence as an *event*—in much the same

way that Jean-Paul Sartre's famous visit to a café in search of his friend Pierre makes possible Pierre's phenomenological absence in *Being and Nothingness*.

12 Lindgren Johnson, private correspondence, Oct. 8, 2023.

13 For a critique of Singer's utilitarianism, see Alice Crary and Lori Gruen, *Animal Crisis: A New Critical Theory* (Cambridge, UK: Polity Press, 2022).

14 Buber, 14.

15 Ibid., 15.

16 Barbara Demming, *We Are All Part of One Another* (New York: New Society Publishers, 1984), 176.

CONCLUSION

1 The *Liberator*'s main offices were originally located on Congress Street.

2 "The Liberator," National Park Service, last updated Jan. 16, 2024, https://www.nps.gov, accessed Aug. 9, 2024.

3 "The Liberator," Smithsonian Transcription Center, https://transcription.si.edu, accessed Aug. 9, 2024.

4 Law scholar Gary Francione was the first to popularize the term "abolitionism" to describe the elimination of all forms of animal exploitation.

5 Four years later, when investigators returned to the Agriprocessors plant, animals were still being subjected to illegal cruelties. However, federal authorities raided Agriprocessors not over its treatment of animals, but over dozens of labor violations involving undocumented migrants and exploitation of children. "PETA Reveals Extreme Cruelty at Kosher Slaughterhouse Plants," PETA, accessed May 28, 2021, https://www.peta.org.

6 *The Massachusetts Body of Liberties* (1641), Hanover Historical Texts Project, last modified March 8, 2012, https://history.hanover.edu.

7 Claire Kim, "Abolition," in *Critical Terms for Animal Studies* (Chicago: University of Chicago Press, 2018), 26.

8 After dozens of thoroughbred race horses died at the Santa Anita racetrack, journalist Richard Finnegan observed that "opponents of racing seemed increasingly confident that it would soon go the way of circus elephants, dolphin shows, dog racing, all the discredited animal entertainments." "Can Horse Racing Survive?," *The New Yorker*, May 15, 2021.

9 For an account of the contradictory role of animals in slave narratives, see Lindgren Johnson, *Race Matters/Animal Matters: Fugitive Humanism in African America, 1840–1930* (New York: Routledge, 2018).

10 Marina Bolotnikova, "Activists Acquitted for Taking Piglets from Smithfield Foods," *The Intercept*, Oct. 8, 2022. Only weeks after this legal victory, however, a different court found the same group's founder, Wayne Hsiung, guilty of his involvement in rescuing seventy chickens and ducks from two farms in Sonoma County. Hsiung was sentenced to 90 days in prison and given two years probation.

11 Zipporah Weisberg, "Animal Agency and Multispecies Community at VINE Animal Sanctuary: Impressions, Reflections, and Insights," unpublished paper developed for the Culture and Animals Foundation, Dec. 2022.

12 Author's interview recording #21, VINE Sanctuary, Springfield, Vermont (Aug. 17, 2022).

13 Because many of the animals at VINE suffered violence and psychological abuse in the past, VINE does not generally admit members of the public to the sanctuary, out of sensitivity to the animals' needs.

INDEX

abolitionism: in animal rights movement, 278, 281, 331n4; anti-slavery gradualism and, 277–78, 280–81; slavery and, 277–78, 280–82

Adams, Carol, 140, 160

Adshead, Gwen, 175–76

aestheticization, of violence, 204–6, 316n82, 320n35

agriculture: deforestation and, 27, 36; ecological harms of, 61, 62; meat production and, 7–8; regulation of, 100–101; slavery and, 102; subsidies of, 61, 101. *See also* animal agriculture; farming, small-scale

Agriprocessors, 279, 331n5

American Veterinary Medical Association, 214, 322n62

animal agriculture, 28; abolition movement, 73; antibiotic overuse, 34; biodiversity and, 31, 297n32; capitalism and, 44, 50, 108; climate change and, 27, 39–40, 298n38; consent and, 109–10, 119–25, 127, 279, 310n31; corporatization of, 61; ecological crisis and, 295n16; enlightened omnivorism and, 80; "friendship" and, 116–18, 134; global warming and, 298n38; greenhouse gas emissions and, 32–33, 39, 75, 303n19; human purposes and, 1, 287; industrialization of, 106, 301n2; myth of humane killing, 279–80; mythologizing of, 69, 81, 87, 89–92, 100, 279–80; pan-

demic risk and, 34, 298n41; partnership rhetoric of, 120–21; Pollan and, 31–32, 73, 91, 100, 321n47; regenerative agriculture, 32; regulatory rollback, 306n40; as religion, 92, 305n14; romanticizing of, 27, 107; slavery and, 110–18, 126, 167, 278–79, 283; slavery rhetoric and, 120–25, 128–31, 136, 311n18; sustainability of, 32–33, 68–69, 73, 75, 80, 91, 100, 102–5, 302n17; white sovereignty and, 89–90. *See also* enlightened omnivorism; factory farming; farming, small-scale; meat industry

animal cruelty, 8–9, 11, 62, 129–30; laws against, 259, 279, 329n36, 332n13; on small-scale farms, 76–77; torture, 56; violence against animals, 15–16, 24, 79–80, 123–25, 155–56, 175–76, 179–81, 216, 260–61, 273, 329n29

Animal Farm (Orwell), 117, 212, 310n31, 322n57

animal husbandry. *See* animal agriculture

Animal Liberation (Singer, P.), 54–55, 57, 258, 272

animal rights, 62, 130, 221; abolition movement, 70, 277–78, 281, 283; animal justice, 258–59; empathy and, 261; ethics and, 16; legal rights, 14, 27, 244–47, 259–60, 327n13; mocking of, 180; skeptics of, 260. *See also* personhood animal rights advocacy: animus toward, 10, 11, 280; human rights and, 100, 307n48; movement, co-optation of, 70–72, 80, 302n14; welfarists compared with abolitionists, 70, 278, 283

animal sanctuaries: Rowdy Girl, 312n43; VINE, 135, 166, 284–88, 332n13

animals, nonhuman: Aristotle on, 135, 225, 228, 245; cinematic representations of, 52–53; consciousness of, 226–30, 243; consent and, 109–10, 119–25, 127, 279, 310n31; contempt for, 11–13, 15; contradictory treatment of, 14–15; emotions in, 223, 228, 253, 327n10; empathy in, 181–84, 215–16; empathy with, 171–72; experimentation on, 55, 139, 208, 230–34, 242, 244, 310n28; freedom and, 109–10, 129; individuation of, 48, 250, 254–57, 328n28; intelligence of, 185–87, 230–42, 246–47; language and, 238–39; laws and legal rights for, 14, 27, 244–47, 259–60, 327n13; as machines, 110, 228–29, 241–42, 309n5; memory and, 235–37, 258, 326n55; ontology of, 221–26, 251, 254, 323n4, 327n13; personhood and, 245–52, 259–60, 286, 327n13; plants compared with ontology of, 222–26; play of, 253–54; as property, 14, 27, 110, 128, 244; resistance and escape, 126–27, 129–32, 312nn29–30; as slaves, 4, 11, 15–16, 109, 130–31, 283; as tools, 27, 110, 135, 185, 224; war against, 22, 24, 139, 163, 294n4. *See also* dominion

Animal, Vegetable, Miracle (Kingsolver), 10–11, 68, 72, 148, 197; maternal themes in, 150–51; mocking of vegetarians, 224–25

Anthropocene, the, 30

antisemitism, 209–10, 211, 216

Arendt, Hannah, 95

Aristotle: on animals, 135, 225, 228, 245; on death, 202; on hunting, 139; on love, 265; on slavery, 111–12, 116

Atwood, Margaret, 10

authenticity: capitalism and, 107–8; enlightened omnivorism and, 85–86, 107, 180; in femivore memoirs, 143–44, 147–48, 154, 159, 161; modernity and, 85, 107; nature and, 70, 147–48, 159; of VINE sanctuary, 287

Authorization for the Destruction of Unworthy Life (Binding and Hoche), 191–92

avian influenza. *See* zoonotic disease

Bacon, Francis, 28

bad faith, 152, 209–17; in slavery and domestication, 131

Balcombe, Jonathan, 324n17

Baldwin, James, 152

Barwick, Emily Moran, 178

Beston, Henry, 243

Bill and Lou (oxen), 134–36, 166, 284

Binding, Karl, 191–93, 199, 200

biodiversity: animal agriculture and, 31, 297n32; capitalism and, 29; ecological collapse, 20–22, 31–32

bird intelligence, 237–38, 325n50

The Birds (film), 52–53

Bittman, Mark, 39, 73

Blade Runner (film), 174

Blut und Boden (blood and soil), 204

Bost, Jay, 74–76, 190–91

Bourdain, Anthony, 4, 180

bovine spongiform encephalopathy (BSE), 58–59

Brethren of Purity, 127–29, 311n22

Brown, Harold, 185–87

Brown, Jenny, 166, 316n83

BSE. *See* bovine spongiform encephalopathy; mad cow disease

Buber, Martin, 267; anthropocentrism of, 330n2; compassion and, 274; *I and Thou*, 263, 265; *I-It* relationships, 263, 264–65, 273; *I-Thou* relationships, 263–64, 266, 273–75, 287

Buddhism, 56, 261, 300n28; compassion in, 187–88

Budiansky, Stephen, 119

Bundy, Ammon and Cliven, 97

Burger King, 141, 313n4

Bush, George W., 60, 81, 101, 304n33

CAFO. *See* Concentrated Animal Feeding Operations

Canadian sled dog massacre, 190

capitalism: animal agriculture and, 44, 50, 108; animal economy and, 43; animal exploitation and, 103–6; biodiversity and, 29; capitalist state, 45, 79, 303n28, 306n36; consumer desires and, 29; ecological crisis and, 28–30; environmental regulation and, 29; extermination crisis and, 27–28, 295n16; historical origins of, 28; human supremacy and, 140; industrialization and, 27; *The Jungle* critique of, 49; labor and, 28; machinic culture and, 37; masculinity and, 157; nature and, 28–29, 37; populist agrarian movements and, 306n36; small farms compared with large farms and, 103–6; speciesism and, 26–30; temporality of, 28, 29–30

Capper, Judith, 102–3, 164

Carpenter, Novella: farming memoir, 151, 152, 154–55, 156; killing in, 154–55

Carson, Rachel, 24, 53

Cartesianism, 229, 326n62

The Case of Animals vs. Man Before the King of the Jinn (Brethren of Purity), 127–29, 311n22

category errors, 224–25

Cavalieri, Paola, 327n13

cellular meat, 34–35; critique of, 298n42

Chicago Yards, 46, 198–99, 301n2

chickens, empathy in, 321n42

Chipotle, 77–78

climate change, 1, 21, 283–84; animal agriculture and, 27, 39–40, 298n38; ecological collapse and, 20–22, 31–32; extinction events and, 27; greenhouse gas emissions and, 32–33, 39, 75, 303n19; mass die-offs, 23–24

cognitive ethology, 172

colonialism, 28, 44, 89, 102; rape and, 140; zoonotic disease and, 43

community, interspecies, 16, 294n18

companion animals, 14–15, 267–72, 330nn10–11

Concentrated Animal Feeding Operations (CAFO), 213, 322n60

consciousness, 13; animal, 226–30, 243; freedom and, 259; human, 229–30; intentionality and, 252–54, 328n17; openness of, 256–57; plants, absence in, 226; qualities of, 250; as singularity, 254–57, 267; temporality and memory, 250, 258–59; vulnerability and, 250, 251–52. *See also* personhood

consent: animal resistance and, 126–27, 129–32, 312nn29–30; of animals to agriculture, 109–10, 119–25, 127, 279–80, 310n31; rape culture relation to, 121–22

conservation: hunting as, 211; limits of, 25–26; wildlife management, 211

COVID-19, 213–14; mink slaughter, 9

cows: BSE and, 58–59; Harold Brown and Snickers, 186; Pollan on, 170, 185–86; rape of, 79; separation trauma and, 55, 133; skinned alive, 9

Crary, Alice, 331n13

Darwin, Charles, 13, 181, 229; on animal memory, 236; on animals as slaves, 109

Davis, Camas, 144, 316n75

Davis, Karen, 206, 256, 319n12, 321n42

Dawkins, Richard, 229

death, 20–21; harm of, 201–2; life conflated with, 157–58; in omnivore discourse, 202–6

Deckha, Maneesha, 327n13

"Defending Your Dinner" contest (*New York Times*), 72–76, 190–91

democratic socialism, 308n65

Derrida, Jacques, 215

DeSantis, Ron, 97–98

Descartes, René, 228; Cartesianism, 229, 326n62

de Waal, Frans, 184, 232, 254

Dew, Thomas, 116, 131, 312n37

Dick, Philip K., 173–74

Diet for a Small Planet (Lappé), 53–54, 57, 67, 300n26

diet, meat-based, 2–3, 41, 63, 299n5; "flexitarian," 73, 81, 208; protein and, 211, 322n56; water consumption and, 31, 32. *See also* meat-eating

diet, plant-based, 298n37; ecological and health advantages of, 32–33. *See also* veganism; vegetarianism

Do Androids Dream of Electric Sheep? (Dick), 173–74

dogs, 189–90, 327n10

domestication, animal, 3, 122; Pollan on, 4, 310n1, 311n3; slavery and, 4, 11, 130–31; violence of, 27. *See also* animal agriculture; consent

dominion, 27, 30, 110; abolitionism and, 278; Biblical, 228–29; as natural right, 120; Nazism and, 320n30; "new meat" and, 114; slavery and, 113–14, 120; species right, 259. *See also* speciesism; worthlessness

Donaldson, Sue, 245–46, 257, 329n38

donkeys, empathy in, 172–73

Donne, John, 274

eating animals: cognitive dissonance around, 11; as natural, 14–15. *See also* diet, meat-based; meat-eating

ecological collapse, 20–22; role of animal system in, 31–32. *See also* environmental movement

Effective Altruism, 302n14

Eichmann, Adolph, 197, 321n45

empathy: animal ethics and, 257, 272–73; animal rights and, 261; in animals, 181–84, 215–16; with animals, 171–72; autism and, 177–78; in chickens, 321n42; in donkeys, 172–73; ethics and, 257, 272–73; Golden Rule, 261, 329n40; "Harry Lime Disease" and, 170–72; love and, 266–73; phenomenology of, 261, 329n40; Pollan and, 170–71, 186; psychopathy and, 174–79, 187, 317n8; sociopathy and, 174, 177; vulnerability and, 174–77, 185

An Enemy of the People (Ibsen), 280

enlightened omnivorism, 16, 64, 72–76, 78–79, 304n1; animal death and, 202–4; authenticity and, 85–86; class and, 86; conservatism of, 81, 86; legitimizing of animal agriculture, 80; mass killing and, aestheticization of, 205–6; myth of humane killing, 259, 279; nationalism and, 86; nature and, 85; Nazism and, 207–8; Orwellian language of, 202; social justice and, 86. *See also* Pollan, Michael

environmental movement: Carson and, 24, 53; failure of, 25–26, 295n9; "invasive" species and, 260–61; mass extinction and, 25–26, 295n9; vegetarianism and, 1, 2 "ethical meat," 74–75, 118; critics of, 73

ethics: animal, 16, 72–73, 257–61; of animal experimentation, 230–34, 242; animal rights and, 16; empathy and, 257, 272–73; feminist, 329n40; flexitarian diets, 81; of food policy, 67; of killing, 16, 257–58; of meat-eating, 39–40, 72–76; Nussbaum and, 258–59; utilitarian, 257–58, 272–73; vulnerability and, 261

eugenics, 191–92, 207, 322n64

euphemism, 78, 153, 211

euthanasia, discourse of: in Canadian sled dog massacre, 190; in Holocaust, 191–94; in Nussbaum's ethics, 329n33

evil, radical, 1, 216

existential purpose, 216, 273, 282. *See also* authenticity

experimentation, animal, 55, 139, 208, 244, 310n28; ethics of, 230–34, 242

exterminationism, 21–22, 36

extinction, mass, 19–23; chemical causes, 24–26; climate change and, 27; environmentalism and, 25–26, 295n9; human settlement and, 26–27; hunting and, 27, 30, 296n22

factory farming, 51, 61–62; aquaculture, 78; femivorism and, 163–66; in *The Omnivore's Dilemma*, 67; small-scale farming contrasted with, 69; sustainability of, 80, 302n17. *See also* animal agriculture

Faludi, Susan, 160–61

FAO. *See* Food and Agricultural Organization

farming. *See* agriculture; animal agriculture; factory farming

farming, deforestation and, 27, 36

farming, small-scale, 63–65, 72; animal agriculture and, 68–70; animal cruelty and, 76–77; capitalism and

large-scale farming compared with, 103–6; factory farming contrasted with, 69; humane farming, myth of, 131–32; libertarianism and, 92–93, 95–96, 101, 306n30, 306n33; myth of, 103–6, 131–32; reactionary politics and, 97–98, 102–3

fast food culture, 51, 61

The Feminine Mystique (Friedan), 144, 313n11

feminism: animal advocacy and, 284–85; ecofeminism, 160; feminist care ethics, 329n40; femivorism and, 159–66, 315n72; hunting and, 142; liberal, 160–61; radical, 159–60; speciesism and, 160

"The Femivore's Dilemma" (Orenstein), 148, 314n25, 315n72

femivorism, 142, 314n25; authenticity and, 143–44, 147–48, 154, 159, 161; author demographics, 144, 313n11; domesticity and, 161–62; eroticism and, 156–58; factory farming and, 163–66; feminism and, 159–66, 315n72; hunting and, 154, 156, 163; masculinity and, 162–63, 316n75; mastering of animals and, 145–47; maternal and natalist themes of, 146–53; memoirs, 86, 121, 143–58, 311n18, 316n73; militarism and, 162–63; neo-liberalism and, 161; psychopathy and, 179; sentimentality and, 152–53, 158, 169; violence and, 133, 151, 152–53, 155–56, 157, 161–62, 178; vulnerability and, 155–56

Feuerbach, Ludwig, 266, 330n5, 330n7

fish: extermination of, 8, 293n5; human friendships with, 272; individuality in, 255; memory in, 236–37; Nussbaum on, 258–59, 329n34; pain in, 258–59, 329n35; senses of, 230–31; tool use in, 233 fishing industry, 31; ecological crisis and, 295n16; "humane" meat myth, 78; morbidity and, 7–9, 293n5

flexitarianism, 73, 81, 208

Foer, Jonathan Safran, 39, 72–73

Food and Agricultural Organization (FAO): lobbying of, 33–34, 298n39; reports, 31, 33

Foster, John Bellamy, 296n20

Fowler, Bathsheba, 277

Francione, Gary, 327n13, 331n4

freedom: animals and, 109–10, 129; consciousness and, 259; personhood and, 245

Freud, Sigmund, 12–13

Friedan, Betty, 144, 313n11

Friend, Catherine, 81, 99; on animal death, 150, 152; on domestication, 122; farming memoir, 148–49, 151–52, 153, 155, 162; maternal themes of, 151–52; on violence, 153, 155

friendships, interspecies, 185–86

Fugitive Slave Act (1850), 282–83

GAP. See Global Animal Partnership program

Garrison, William Lloyd, 277–78, 280–81

gas chambers: in meat industry, 195; in Nazi Germany, 96, 192–95

gender: domesticity and, 161–62; meat economy, role of women in, 141–43, 313n7; patriarchy, 5–6, 162; veganism and, 141, 166, 316n84. See also femivorism; masculinity

genocide, 12, 38; animal tropes and, 294n14; Nazism and, 192–95, 197–99, 204–7, 208; origin of term, 21–22; treatment of animals as, 21–22, 38

Gigliotti, Carol, 253

Global Animal Partnership program (GAP), 71, 120–21

global warming. See climate change

Godwin, Benjamin, 123–25

Goebbels, Joseph, 204, 208, 213

Goodall, Jane, 53, 108, 232–33

Gottlieb, Roger, 330n9

Grandin, Temple: animal slaughter as "religious," 305n14; autism and, 165, 319n11; gas chambers, advocacy of, 195–96; "humane" animal killing techniques, 164–65, 177, 196–97, 198; ramp design praise and, 316n82; utilitarianism and, 257

Green Mountain College, Bill and Lou controversy at, 134–36, 166, 284

Green Revolution, 50

Gruen, Lori, 302n14

Guthman, Julie, 67, 98

H5N1 virus (avian influenza). See zoonotic disease

Hall, Prince, 277

Harper, Breeze, 73

Harper, William, 113–14, 136, 320n30

"Harry Lime Disease," 170–72

Hartsock, Nancy, 157

Hasidism, 263

Hawking, Stephen, 38

Heifer International, 108

HeliBacon, 139, 140, 313n1

Hemingway, Ernest, 144, 266

Herman, Judith, 181

Himmler, Heinrich, 197, 198, 206, 321n47

Hitchcock, Alfred, 52

Hitler, Adolf, 192–93, 198; flexitarianism of, 208; vegetarianism of, 207–8. See also Nazism

Hobbes, Thomas, 119–20, 223

Hoche, Alfred, 191–93, 199, 200

Holocaust, 195, 197–99, 203–5, 209, 212–14; euthanasia discourse, 191–94. See also genocide; Nazism horses, 44, 299n13; auction of, 167–68; racing, 282, 331n8

Höss, Rudolf, 194, 197, 205

HSUS. *See* Humane Society of the United States

human-animal divide, 13–14; racism and, 12, 294n15. *See also* speciesism

"humane" animal killing, 189–92, 195–97, 199, 201, 214; animal agriculture and, 279–80; enlightened omnivorism and, 259, 279; humane death, 203; "humane" meat, 71, 73, 76–81, 121, 131–32, 198, 279; Nazism and, 206–7

Humane Society of the United States (HSUS), 71–72, 302n16; Meatless Mondays campaign, 102

human rights: animal advocacy and, 100, 307n48; personhood and, 246

human supremacy: animal agriculture and, 40; capitalism and, 140; evolutionary theory and, 229; human species right, 259–60; meat-eating and, 40; PETA and, 55; speciesism and, 13–14, 22, 210, 214, 216–17. *See also* dominion; speciesism

hunting: as alternative to farming, 308n63; bad faith of, 211; canned hunts, 154; as "conservation," 211; as feminist, 142; in femivore memoirs, 154, 156, 163; malignant narcissism and, 273; masculinity and, 139, 178, 313n1; mass extinction and, 27, 30, 296n22; McCaulou, 142, 154, 156, 163, 222; in *The Omnivore's Dilemma*, 176–77; psychopathy and, 176; vulnerability and, 121; of whales, 44, 282

Husserl, Edmund, 328n17

I and Thou (Buber), 263; love in, 265

Ibsen, Henrik, 280

In Defense of Food (Pollan), 63

industrialization: animal agriculture and, 106, 301n2; animal die-offs and, 25; capitalism and, 27; extermination and, 27–28, 295n16; wage slavery and, 131

inequality, 1, 185, 281–82; ecological pressures of, 29; locavorism and, 98, 108

insect intelligence, 240–42

intelligence: animal, 185–87, 230–42, 246–47, 318n40, 326n55; bird, 237–38, 325n50; human, 232; insect, 240–42; types of, 232

Interstellar (film), 37–38

invasive species, 260

isolationism, 93–94, 95

"is-ought" fallacy, 6

Itani, Junichiro, 254

Jackson, Wes, 110, 143

Jainism, 56

January 6, 2021 attacks, 97

Jefferson, Thomas: agrarian mythos of, 91–92; isolationism of, 93–94; on liberty, 120; populist localism of, 99; romantic image of farmers, 91–92, 101–2; slavery and, 117, 133, 185; white supremacy of, 185

Jensen, Derrick, 103, 202, 222

Johnson, Lindgren, 272, 331n9

Jones, Miriam, 284

jones, pattrice, 166, 284–85

The Jungle (Sinclair), 47–48, 51, 61, 300n18; capitalism critique in, 49; legacy of, 50

Kaminer, Ariel, 73, 107

Kant, Immanuel, 67, 261; conception of persons, 245–46, 249–50, 327n8

Katzen, Mollie, 142, 154, 158–59

Keith, Lierre, 10, 103, 116; on animal "partnership," 120, 122–23; on cycle of life, 202, 203–4

Khan, Genghis, 86, 304n3

Kheel, Marti, 139, 160

Kimball, Kristin: on being eaten, 315n67; on death, 315n67; on meat-eating, 163; memoir, 133, 146, 153, 156–57, 162, 311n18; patriarchy and, 162; violence in, 133, 153, 178

Kingsolver, Barbara: on animal rights, 130; on animals as property, 110; category errors of, 224–25; maternal themes of, 150–51; mocking of vegetarians, 224–25. See also *Animal, Vegetable, Miracle*

Ko, Aph, 294n15

Kolbert, Elizabeth, 295n16

Ko, Syl, 12

Kuhse, Helga, 199–201

Kymlicka, Will, 245–46, 257, 329n38

land grant colleges, 45, 50

language: animals and, 239, 264; Orwellian, 15, 42, 71, 157, 202; speciesism and, 14

Lappé, Frances Moore, 53–54, 57, 67, 300n26

LaVeck, James, 70–71

laws and legal rights: animal cruelty, 259, 279, 329n36, 332n13; for animals, nonhuman, 14, 27, 244–47, 259–60, 327n13; Fugitive Slave Act, 282–83; Nazism and animal, 207. See also human rights

Leigh, Meredith, 157–58

Lemkin, Raphael, 21–22, 38

Leopold, Aldo, 74

Levinas, Emmanuel, 174, 212

Levi, Primo, 212

The Liberator (abolitionist newspaper), 277, 280–81

libertarianism, 10; meat-eating and, 102–3; of *The Omnivore's Dilemma*, 67; Salatin and, 92, 95; small-scale

farming and, 92–93, 95–96, 101, 306n30, 306n33

Light, Andrew, 39, 73

Limbaugh, Rush, 40

Livestock's Long Shadow (FAO study), 31; harassment of authors of, 33

lobbying: animal, 33–34, 164; of FAO, 33–34, 298n39. See also environmental movement

locavorism, 64, 311n18; animal death and, 203, 320n30; class and, 86; as conservative movement, 102–3; contradictions of, 65–66; inequality and, 98, 108; malignant narcissism and, 273; myth of human beneficence, 132–34; nativist politics of, 98–99; Pollan on, 66–67, 102; social justice and, 65; as white movement, 102

Locke, John, critique of Hobbes, 120

love, 330n5; for animals, 14–15; grief and, 273; as *I-Thou* relationship, 265, 271–72; singularity and, 265–66; utilitarianism and, 272–73; as way of knowing, 266; worthiness of animals revealed by, 265–66, 272, 274

Macbeth (Shakespeare), 151

Mackey, John, 71

mad cow disease (BSE), 58–59

male domination, 5–6, 162

Marcuse, Herbert, 157

Marino, Lori, 327n10

Marxism, ecological, 30

Marx, Karl, 304n1

Marx, Leo, 99

masculinity: in Burger King "Manthem" advertisement, 141, 313n4; capitalism and, 157; control of nature and, 28; femivore memoirs and, 162–63, 316n75; hunting and soldiering and, 139, 178, 313n1; meat-eating and, 139–42, 313n4, 313n7, 315n60; Pollan and, 90, 176, 178; ranching and, 14, 299n14; violence and, 140

mass mortality events, 20–21

McCaulou, Lily, 142, 154, 156, 163, 222

McCorkindale, Susan, 145, 150, 163

McMinn, Suzanne, 311n18; farming memoir, 146–47, 149, 156, 163

McWilliams, James, 75

meat: associated with tradition, 2, 102–3; cellular, 34–35, 298n42; definitions of, 41–42; "humane," 71, 73, 76–81, 121, 131–32, 198, 279; "naturalness" of, 3–5; "new meat," 69–70, 76, 107, 114; postwar expansion of, system, 50–55, 61

meat-eating: bad faith of, 211; disease and, 57–59; entitlement and, 3–4; ethics of, 39–40, 74–76; humanness and, 4; human supremacy and, 40; libertarianism and, 102–3; masculinity and, 140–42, 313n4; naturalization of, 2–5, 40, 158–59; Pollan on, 4

meat economy, role of women in, 141–43, 313n7

meat industry, 31; cellular meat, 34–35, 298n42; child labor in, 50; environment and, 59; food insecurity and, 59; greenhouse gas emissions, 32–33, 75, 296n27, 303n19; health and, 59; Nazism compared to, 189; post-World War II, 50–51, 59; PTSD in, workers, 50; regulation of, 42–43, 58, 299n9

Meatless Mondays campaign, 102

Meijer, Eva, 294n18

Melville, Herman, 88, 130

memoirs, femivore, 86, 121, 143–58, 311n18, 316n73

Merleau-Ponty, Maurice, 187, 241

Metamorphoses (Ovid), 56

Midgley, Mary, 229

Millett, Kate, 167–69

mink slaughter, COVID-19 and, 9

mirror test, 247–49, 327n9, 327n10

Moby-Dick (Melville), 88, 130

Montaigne, Michel de, 238–39, 252

Moosewood Cookbook (Katzen), 142, 154, 158–59

Mumford, Lewis, 64

Mussolini, Benito, 212, 320n35

Nagel, Thomas, 226–27

nativism, 98–100

naturalistic fallacy, 4–5

Nazism: agricultural background of, 207; animal welfare laws of, 207; artificial foods, aversion to, 321n47; Blut und Boden (blood and soil), 204; dominion and, 320n30; enlightened omnivores and, 207–8; eugenics program, 192, 207, 322n64; gas chambers and, 96, 192–95; "humane" genocide rhetoric of, 192–95, 197–99, 206–7, 208; mass killing and, 192–93; meat industry compared to, 189; natural foods and, 207–8; "natural" genocide justification under, 204–5; T4 euthanasia program, 192–94; violence, aestheticization of, 204–5, 320n35

neoliberalism, 67, 107; femivorism and, 161

Nestlé, 31

New Atlantis (Bacon), 28

Newkirk, Ingrid, 55

"new meat" renaissance, 69–70, 76; dominion and, 114; modernity and, 107

New York Times, 72–76, 190–91

NhRP. See Nonhuman Rights Project

Nibert, David, 299n11

Niman, Bill and Nicolette, 105, 308n60

1984 (Orwell), 202

Nonhuman Rights Project (NhRP), 246–47

Nussbaum, Martha, 258–59, 329nn33–34

The Omnivore's Dilemma (Pollan), 59, 61–62, 64, 72, 300n26; animal slaughter in, 67; factory farming in, 67; grass in, 88–89, 304n7, 305n10; hunting in, 176–77; libertarianism of, 67; locavorism in, 66–67; pastoralism of, 87–90; reception of, 63; Salatin in, 90–97, 104, 110, 305n19, 307n50

omnivorism: naturalization of, 4–5; "new," 79. *See also* enlightened omnivorism

ontology, animal, 221, 251, 254, 323n4, 327n13; plants compared with, 222–26

Open Road mythology, 89–90

Orenstein, Peggy, 142; "The Femivore's Dilemma," 148, 314n25, 315n72

organic food industry, 65

Ortega y Gassett, José, 121

Orwell, George, 157; *Animal Farm*, 117, 212, 310n31, 322n57; *1984*, 202; on totalitarianism, 202, 212

Orwellian language: in *1984*, 202; reconciliation of antithetical concepts, 15, 42, 71, 157

Ovid, 56

oxen, 134–36, 166, 284

Pacheco, Alex, 55

pandemics. *See* zoonotic disease

pastoralism, 11, 85, 304n4; history of, 86, 87; New American Pastoral, 86; of *The Omnivore's Dilemma*, 87–90

patriarchy, 5–6, 162

Patterson, Charles, 208, 215

People for the Ethical Treatment of Animals (PETA), 55

Perdue: child labor and, 49–50; hybrid plant-animal products of, 302n17

personhood: animals and, 245–52, 259–60, 286, 327n13; autonomy and intentionality relation to, 250, 252–54, 328n15; consciousness relation to, 250–52, 257; freedom and, 245; human rights and, 246; Kantian, 245–46, 249–50, 327n8; mirror test, 247–49, 327n9; new approach to, 249–53; reason and, 245–46; vulnerability and, 253

pesticides, 24

PETA. *See* People for the Ethical Treatment of Animals

plant-animal hybrid products, 302n17

Plato, 115

Plutarch, 126

Pollan, Michael, 39, 60–62, 64, 322n60; animal agriculture, defense of, 31–32; on animal and plant protein conversion efficiencies, 305n10; on animal intelligence, 185, 318n40; on animal liberation, 131; on animal liberty, 110, 114; animal ontology and, 221, 254, 323n4; corporate agriculture, critique of, 91, 301n2, 321n47; *In Defense of Food*, 63; on domestication, 4, 310n1, 311n3; domestication as slavery, rejection of, 4; empathy for animals, lack of, 170–71, 186–87; on hunting, 176–77; on locavorism, 66–67, 102; mass killing, aestheticization of, 205–6; meat-eating and, 4; myth of sustainable animal agriculture, 73, 100; on ontological indeterminacy of nonhuman animals, 323n4; organic foods industry, critique of, 65; toxic masculinity of, 178; utilitarianism and, 257; veganism, attack on, 102; on working animals, 112. See also *The Omnivore's Dilemma*

population growth, human, 29, 296n20

populism, agrarian: capitalism and, 306n36; cultural conservatism and, 98–100 post-traumatic stress disorder (PTSD): in animals, 25, 133, 216; in slaughterhouse workers, 50

Prentice, Jessica, 64

psychopathy, 171, 316n2; empathy and, 174–79, 187, 317n8; femivore memoirs and, 179; hunting, 176; serial killers, 178–79

PTSD. *See* post-traumatic stress disorder

Pythagoras, 56–57

racism, 1; anti-Asian, 141; fetishization of animal breeds and, 311n18; human-animal divide and, 12, 294n15; Jefferson white supremacy and, 185; Salatin and, 99–100

radical evil, 1, 216

ranching, 44–45; masculinity and, 14, 299n14

rape: colonization and, 140; of cows at US Meat Animal Research Center, 79; culture and consent, 121–22; "rape rack" in monkey experiments, 55; in slavery, 124

Regan, Tom, 73, 250

regulation: of agriculture, 100–101; animal and food safety, 97, 306n40; environmental, 24, 29; language of, 42; of meat industry, 42–43, 58, 299n9

relationality, 263–66; with animals, 271

religion, 92, 94–95, 305n14. *See also* Buddhism

Republic (Plato), 115

resistance, animal, 126–27, 129–32, 312nn29–30

Rich, Adrienne, 159

Riley, Elizabeth, 277

Rodale, J. I., 143

Rowdy Girl animal sanctuary, 312n43

Rudy, Kathy, 116, 121, 123, 310n2, 310n28, 320n30

rural renaissance, 65

Salatin, Joel: on beneficence of animal agriculture, 132; on cycle of life, 202; evangelical Christianity of, 92, 94–95; isolationism of, 93–94, 95; mass killing, aestheticization of, 205; in *The Omnivore's Dilemma*, 90–97, 104, 110, 305n19, 307n50; "partnership" with animals, 120; politics of, 93, 94–97, 98–100, 101, 306n30, 306n33; racism of, 99–100; on small-scale farming, myth of, 104

Sampson, Dede, 64

sanctuaries, animal. *See* animal sanctuaries

Sanders, Brenda, 166

Sartre, Jean-Paul, 209, 216–17, 330n11; on bad faith, 210–11

Schmitt, Carl, 204, 322n59

Scruton, Roger, 81, 304n34

self-deception, 1–2, 16. *See also* bad faith; Sartre, Jean-Paul

sentimentality: in femivore memoirs, 152–53, 158, 169; in locavore discourse, 132–33; veganism and, 152

September 11 attacks, 60, 61, 66, 81

Shakespeare, William: *Macbeth*, 151; *Twelfth Night*, 57

Shapiro, Paul, 72, 302n17

Sierra Club, 26, 260

Silent Spring (Carson), 24, 53, 66

Sinclair, Upton, 46–51, 61, 300n18

Singer, Isaac Bashevis, 189, 214–15

Singer, Peter, 39; *Animal Liberation*, 54–55, 57, 258, 272; "conscientious omnivores," endorsement of, 257; on ethics of killing animals, 73, 201–2, 257–58; on euthanizing disabled infants, 199–201; on speciesism, 7; species right and, 259; utilitarianism of, 54–55, 199–202, 257, 272, 302n14

Skinner, B. F., 323n13

slaughterhouse workers, 50

slavery, 6–7, 43; abolition movement, 277–78, 280–82; agriculture and, 102; animal, 4, 11, 15–16, 109, 130–31, 283; animal agriculture and, 110–18, 120–26, 128–31, 136, 167, 278–79, 283, 311n18; as beneficent, 320n30; Darwin on animals and, 109; domestication and, 4, 11, 130–31; dominion and, 113–14, 120; friendship and, 116–18; Fugitive Slave Act, opposition to, 282–83; hierarchy and, 111–12, 114; Jefferson and, 117, 133, 185; as natural, 111–14, 116, 309n18, 309n24; racial, 113–14, 115–16; rape in, 124; wage labor and, 131

sled dog massacre, 189–90, 327n10

Smuts, Barbara, 255–56

sociopathy, 316n2; empathy and, 174, 177. See also psychopathy

speciesism, 54, 293n4; capitalism and, 26–30; feminism and, 160; human identity and, 7, 12–13; human supremacy and, 13–14, 22, 210, 214, 216–17; language and, 14

species right, 122, 259

Spinoza, Baruch, 187

Stallwood, Kim, 166

Stanescu, Vasile, 98, 297n33, 304n34, 313n5

Stangneth, Bettina, 205, 321n45

Stein, Edith, 173, 184

stockyards, in Chicago, 46, 198–99, 301n2

suffering, animal: Nazi laws to prevent, 207; necessary compared with "undue," 9, 12–14, 30, 114, 190, 280

sustainability: of animal agriculture, 32–33, 68–69, 73, 75, 80, 91, 100, 104–5, 302n17; of factory farming, 80, 302n17; at Green Mountain College, 134–36

Suzuki, David, 295n9

technology: alienation from nature and, 36–38; animal extermination role of, 8, 37; feminism and, 159; Salatin farm use of, 94

temporality: animal, 235–36, 238; of capitalism, 28, 29–30; consciousness and, 250, 258–59

terrorism, 60, 61, 66, 81

The Third Man (film), 170–71

Thoreau, Henry David, 35–37

torture: of animals, 56; in War on Terror, 60

totalitarianism, 192, 202. See also Nazism

Tribe, Laurence, 246

Trump, Donald, 11; farmer support for, 100

Twelfth Night (Shakespeare), 57

US Department of Agriculture (USDA), 2, 45, 96, 307n50

US Meat Animal Research Center, 79–80

utilitarianism, 54; critique of, 199–202; ethics of, 257–58, 272–73; love and, 272–73; of Pollan, 257; of Singer, 54–55, 199–202, 257, 272, 302n14

Van Wing, Sage, 64

veganism, 10, 33, 54, 102; effeminacy and, 141; gender and, 141, 166, 316n84; geoengineering and, 32; greenhouse gas emissions, 32; health benefits of, 57; industrialized agriculture and, 62–63; morality and, 1; protein and, 322n56; sentimentality and, 152; stigmatization of, 1; as unnatural, 4; water consumption and, 32

vegans: animus toward, 10, 11, 224, 294n10; demographics of, 63; mockery of, 211, 280; "pathological," 163

vegetarianism, 53–54; Eastern tradition, 55–56; environmentalism and,

1, 2; health benefits of, 57; history of, 55–57; industrialized agriculture and, 62–63; *Moosewood Cookbook* and, 142, 154, 158–59; objections to, 322n56; Western tradition, 56–57

vegetarians: animus toward, 10; demographics of, 63

Vettese, Troy, 43–44

VINE animal sanctuary, 135, 166, 284–88, 332n13

violence: aestheticization of, 204–6, 316n82, 320n35; against animals, 15–16, 24, 79–80, 123–25, 155–56, 175–76, 179–80, 216, 260–61, 273, 329n29; of domestication, 27; euphemizing of, 78, 153, 211; in farming memoirs, 153, 155–56; of food production, 8–9; masculinity and, 140; in wildlife management, 211. *See also* animal cruelty; worthlessness

vulnerability: consciousness and, 250, 251–52; empathy and, 174–77, 185; ethics and, 261; in femivore memoirs, 155–56; friendship and, 117; "humane" meat and, 73, 121, 198; hunting and, 121; kinship and, 202–3; morality and, 212, 261; personhood and, 253; rights and, 259

Wadiwel, Dinesh, 294n4, 296n24

Walden (Thoreau), 35–37

Wallace, David Foster, 7

War on Terror, 60

Weaver, Jim, 66, 98, 122, 197

Weisberg, Zipporah, 284

whales: hunting of, 44, 282; resistance of to being hunted, 130; transmission of culture, 13

Whistler Outdoor Adventures, sled dog massacre, 189–90, 327n10

White, E. B., 87–88, 304n6

Whole Foods Market: animal compassion campaign, 71–72, 78; Global Animal Partnership program, 120–21

wildlife management, 211

Wirz, Fritz, 204, 321n47

Wise, Steve, 328n15

Woginrich, Jenna, 112, 305n14; on animal death, 189; on "barnheart," 145; farming memoirs, 86, 121, 145, 146; on myth of beneficence, 132; violence and, 155–56

women. *See* feminism; femivorism; gender

Woolf, Virginia, 142

worthlessness: of human lives, 190–92, 200, 209–10, 212–13; of nonhuman animal lives, 9, 12–13, 14, 30, 76, 81, 209–10, 215–17, 221, 245, 248, 258

zoonotic disease: avian influenza, 11, 21, 34, 58, 101, 307n52; emerging diseases, 34, 298n41; European colonization of Americas and, 43

ABOUT THE AUTHOR

JOHN SANBONMATSU is Professor of Philosophy at Worcester Polytechnic Institute, in Massachusetts. He is the author of *The Postmodern Prince* and editor of *Critical Theory and Animal Liberation*. He lives in the Boston area. For more information, go to www.JohnSanbonmatsu.com.